# GEOGRAPHIES OF HEALTH AND DEVELOPMENT

T0298871

# Geographies of Health

Series Editors

Allison Williams, Associate Professor, School of Geography and Earth Sciences, McMaster University, Canada

Susan Elliott, Professor, Department of Geography and Environmental Management and School of Public Health and Health Systems, University of Waterloo, Canada

There is growing interest in the geographies of health and a continued interest in what has more traditionally been labeled medical geography. The traditional focus of 'medical geography' on areas such as disease ecology, health service provision and disease mapping (all of which continue to reflect a mainly quantitative approach to inquiry) has evolved to a focus on a broader, theoretically informed epistemology of health geographies in an expanded international reach. As a result, we now find this subdiscipline characterized by a strongly theoretically-informed research agenda, embracing a range of methods (quantitative; qualitative and the integration of the two) of inquiry concerned with questions of: risk; representation and meaning; inequality and power; culture and difference, among others. Health mapping and modeling has simultaneously been strengthened by the technical advances made in multilevel modeling, advanced spatial analytic methods and GIS, while further engaging in questions related to health inequalities, population health and environmental degradation.

This series publishes superior quality research monographs and edited collections representing contemporary applications in the field; this encompasses original research as well as advances in methods, techniques and theories. The *Geographies of Health* series will capture the interest of a broad body of scholars, within the social sciences, the health sciences and beyond.

*Also in the series*

Soundscapes of Wellbeing
in Popular Music
*Gavin J. Andrews, Paul Kingsbury and Robin Kearns*

Mobilities and Health
*Anthony C. Gatrell*

Space, Place and Mental Health
*Sarah Curtis*

Healing Waters
Therapeutic Landscapes in Historic and Contemporary Ireland
*Ronan Foley*

# Geographies of
# Health and Development

*Edited by*

ISAAC LUGINAAH
*The University of Western Ontario, Canada*

RACHEL BEZNER KERR
*Cornell University, USA*

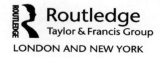

Routledge
Taylor & Francis Group

LONDON AND NEW YORK

First published 2015 by Ashgate Publishing

2 Park Square, Milton Park, Abingdon, Oxfordshire OX14 4RN
711 Third Avenue, New York, NY 10017

*Routledge is an imprint of the Taylor & Francis Group, an informa business*

First issued in paperback 2018

**British Library Cataloguing in Publication Data**
A catalogue record for this book is available from the British Library.

**The Library of Congress has cataloged the printed edition as follows:**
Geographies of health and development / [edited] by Isaac Luginaah and Rachel Bezner Kerr.
    p. ; cm. -- (Ashgate's geographies of health series)
  Includes bibliographical references and index.
  ISBN 978-1-4094-5457-1 (hardback)

    I. Luginaah, Isaac N., editor. II. Bezner Kerr, Rachel, editor. III. Series: Ashgate's geographies of health series.
    [DNLM: 1. Delivery of Health Care. 2. Developing Countries. 3. Geography, Medical. 4. Health Status Disparities. 5. Socioeconomic Factors. WA 395]
    RA441
    362.1--dc23

                                                                    2014033740


ISBN 978-1-4094-5457-1 (hbk)
ISBN 978-1-138-54695-0 (pbk)

# Contents

# List of Figures

# List of Tables

# Notes on Contributors

**Rachel Bezner Kerr, PhD** is an Associate Professor in the Department of Developmental Sociology at Cornell University. Her research interests converge on the broad themes of sustainable agriculture, food security, health, nutrition and social inequalities, with a primary focus in southern Africa. She uses principles of participatory action research in her work.

**Elijah Bisung** is a PhD candidate from Ghana studying in the Department of Geography, University of Waterloo. His research interests span the environment and human development.

**Hans-Georg Bohle, PhD** who passed away in September 2014, was a German geographer and development researcher. He was chair of development geography in the Geography Department of Bonn University. He published widely on issues of vulnerability, human security and resilience, with special emphasis on food, water and health in South Asia.

**Abel Chikanda, PhD** is a Project Manager at the Balsillie School of International Affairs in Waterloo, Ontario. He is an active member of the Southern African Migration Programme (SAMP) which regularly conducts applied research on migration and development issues in southern Africa.

**Lauren Classen, PhD** received her doctorate in Anthropology from the University of Toronto. Her research interests include the social life of development programmes and child/youth health in African contexts. Most recently her work has examined how young people in rural Malawi engage with and employ global health discourses.

**Jenna Dixon, PhD** is a Postdoctoral Fellow in the Department of Geography and Environmental Management, University of Waterloo. Her research interests focus on the provision of health care to women in resource-poor settings.

**Belinda Dodson, PhD** is an Associate Professor of Geography and Director of the Graduate Program in Migration and Ethnic Relations at Western University in London, Ontario. Her research examines the intersection of migration, gender and development, with a regional focus on Southern Africa.

**Jane Ebeniro** completed an MSc in Applied Geography at the University of North Texas. Jane conducted the field work for this for her MSc thesis. Jane is currently pursuing a dual master's degree in Health Systems Management and Business Administration at Texas Woman's University in Dallas, Texas.

**Susan J. Elliott, PhD** is a Professor in the Department of Geography and Environmental Management and Dean of Applied Health Sciences at the University of Waterloo. Her research interests involve environment and health as well as population health.

**Christina Ergler, PhD** is a lecturer in Social Geography at Otago University. Her research interests are at the intersection of geography, sociology and public health and centre on how physical, social and symbolic environments shape and are shaped by the way people play, live, age fall ill and get better in particular places.

**John Eyles, PhD, FRSC** is a social and policy scientist working at McMaster University. He is also cross-appointed in the Centre for Health Policy in the School of Public Health at the University of Witwatersrand. His research interests include environmental health as well as the distribution of health inequities and the mechanisms for resource reallocation in health care.

**Jana Fried, PhD** is a postdoctoral fellow at the Social Sciences Research Laboratories at the University of Saskatchewan. She is a geographer whose research interest range from development and health geography with a particular focus on Southern Africa to public perceptions of natural resource extraction and nuclear energy production.

**Gavin George, PhD** is a Senior Research Fellow at the Health Economics and HIV and AIDS Research Division at the University of KwaZulu-Natal. Gavin has completed numerous studies in the field of HIV/AIDS and Health Economics. These have been undertaken on behalf of UN agencies, governments, funders as well as big business.

**Dr Trevor Hancock** is a Professor of Public Health at the University of Victoria. He is a founder of the now-global Healthy Cities movement, the Canadian Association of Physicians for the Environment and the Canadian Coalition for Green Health Care, and was the first leader of the Green Party in Canada.

**Jacqueline P. Hellen** is a graduate student at Tulane University School of Public Health and Tropical Medicine. Besides her work in India, Jackie has focused on researching family planning programs in sub-Saharan Africa, particularly in the Democratic Republic of Congo and Burkina Faso.

**Robert Huish, PhD** is Assistant Professor at Dalhousie University in International Development Studies. His research encompasses approaches to global health equity through comprehensive development. He is the author of *Where No Doctor Has Gone Before: Cuba's Place in the Global Health Landscape*. He teaches courses on Global Health, Activism, and Development.

**Robin Kearns, PhD** is Professor of Geography at the University of Auckland. His research interests span social, cultural and health geography with publications exploring links between culture, place and health. Robin edits three journals; *Health & Place*, *Health and Social Care in the Community*, and the *Journal of Transport and Health*.

**Sarah Lovell, PhD** is a Health Geographer at the Dunedin School of Medicine. Her research interests focus on health inequalities. Her recent work includes examining issues of access to healthcare, the use and efficacy of community capacity building strategies in health sector responses to climate change.

**Isaac Luginaah, PhD** is an Associate Professor and a Canada Research Chair in Health Geography, Western University. His research includes health impacts of environmental exposure and population health. He is currently Editor for the *African Geographical Review*. He has published several articles in peer review journals.

**Florence M. Margai, PhD** was a Professor and Associate Dean at Binghamton University. She specialised in geospatial analysis of environmental health hazards. She worked with non-profit organizations in the US and Africa and assisted with disease intervention, sustainability and capacity development initiatives. She published three books, and several scientific articles.

**Jacob B. Minah, MD** is a retired paediatrician and homeopath in Steinheim, Germany where he maintained a private practice for over 20 years. He travels regularly to Africa to render humanitarian assistance. He is the founder of a non-profit organisation, MALAMED, that promotes research and development of alternative therapies for malaria.

**Paul Mkandawire, PhD** is Assistant Professor of Health and Human Rights in the Institute of Interdisciplinary Studies at Carleton University. His broad area of research is in the domain of social and environmental determinants of health and the role of scientific evidence in global public health policy.

**Pat Neuwelt, MD, PhD, FRNZCGP, FNZCPHM** is a Senior Lecturer in public health at the University of Auckland. A public health medicine physician, her research focuses on addressing structural (policy, system) barriers to primary health care access for indigenous and other disadvantaged populations.

**Ashley Ning** completed a Masters in Geography at the University of Toronto. Her research interests include issues related to the mobilities of Aboriginal youth, and the related impact on health and social support.

**Joseph R. Oppong, PhD** is a Professor of Geography and Associate Dean for Research and Professional Development at the University of North Texas. Dr Oppong's research centres on Medical Geography, particularly on HIV/AIDS and tuberculosis genotypes, and racial/ethnic disparities in health. Dr Oppong is currently the US representative to the International Geographers Union.

**Bimal Kanti Paul, PhD** is a Professor of Geography at Kansas State University. He has published widely on topics related health and environmental disasters. He is currently editor of the *Geographical Review*. He published a book entitled *Environmental Hazards and Disasters: Contexts, Perspectives and Management* in 2011.

**Michael Pennock MASc** is a population health epidemiologist based in Victoria, British Columbia. Formerly the Research Director of the Population Health Research Unit at Dalhousie University, Mike is currently working with the BC Ministry of Health where he is responsible for the Population Health Surveillance and Epidemiology program.

**Blake Poland, PhD** is Associate Professor at the Dalla Lana School of Public Health, University of Toronto. His research has focused on the settings approach to health, the health of marginalised groups, and the sociology of tobacco control. Recently his work involves

*Geographies of Health and Development*

environmental health promotion and building community resilience for the transition to a post-carbon society.

**Tim Quinlan, PhD** has a part time-post at the Athena Institute, Free University, Amsterdam, and is a Research Associate at the Health Economics and HIV/AIDS Research Division, University of KwaZulu-Natal. He trained as an anthropologist, was involved in environmental studies for 12 years, followed by health-focused research since 2002.

**Candice Reardon** completed a Masters in Health Promotion at the University of KwaZulu-Natal. She is a researcher at the Health Economics and HIV/AIDS Research Division. Candice's research interests include issues related to the sexual and reproductive health of young people, health care systems and access to health care.

**Mark W. Rosenberg, PhD** is a Professor of Geography and a Canada Research Chair in Development Studies at Queen's University, Ontario. His scholarship has received an extensive list of awards. In 1999, Dr Rosenberg received the Canadian Association of Geographers' Award for Service to Geography. Dr Rosenberg's leadership within Health Geography is renowned.

**Patrick Sakdapolrak, PhD** is a post-doctoral researcher at the Department of Geography, University of Bonn. He was educated at Department of Geography, University of Heidelberg, Germany and at the University of Wollongong. He holds a PhD from University of Bonn. His current research focuses on social vulnerability.

**Ted Schrecker, PhD** left Canada in 2013 for a position as Professor of Global Health Policy at Durham University. A political scientist by background, he worked for many years as a legislative researcher and consultant, and was actively involved with the work of the WHO Commission on Social Determinants of Health.

**Corinne J. Schuster-Wallace, PhD** is a Program Officer for the Water-Health Nexus at the United Nations University Institute for Water, Environment and Health. Her research interests involve tool development, capacity building and science-policy bridging around water-health issues.

**Lizzie Shumba** is the Coordinator for the Soils, Food and Healthy Communities project in Ekwendeni, Malawi. Lizzie holds a diploma in nutrition from the Natural Resources College in Lilongwe, and is currently completing a degree at the Lilongwe University of Agriculture and Natural Resources, in Middle Extension and Nutrition.

**Vandana Wadhwa, PhD** is President/CEO of Meridian Research & Consulting, Inc., and Visiting Scholar at Boston University. She engages in theoretical and applied research on health and disability, gender, development, and social justice. She is the current Chair of the Asian Geography Specialty Group of the Association of American Geographers.

**Kathi Wilson, PhD** is a Health Geographer and an Associate Professor at the Department of Geography and Program in Planning, University of Toronto. Her research focuses on understanding the links between health and place; and the inequalities in access to health care as they pertain to Aboriginal populations and recent immigrants.

# Preface

This collection brings together two sets of research interests for both editors. For Luginaah, it joins his interests in health geography. For Bezner Kerr, it puts front and centre her interest in development geography. In the past couple of years we have been working together with the aim of bringing together issues related to the inextricable links between the geographies of health and development. To help us with this, we invited an international group of scholars who submitted abstracts which were reviewed and those selected were then asked to submit their papers which were reviewed by the editors and in some cases by independent reviewers. The 17 chapters in this book extend our understanding of the links between health and development in a globalising world.

Gratitude is extended to all contributors, who worked diligently to submit their work in a timely manner and who incorporated editorial comments – large and small, with great generosity. We feel greatly rewarded to have worked with all our contributors and thank them for many insights shared through their work.

Many hands were involved in this book, but the assistance of one person – Jenna Dixon – then a graduate student in the Department of Geography, Western University, immeasurably eased the job of editing this collection. She worked diligently in the preparation of this collection, carrying the vast majority of responsibility for correspondence with all contributors, and giving the detailed attention required to formatting and style requirements. We will also like to thank Sarah Mason, Nandini Thogarapalli, Shirley Ngai, Andrea Rishworth, Jenna Mason and Caren Raedts for their editorial support.

Heartfelt gratitude to all members of immediate families of Luginaah and Bezner Kerr who have allowed the mental space and time to devote to this project, and who have ensured the balance needed for effective work.

Isaac Luginaah, London, Ontario
Rachel Bezner Kerr, Ithaca, New York

# List of Abbreviations

| | |
|---|---|
| AAPIO | American Association of Physicians of Indian Origin |
| ACT | Artemisinin Combination Therapy |
| AHP | African Health Placements |
| AIDS | Acquired Immunodeficiency Syndrome |
| APSU | Arsenic Policy Support Unit |
| ART | Anti-Retroviral Therapy |
| BAMWSP | Bangladesh Arsenic Mitigation and Water Supply Project |
| BGS | British Geological Survey |
| CCAP | Church of Central Africa Presbyterian |
| COI | Cost of illness |
| CSW | Commercial Sex Worker |
| CVD | Cardiovascular Disease |
| DCH | Dhaka Community Hospital |
| DDT | Dichlorodiphenyltrichloroethane |
| DHS | Demographic and Health Survey |
| DOTS | Directly-Observed Therapy (short course) |
| DPHE | Department of Public Health and Engineering |
| DSDH | Commission on the Social Determinants of Health |
| DTW | Deep Tube Well |
| DW | Dug Wells |
| EEA | European Economic Area |
| ELAM | Escuela Latinoamericana de Medicina |
| EROI | Energy Return on Investment |
| FANTA | Food and Nutrition Technical Assistance Project |
| FGD | Focus group discussion |
| FSW | Female sex worker |
| FWHS | Rain Water Harvesting System |
| GCIM | Global Commission on International Migration |
| GDP | Gross Domestic Product |
| GIPA | Greater Involvement of People living with HIV/AIDS |
| GIS | Geographic Information System |
| GMC | General Medical Council |
| GNP | Gross National Product |
| GP | General Practitioner |
| HCWH | Health Care Without Harm |
| HEALS | Health Effects of Arsenic Longitudinal Study |
| HFIAS | Household Food Insecurity Access Scale |
| HIV | Human Immunodeficiency Virus |
| HPCSA | Health Professions Council of South Africa |
| HRH | Human Resources For Health |
| ICU | Intensive Care Unit |

| | |
|---|---|
| ID | Identification |
| IDI | In-depth interview |
| IEA | International Energy Agency |
| IMF | International Monetary Fund |
| IOM | International Organization for Migration |
| IPAM | Implementation Plan for Arsenic Mitigation |
| IRS | Indoor Residual Spraying |
| ISRDS | Integrated Sustainable Rural Development Strategy |
| ITN | Insecticide Treated Nets |
| KBHC | Kroo Bay Health Center |
| LDCs | Least Developed Countries |
| LDDC | London Docklands Development Corporation |
| LMICs | Low and middle income countries |
| MDGs | Millennium Development Goals |
| MDR | Multidrug-Resistant |
| MHFW | Ministry of Health and Family Welfare |
| MIDA | Migration for Development in Africa |
| MIT | Massachusetts Institute of Technology |
| MOU | Memorandum of Understanding |
| MPI | Multidimensional Poverty Index |
| MSM | Men who have sex with men |
| NACP | National AIDS Control Programme |
| NEPAD | New Partnership for Africa's Development |
| NGO | Non-Governmental Organization |
| NHIS | National Health Insurance Scheme |
| NHS | National Health Service |
| NPAM | National Policy for Arsenic Mitigation |
| OECD | Organisation for Economic Co-operation and Development |
| OFW | Overseas Filipino worker |
| OPEC | Organization of the Petroleum Exporting Countries |
| OSD | Occupational Specific Dispensation |
| PLAB | Professional and Linguistics Assessments Board |
| PLHA | People living with HIV/AIDS |
| PMTCT | Prevention of Mother to Child (HIV) Transmission |
| PPB | Parts per billion |
| PRSP | Poverty Reduction Strategy Program |
| PSBC | Public Service Bargaining Chamber |
| PSF | Pond Sand Filter |
| RBM | Roll Back Malaria |
| SAP | Structural Adjustment Program |
| SD | Standard deviation |
| SDH | Social determinants of health |
| SEM | Simultaneous equation model |
| SES | Socio-economic status |
| SFHC | Soils, Food and Healthy Communities |
| SHI | Social Health Insurance |
| SOES | School of Environment Studies |
| SSA | sub-Saharan Africa |

| STD | Sexually transmitted disease |
| STI | Sexually transmitted infection |
| T2D | Type II Diabetes |
| TB | Tuberculosis |
| TG | Transgender |
| TGSW | Transgender sex worker |
| TPF | Three Pitchers Filter |
| TRIPS | Trade-Related Aspects of Intellectual Property Rights |
| TW | Tube Well |
| UK | United Kingdom |
| UNDP | United Nations Development Program |
| UNICEF | United Nations Children Fund |
| US | United States |
| USA | United States of America |
| UWR | Upper West Region of Ghana |
| WHO | World Health Organization |
| WTO | World Trade Organization |
| WTP | Willingness to Pay |
| WWII | World War Two |
| XDR-TB | Extensively Drug Resistant Tuberculosis |

# Chapter 1
# Introduction

Isaac Luginaah, Rachel Bezner Kerr and Jenna Dixon

## Introduction

Health/medical geography is a sub-discipline of human geography that involves the application of geographical perspectives, information, and methods to the study of health, disease, and health care. Initially called medical geography, the sub-discipline has since been broadened to include the full spectrum of health, health promotion and disease prevention, through to disease and risk mapping. Health geography can provide a spatial understanding of a population's health, the distribution of disease in an area, and the environment's effect on health and disease, while also offering an understanding and insight into the influence of culture, inequality and representation on place and health.

Geography offers a unique lens to the study of health by not only focusing on the distributive features of disease and disease services (traditionally conceptualised as space), but also broadening the discussion to more complex notions of place; with this, health related phenomenon is understood through a give-and-take relationship between people and their settings and thus an analysis of health must integrate both contextual and compositional factors. As the field of health geography has widened and established itself as an important contender in academic and policy circles, so too have the topics of research increased. While the discipline has always remained concerned over questions of inequality and health, this concern has manifested itself into a multitude of new and innovative research programs. Most notably, discussions of inequality and health have become a salient element in development studies. Developing countries, historically embedded in unequal global relationships and composed of unique cultural identities and histories, face special circumstances in defining, establishing, and maintaining 'health'. To date conversations about the geographies of health in development have been limited and do not reflect the importance of the budding scholarship across the world on the subject.

## What is Development?

Development itself is a somewhat ambiguous term that has different meanings to different people. Other common terms, such as 'Developing World', 'Third World' or 'Global South' have similar ambiguity and some have objected to their appropriateness. While we will not go too much further into this debate on nomenclature, the reader should be aware of this background, and know that there are other excellent sources out there that explore the contestation over terminology (see for example: Chant and McIlwaine 2009; Potter et al. 2008). Instead here we highlight the terminology in order to provide some background as to the focus of this book. The Developing World (or Third World or Global South) is an abstract idea that divides the world into different spatial ranges ranked by levels of economic wealth and development. The actual term 'underdeveloped' is traced back to a post-WWII speech by American President Harry S. Truman which recognised the difference between the 'underdeveloped' and the 'prosperous' regions of the world. The post-war belief was that the absence of colonialism meant that, theoretically, all the countries of the world could bring themselves up the ladder to become developed (prosperous) countries.

Undeniably a great deal of writing and study has happened since that time, and geographers now highlight the fact that the hardships of the developing world are deeply rooted historical conditions, such as slavery and colonialism, as well as contemporary exploitation, unequal access to resources and undue adversities that others do not deal with. Yet within developed countries, the emergence of the inequalities debate (Townsend and Davison, 1982) and work on minority groups, e.g., Aboriginals, have also brought to the fore questions about development within developed countries. So, then, what is development? Traditionally definitions have tended to focus on economic measurements, such as a country's gross domestic product (GDP), however these definitions are quite limited in their understanding of human well-being. Here we like Sen's (2000) definition, which steps away from solely economic measures and argues that development is a removal of various types of 'unfreedoms' which leave people without choice and agency in their own lives:

> The removal of substantial unfreedoms ... is constitutive of development ... The intrinsic importance of human freedom, in general, as the preeminent objective of development is strongly supplemented by the instrumental effectiveness of freedoms of particular kinds to promote freedoms of other kinds ... For example, there is strong evidence that economic and political freedoms help to reinforce one another ... Similarly, social opportunities of education and *health care*, which may require public action, complement individual opportunities of economic and political participation and also help to foster our own initiatives in overcoming our respective deprivations. If the point of departure of the approach lies in the identification of freedom as the main object of development, the reach of the policy analysis lies in establishing the empirical linkages that make the viewpoint of freedom coherent and cogent as the guiding perspective of the process of development. (Sen, 2000, xxi, emphasis added)

Note now the parallels between Sen's vision of development, and the World Health Organization's conceptualisation of how health and development meet: 'Better health is central to human happiness and well-being. It also makes an important contribution to economic progress, as healthy populations live longer, are more productive, and save more' (WHO, 2013). Both definitions are grounded in the idea that human well-being is interconnected with numerous facets of life. While economics is important, other aspects (in this case: human health) are also very important. As well, the increase in one aspect tends to lead to an increase in other aspects.

Again we ask, *what is development and what is development geography?* For the purposes of this book we are defining development on two levels. First, it is a *spatial* focus. Development tends to focus its study on certain areas of the planet (i.e., Latin America, sub-Saharan Africa and so on). However, it is not limited to these areas, and many 'development' questions arise in the spatial context of developed countries (or the Global North/the First World). For instance, although Canada enjoys some of the highest living standards in the world, its aboriginal population is still suffering from the colonial legacy and one of the consequences of this are living conditions that many deem to be 'Third World' (Young, 1995). This then bring us to the second level of our definition: an *equality* focus. Development focuses on contexts of inequality, exploitation, inability to access resources and global power imbalances. Or to say otherwise, development questions arise when 'unfreedoms' are occurring, as described by Sen (2000) above. Development geography thus attends to both the geographical *and* social location of subjects.

## Geographies of Health and Development

While an admittedly widespread foundation, development geography has always been an interdisciplinary field, and indeed few of the early development geographers identified themselves as such (it was not until the early 2000s that the American Association of Geographers even formed a speciality group for the area). In many ways the convergence of the geographies of health and development is a natural one, as at their core these disciplines focus on many overlapping issues. Namely, both disciplines have a keen sense for inequality and highlighting its societal fallout. However, the merging of the two areas is 'more than the sum of its parts', or so to speak. Health and development are interactive and work in conversation to build a single sub-discipline: the Geographies of Health and Development. This book provides a look into the uniqueness of that sub-discipline, paying particular attention to both the novel insights and the accompanying challenges that are occurring on this plane of investigation.

The most obvious grounding of the sub-discipline is the explicit causal relationship between health and development (or put inversely, the relationship between ill-health and underdevelopment) as illustrated in Figure 1.1. Poor health can hurt development efforts. Economically, for example, sick citizens do not make for a productive workforce and countries ravaged by HIV/AIDS have drastically reduced labour supplies. On a household scale, households often risk going into debt in order to pay for health care or to cover lost income and as a result children are sometimes pulled from school if their family cannot afford the required payments.

So too can underdevelopment work against health. Basic amenities such as potable water, sanitary facilities, ample nutritious food, well-built residences, and so on, form the basic necessities of health. Historically, when societies acquire these amenities morbidity and mortality rates drop right down as communicable diseases are more easily controlled. Additionally, developed countries have enough wealth to provide national access to health care, further improving the health of their citizens; and the health care available is of high quality with modern technology and an ample supply of health workers. In underdeveloped countries with low tax bases, it becomes extremely hard to finance basic health care and other public health initiatives. Even immunisation programs with well proven long term health improvements in controlling infectious disease must rely on foreign donors for financing. Correspondingly, development translates into increased population education which improves health literacy and behaviours and therefore the country's overall health status.

While the geographies of health and development form a natural bond, there are simultaneously many challenges encountered by researchers working around this nexus; this is especially the case when health geographers are moving to work in a context outside of the discipline's traditional domains. The first challenge to confront health geographers in developing contexts is the striking differences in mortality and morbidity statistics when compared to that of developed countries. Health problems in a developing context take on either much higher rates of prevalence or tackle different types of diseases all together, as a result of the varied environmental, cultural, structural and economic vulnerabilities of the

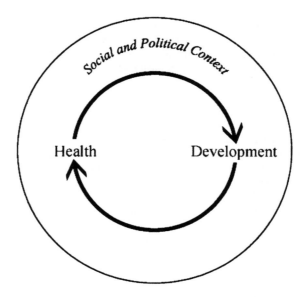

**Figure 1.1      Geographies of Health and Development**

people they impact. In *Part I* of this book, we begin by exploring some of the circumstances surrounding the distinctive health inequities currently facing many developing countries, including malaria, maternal mortality and HIV/AIDS.

While health care has been argued to be a tool to both reducing the burden of these diseases and to improving people's economic circumstances, the access and utilisation of health care also confronts unique problems in developing countries. *Part II* of this book outlines how matters of physical access, human resource shortages, emotional and cultural comfort and, perhaps most importantly, the challenges of financing, together shape the access and utilisation of health care for people of developing countries. The authors in this section all put forward the argument that effective health care must be tailored to the population they serve, emphasising appropriate and personally empowering care.

*Part III* of this book approaches health challenges from a more traditionally 'development geography' perspective. Here, we understand human health and the ecological surroundings to be two different sides of the same coin. Thus as many others have documented the environmental decline facing developing countries, this book examines how the environment interacts to influence the health of the people that live in these locations. This includes discussion around challenges of food (in)security, and the importance of clean and uncontaminated water for health.

Finally, many of the development and health problems highlighted in the previous three sections are brought to a head when placing development within a broader discussion on globalisation in *Part IV*. As the world becomes more connected and the national border holds less significance, people are simultaneously urbanising at a dramatic rate. As global cultures and economies become highly integrated, the urban setting, accordingly, becomes the nexus of many financial and health changes. Together, these trends increase the significance of global and international policy decisions on the lived experience of the people in developing countries. The final section of this book explores the influence of globalisation on health, specifically within the urban environment, against the backdrop of global health policy.

## Overview of Book

*Part I: Disparities in Health Outcomes and the Challenges to Health Equity*

Margai and Minah (Chapter 2) provide a contextualised presentation of malaria risk factors, treatment seeking practices and intervention efforts in poor communities in Sierra Leone. Current challenges in public health with regards to the prevention, management and treatment of malaria is well described, with emerging intervention strategies highlighted. The chapter describes the impact of malaria in poor settings, drawing attention through a case study which illustrates the efforts and challenges to reducing the global burden of malaria. Whilst Sierra Leone was highlighted in this chapter, the arguments and lessons learned can be applied to any number of nations that experience the burden of malaria.

Oppong and Ebeniro (Chapter 3) examine the geography of maternal mortality in Nigeria and argue that adverse life situations such as maternal death do not affect populations uniformly, but vary with social and economic factors in place of residence. The examination of vulnerabilities spatially, is crucial to the prevention and control of maternal health risks and mortality. The chapter recommends targeting vulnerable populations and places with health education as an important strategy for reducing maternal mortality in Nigeria and elsewhere. However, this must be supplemented with poverty reduction, improved access to health care and cultural reform including changing some of the religious laws and practices.

Hellen and Wadhwa (Chapter 4) highlight the structural violence that may be engulfing sex work in Pune, India. The work is based on a study that aimed at understating the impact of India's National AIDS Control Organization's strategy of using NGOs to reach out to people living with HIV/AIDS and among in high-risk populations such as commercial sex workers. They argue that while prevention efforts in Pune may be insufficient due to scarce mobilisation and education, especially in the case of the female sex worker population; the results nonetheless offer a helpful window into some of the realities associated with attempting to control the HIV epidemic in India. Resultantly, the data are useful in highlighting impediments to effective prevention efforts; the study proposes suggestions to help address them.

Wilson, Rosenberg and Ning (Chapter 5) address the health and development challenges among Aboriginal peoples not only in Canada, but also in the United States, New Zealand and Australia. The chapter argues that while the gaps in health status between Aboriginal and non-Aboriginal populations have narrowed in terms of health status and social and economic development, the improvements have been uneven and new inequalities in health and well-being have emerged. For example, while differences in life expectancy have narrowed between Aboriginal and non-Aboriginal populations in Canada, young Aboriginal adults are disproportionately represented among those with HIV/AIDS. Furthermore, although educational attainment is slowly improving among Aboriginal students, young Aboriginal adults are disproportionately represented in the prison system in Canada. This chapter explains these gaps through both historical and current lenses of racism and racist strategies that hold back widespread improvements in health and the development of Aboriginal Peoples.

*Part II: Health Access and Utilisation in Developing Countries*

Dixon and Mkandawire (Chapter 6) examine arguments against health insurance financing, especially in developing countries, as these have been underpinned by a narrow conceptualisation of health that does not fully reflect the political ecologies and spatial contexts within which diseases have flourished. Drawing on the social determinants of health framework, and using Ghana's Upper West Region as a case study, the chapter critically engages with the literature on health insurance and argue for alternative assumptions on the meaning of 'health' in health insurance. This chapter challenges traditional reductionist approaches to health financing and emphasises a greater collective responsibility for societal well-being in developing contexts.

Eagler, Sakdapolrak, Bohle and Kearns (Chapter 7) investigate health care preferences among poor urban dwellers in Chennai, India. Based on field work, this chapter examines the ability of poorer urban residents to access health care and why they express what might appear to be a paradoxical preference for private health care. This chapter uses a space-centred approach to offer a geographical perspective on the health care landscape of Chennai and how providers and urban poor users present and negotiate the complex nature of entitlements to health care in this emerging mega city. Although discussions of health insurance issues in developing countries are beginning to emerge in health geography literature, what is presented in this chapter is new and captivating.

George, Reardon and Quinlan (Chapter 8) examine the changing human resource needs in Africa as a result of the burden of disease and as health care strategies evolve. The focus of this chapter is a discussion on the a need for a consistent focus on how to build up and sustain the human resources necessary to provide health care in an equitable manner, albeit with unequal distribution of human resources between urban and rural centres and between the public and private health sectors. This chapter seeks to qualify what is commonly perceived to be a problem of staff shortages: a lack of the required number of service delivery staff such as doctors and nurses to serve the health care demands of a national population. A nuanced exploration of the anomalies in a large yet fragmented body of information on the human resource challenges is provided to illustrate the actual nature of the staff shortage problem in sub-Saharan Africa.

Huish (Chapter 9) provides an interesting contribution to the understanding of how ethics in health-worker education matter in bolstering or weakening health-care systems. This chapter compares national-level training programs by using case studies from Cuba and the Philippines. The case studies provide intriguing findings whereby while in Cuba health education has a dedicated focus on service provision to the poor, community-based practice through disease prevention and health promotion, and ultimately a consciousness of the need to deliver health-care to some of the poorest places in the world; in the Philippines, there is a conscious ethic within institutions and on a national level to encourage outmigration for the sake of garnering economic remittance. This chapter provides for the reader an opportunity to examine ways in which medical education can be an empowering force to embolden the strength and capacity of health care systems in the context of development.

*Part III: Environmental Influences on Health and Development*

Classen, Bezner Kerr and Shumba (Chapter 10) draw attention to the complex factors influencing rural youth food and nutrition research, and the need for creative methods for engaging young people in social and health research. Using field work data from Malawi, this chapter shows that understanding the particularities of shifting youth labour, mobility and social relations in the contemporary climate of market liberalisation and an expanding socioeconomic divide is critical to developing appropriate food security and nutrition programming for rural youth.

Pennock, Poland and Hanncock (Chapter 11) provide an intriguing account of the effects of rising energy prices and growing energy insecurity associated with a tightening of global oil supplies. This chapter considers what 'peak oil' might mean for the future of globalisation, 'development', and discourses of economic growth and 'progress'. The reader is asked to question what it may take to plan for future high cost in energy and impact on the social determinants of health of disadvantaged populations.

Schuster-Wallace, Elliott and Bisung (Chapter 12) discuss the linkages between water environment and health, and present the water-health nexus as represented by the intersection between the bio-physical system, the hydrosocial system, and human health. Using examples from rural communities in Kenya and elsewhere, this chapter also examines these linkages from the perspective of individuals and communities where lack of access to safe water and the consequent burden of poor health are a reality. The reader is provided with the facilitators and barriers to ownership and sustained management of water resources for health.

Paul (Chapter 13) provides a critical overview of health effects of arsenic poisoning of underground water in Bangladesh, and queries why some development programs may often have negative implications on human health. The reader is taken through the historical processes that have resulted in tubewell water becoming the greatest health threat to the people of rural Bangladesh because of arsenic poisoning of such water sources. This chapter outlines how many Bangladeshis are suffering from arsenic-related diseases ranging from melanosis to skin and various cancers.

*Part IV: Globalisation and Urbanisation: Global Policy Consequences on Local Health Problems*

Fried and Eyles (Chapter 14) make an important case that tuberculosis may be an indicator of and a barrier to development, with the causes of tuberculosis linked to poverty and lack of development and its impacts challenging past and future development gains. This chapter points out the re-emergence of tuberculosis in the late twentieth century, the rapid increases in multi-drug resistant and extremely drug-resistant tuberculosis variants, its relationship to HIV/AIDS and alarming global numbers as critical points that deserve attention by geographers involved in health and development work.

Lovell and Rosenberg (Chapter 15) provide interesting arguments on how global economic forces are shaping health and health care and the progress geographers have made in examining these relationships. The reader is provided a discussion of the contested nature of globalisation, contextualising the processes which currently have implications for human health. This chapter examines the relationship between economic development and health and examine the impacts free trade has had on the health of populations; and argues that the role of globalisation with its emphasis on free trade and economic development marginalises the importance of health and social development and turns health into just another commodity to be traded on the global stage.

Schrecker (Chapter 16) discusses how contemporary geographies of health and development must incorporate new understandings of globalisation. The reader is taken through how globalisation magnifies and transforms the juxtapositions of wealth and privatisation by gradually detaching economic opportunities from national boundaries, with its influence penetrating deeply into the organisation of economies and societies within national borders: hence, local depth. This chapter also discusses processes of reterritorialisation that link the global and the local.

Chikanda and Dodson (Chapter 17) provide an interesting contribution to the understanding of the geography of health and development by examining the movement of health professionals out of Africa, the impact this creates on the declining quality of health care in the continent, and the important role the 'diasporas' can play in the development of their countries of origin. Using Zimbabwe as a case study, the chapter makes an assessment of the merits of adopting diaspora engagement initiatives as a way of utilising the skills and professional expertise of Africa's emigrant medical professionals.

The contributions in this book provide a variety of stories of the geographies of health and development. From the chapters, it is apparent how health and development interconnect. The geographies of health and development is an emerging sub-discipline, tying in with many of the conceptual, theoretical and practical components of other disciplines working in health, health care, economics, and international development. Further, notions of space and place are of upmost importance as both the local and global scales heavily influence geographies of health and development. Spatially and theoretically grounded in geography, this collection offers a fresh perspective on the dialectic relationships between health and development, and together finds a home within the series *Geographies of Health*.

### References

Chant, S. and McIlwaine, C. 2009. *Geographies of Development in the 21st Century: An Introduction to the Global South*. Massachusetts: Edward Elgar Publishing Inc.

Potter, R., Binns, T., Elliot, J.A. and Smith, D. 2008. *Geographies of Development*, 3rd Edition. Harlow: Pearson Education.

Sen, A. 2000. *Development as Freedom: Human Capability and Global Need*. New York: Anchor Books.

Townsend, P. and Davison, N. 1982. *Inequalities in Health: The Black Report*. Harmondsworth, Middlesex: Penguin.

WHO. 2013. *Health and development*. World Health Organization. Available at: http://www.who.int/hdp/en/.

Young, E. 1995. *Third World in the First: Development and Indigenous Peoples*. New York: Routledge.

# PART I
# Disparities in Health Outcomes and the Challenges to Health Equity

# Chapter 2

# Malaria Risk Profiles, Treatment Seeking Practices and Disease Intervention Efforts in Poor Communities: A Case Study in Sierra Leone

Florence M. Margai and Jacob B. Minah

## Introduction

In an era in which many developing countries are undergoing epidemiological risk transitions, malaria remains atop the world's deadliest infectious diseases, claiming the lives of up to one million people each year. Despite intense efforts to curb the global burden of the disease, it is still one of the leading causes of mortality in low-income countries accounting for at least 5.2 per cent of the death toll (WHO 2011). And nowhere are these conditions more serious than in sub-Saharan Africa (SSA) where 90 per cent of the deaths occur alongside adverse health complications such as poor reproductive outcomes, cognitive and neurological impairments, and other developmental delays in young children (Guyatt and Snow 2001; Holding and Kitsao-Wekulo 2004; Samba 2004). The changing global climate, armed regional conflicts, the HIV/AIDs pandemic, and rising levels of poverty have all contributed to the persistence of this disease in the region (Minah and Margai 2008; Stratton et al. 2008).

The quest for more enduring and efficacious therapies for malaria continues in earnest along several scientific fronts as *Plasmodium falciparum*, the most fatal of the four parasitic species, unremittingly morphs into newer and more resistant strains. Amidst these scientific pursuits, the political and scholarly discourse on disease management strategies continues, as policy makers weigh in on the approaches that work best in resource-poor settings and how to fit these into the grand scheme of national health and economic reform policies. Questions relating to the prioritisation of various intervention strategies, and the sustainability of these programs within an era of economic downturns and limited fiscal budgets have been hotly debated (Gallup and Sachs 2001; Sachs and Malaney 2002; Malaney et al. 2004; Worrall et al. 2005; Castro and Fisher 2012). The scientific literature is replete with specific questions relating to the nature, direction and strength of the association between poverty and malaria: Is the relationship causal and/or bidirectional? If causality exists, what are the implications for malaria control efforts? If poverty is a significant cause of malaria, will poverty alleviation policies significantly reduce the disease burden? On the contrary, if the relationship is bidirectional, with malaria being the most influential cause of poverty, will disease prevention strategies be effective tools of development to permanently lift these countries out of poverty?

The purpose of this chapter is to critically examine these issues based on evidence compiled in the literature during the past decade. We will also assess the malaria control/elimination strategies that are currently in place within African countries, and their effectiveness in light of the target dates established by global funding agencies. Then, using a case study, we will illustrate the health challenges and treatment seeking practices among local residents in a low-income community in Sierra Leone, and the results of an intervention study aimed at reducing the disease burden.

## Causal Linkages between Malaria and Poverty in Sub-Saharan Africa

Within the context of development and health, malaria offers a classic illustration of the close correspondence between poverty and disease. Scientists have long described malaria and poverty as inextricably linked with distinct associations observed on maps revealing high levels of endemicity in poor regions. Globally, the disease is endemic in about 106 countries, notably poor countries, and 48 of these countries are in SSA. While a host of physical environmental factors are partly to blame for the historical and current distribution of the disease, during the past decade, many scholars have proceeded to critically examine the relationships between socio-economic status (SES) and the persistence of the disease using economic and spatial analytical models (Gallup and Sachs 2001; Cropper et al. 2004; Castro and Fisher 2012).

In a seminal paper first produced by Sachs and Malaney (2002), the relationship between poverty and malaria was characterised as both causal and bidirectional, with the link from malaria to poverty deemed to be more powerful than the other way around. Their findings were based in part on earlier economic assessments of the cumulative effects of malaria, in which the disease was found to reduce the Gross National Product per capita by more than 50 per cent in high risk malarious countries when compared to non-malarious countries (Gallup and Sachs 2001). In a subsequent study, Malaney et al. (2004) examined the diverse mechanisms through which malaria can negatively impact the long term economic development of a country. Since previous studies had focused primarily on microeconomic methods such as Cost of Illness (COI), Willingness to Pay (WTP) and production finance, Malaney et al. (2004) called for a comprehensive approach that incorporates the ubiquity and endemicity of the disease, and the costs that are borne at all spatial scales including the household, community and national levels. Citing a study that had previously estimated that malaria in Africa costs about US$9.84 per case using the COI method, they found such approaches to be prone to data challenges, and very conservative, producing figures that focus primarily on individual costs, and less useful in the endemic regions. As an alternative, Malaney et al. (2004) proposed the use of a macro approach to uncover the long term economic and social burden of the disease, and parse out the complex nature and strength of the two way causality between malaria and poverty.

Figure 2.1 summarises the principal pathways through which malaria impedes the economic development of countries. The direct costs include private costs that are incurred by individuals and their immediate households. The public costs are incurred within the larger community context including national expenditures on prevention, case diagnosis and treatment. The right side of Figure 2.1 shows the indirect costs. Not surprisingly, these are more diffuse and difficult to calibrate since they consist of both tangible and latent factors such as the perception of health risks in endemic areas. Following the lead by Malaney et al. (2004), one might be able to deconstruct and operationalise these latent factors. For example, the loss of economic productivity can be assessed using metrics that are linked to malaria morbidity, or foregone productivity due to premature death from the disease. Further, individuals who are vulnerable to the disease with repetitive

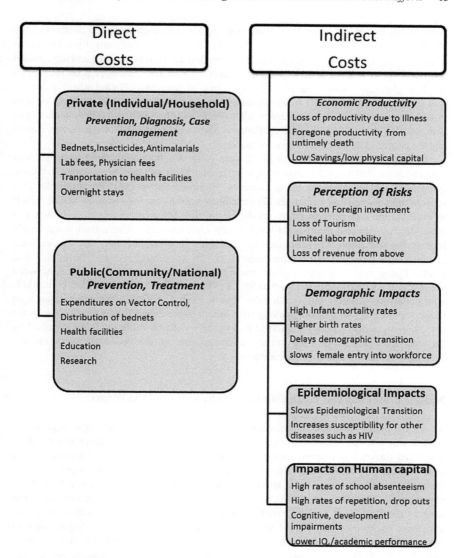

**Figure 2.1    Principal pathways for estimating the costs of malaria morbidity**

episodes are less likely to earn enough income, overall limiting their ability to accumulate financial capital. The perception of disease risk is also likely to impact population mobility and inflow of labour, tourists and potential foreign investors into an endemic region. Demographically, high infant mortality rates in malarious regions may result in higher fertility rates as more women choose to have larger families (as a form of security at old age) limiting or delaying their entry into the workforce. With fewer women in the workforce, the chances of increasing financial capital decline further for these families, contributing to household poverty. Malarious regions with high birth and death rates are also likely to remain entrenched in stage II or III of the demographic transition with limited chances of advancing into the stages that are characteristic of industrialised and modernised societies. The epidemiological impacts of malaria are also worth noting; malarious regions are less likely to follow Omran's (1971) stages of transition. Rather, these countries will remain mired in stage I of the epidemiological transition, with high levels of dual infections associated with other transmissible diseases such as HIV and tuberculosis. These demographic and epidemiological challenges collectively take a toll on the human capital and the overall development of these countries.

In sum, the economic burden of malaria is far-reaching with large scale societal consequences that extend across all spatial levels. Most scholars now agree that these impacts should be assessed using complex multifactorial models. For example, in a recent study, Castro and Fisher (2012) developed a simultaneous equation model (SEM) to evaluate the bidirectional nature of the causal link between poverty and malaria at a multi-disciplinary and multi-scale level. Using childhood data drawn from a nationally representative sample in Tanzania, the variables incorporated into the model were grouped into three categories: the individual and household factors, the human and physical geographical factors, and the macro factors. In the study, the causal link between malaria and socioeconomic status was found to be statistically significant; in households with malarious children, the wealth index was on average 1.9 units lower than those with healthy children. These findings along with others in the extant literature all point to the close correspondence between malaria and poverty with far more evidence supplied on the significant and debilitating impacts of the disease on the social, demographic and economic sectors in low-income countries.

## Malaria Prevention and Treatment: Global Strategies and Challenges

As documented in the preceding section, evidence compiled in recent years suggests that greater emphasis be placed on malaria prevention and treatment therapies as part of an integrated national campaign. Curbing the disease not only serves as a national health care strategy, but it can effectively serve as a poverty alleviation strategy with potentially long term benefits accruing in all sectors of a developing society. Many governments now recognise this important connection, and have joined forces with international organisations such as the Roll Back Malaria program (RBM), and the President's Malaria Initiative, to reform health care policies (Mathanga and Bowie 2007). The global target dates set for controlling malaria have been continually revised, however 2015 is now the official year during which all countries are expected to have significantly reduced the disease morbidity and mortality to near zero levels. Countrywide efforts to achieve these targets revolve around two key strategies: a) prevention, and b) treatment (case management). Figure 2.2 summarises these strategies along with the impediments that hinder full scale implementation. More details are provided below.

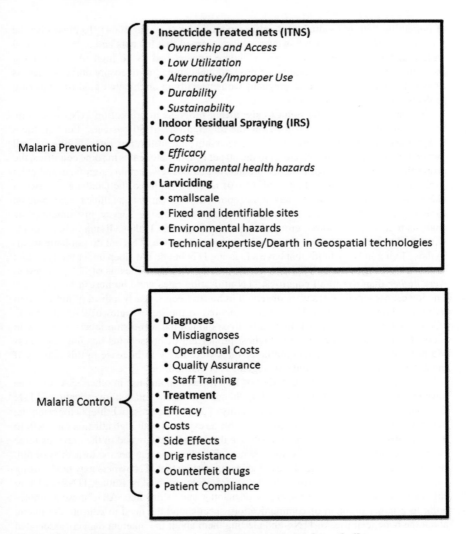

Malaria Prevention
- **Insecticide Treated nets (ITNS)**
  - *Ownership and Access*
  - *Low Utilization*
  - *Alternative/Improper Use*
  - *Durability*
  - *Sustainability*
- **Indoor Residual Spraying (IRS)**
  - *Costs*
  - *Efficacy*
  - *Environmental health hazards*
- **Larviciding**
  - smallscale
  - Fixed and identifiable sites
  - Environmental hazards
  - Technical expertise/Dearth in Geospatial technologies

Malaria Control
- **Diagnoses**
  - Misdiagnoses
  - Operational Costs
  - Quality Assurance
  - Staff Training
- **Treatment**
- Efficacy
- Costs
- Side Effects
- Drig resistance
- Counterfeit drugs
- Patient Compliance

**Figure 2.2    Malaria prevention and treatment approaches: challenges and limitations**

**Malaria Prevention Strategies**

*a. Insecticide Treated Nets (ITNs)*

Malaria prevention has been the most widely adopted strategy gaining worldwide attention and support from nongovernmental organisations and donor agencies that fund vaccine development, and large scale distribution of Insecticide Treated Nets. As early as 2000, ITNs were being described as one of the most efficacious and affordable means of protecting both individuals and entire communities (Lengler 2004). To maximise the full benefits of this approach however, experts warned that the nets had to be distributed widely and the utilisation rates among home owners had to be high. As such, most governments embarked on nationwide promotional campaigns to ensure universal access especially among children and pregnant women, with an anticipated goal of achieving protective coverage of at least 80 per cent.

Reports compiled so far point to significant progress in promoting ITN ownership, however most countries are still below the targeted rate of 80 per cent. Further, there is a persistent mismatch between ITN ownership and utilisation rates. While overall ownership rates appear to inch closer to the 80 per cent targeted rates in some countries, the proportion of owners sleeping under the distributed bednets remains significantly below expectations. For example, Eng et al. (2010) recently explored the challenges between ITN ownership and utilisation rates in five countries with national health care campaigns: Kenya, Niger, Madagascar, Sierra Leone, and Togo. Using survey instruments, the analysis focused on children, grouped into four categories: 1) those living in households with no ITN present; 2) those living in households that own ITNs but do not hang them; 3) those living in households that have a hanging ITN but do not sleep under the ITN; and 4) those sleeping under an ITN. The results confirmed that the levels of ITN *ownership* were *higher* than *use* in all countries. ITN utilisation rates were highest in Madagascar. The lowest ownership rates were observed in Sierra Leone; nearly a third of the children lived in a home without an ITN when compared to the lowest rates of 9.4 per cent in Madagascar (Eng et al. 2010). Ironically, even though the ownership levels were low in Sierra Leone, the country had the highest proportion of households hanging their nets (85 per cent) suggesting that compliance rates were likely to increase in this country if the government were to expand coverage of ITN distribution.

Similar to Eng et al. (2010), studies of ITN ownership and use in other SSA countries have produced comparable findings citing the need for more detailed investigation of ITN distribution strategies, and greater sustainability of these programs. In Ethiopia for example, nets distributed to households are not as durable as expected with high attrition rates within a year (Batisso et al. 2012). Approximately a third of all nets owned in the previous three years are reportedly discarded by homeowners either because they are too torn, dirty or old. In other countries, there is anecdotal evidence suggesting that ITN owners may not be using the nets in the manner prescribed by the governments and NGOs. Rather, ITNs are being sold in the market place as bath sponges, dishcloths, and fishing nets. All of these examples point to a larger problem of communication, specifically, the need to educate the public about the beneficial uses of ITNs, and alerting them about the inherent dangers associated with these alternative uses. National campaigns to expand coverage and ownership of ITNs must be accompanied by behavioural change intervention efforts to promote hanging and the proper use of these bednets.

*b. Larvicides*

Alongside ITNs, national efforts to reduce local malaria transmission entail the use of larviciding. Larval control programs entail the destruction of mosquito larvae by applying insecticides to actual or potential breeding sites (WHO 1996). Challenges associated with this strategy include the inherent risks to non-target organisms in the environment, including humans, and the greater chances of vector resistance with routine use of the insecticides. Larviciding also requires accurate targeting and is recommended mostly in settings where mosquito breeding sites are few, fixed, identifiable, mappable and treatable (WHO 2011). Localities with limited or no access to piped water, poor waste-water or sewage disposal systems are prime candidates for such programs. Participatory mapping approaches using aerial photographs and GIS to generate target areas for mosquito larval control have been proven to be particularly effective in these efforts (Dongus et al. 2007). These geographic technologies have been shown to rapidly and effectively delineate the productive habitats of female anopheles mosquitoes, followed by more targeted spraying of larval sites. Unfortunately, fiscal constraints and the dearth of technical expertise to gather, digitise and analyse the relevant data make it difficult to adopt these geospatial approaches and related strategies for malaria control. Geographers can and should play a critical role in these data acquisition efforts, and the transfer of knowledge and use of these analytical technologies in developing countries.

*c. Indoor Residual Spraying (IRS)*

Given the constraints of larviciding noted above, most SSA countries are advised to utilise the IRS approach for more large scale control of mosquitoes. WHO has recommended about 12 different forms of insecticides with DDT (**d**ichloro**d**iphenyl**t**richloroethane) being the cheapest with a residual efficacy of at least six months. The ban on DDT (under the Stockholm convention) has been temporarily rescinded to allow these countries to mount a quick and effective campaign against malaria, hoping that this will permanently eradicate the disease like it did during the 1960s in temperate regions. However, DDT use is extremely controversial amidst concerns about the long term health effects that have been so widely documented. There are also concerns about the misuse of the chemical in other economic sectors such as agriculture and the possibility of this entering the food chain (Margai 2010). One can only hope that the policy makers in these countries are fully cognisant of the inherent dangers of DDT use, and will use the chemical only as a last resort in the fight against malaria. As with ITN campaigns, the implementation of IRS approaches must be accompanied by full scale communication campaigns to raise awareness about the potential threats of these chemicals to population health and the environment.

**Malaria Control Strategies: Diagnosis and Treatment**

Many SSA countries have adopted WHO guidelines for treating malaria. These strategies begin with the prompt diagnosis and confirmation of the disease either by microscopy or the use of rapid diagnostic test kits. Once a case is confirmed, treatment must follow immediately using an Artemisinin Combination Therapy (ACT). Currently there are five recommended ACTs for SSA and the selection of any of these is based on what is deemed to be the most effective in the selected country. As with malaria prevention efforts, the overarching goal here is to achieve universal access in case management. By 2015, these countries hope to have a 100 per cent confirmation of suspected cases of malaria, followed by 100 per cent treatment of these cases using the most appropriate anti-malarial therapy.

Malaria control initiatives have been riddled with many challenges (see Figure 2.2). One area in particular that demands the most attention is the misdiagnosis of malaria cases due to the lack of resources in the laboratories where diagnostic tests are performed. In a South African case study, parasitologists, Dini and Frean (2003) reviewed the quality of malaria diagnosis in 115 laboratories and found high levels of reporting inaccuracies. One out of every seven blood films were incorrectly interpreted leading to an unacceptably high error rate of 13.8 per cent. Similar problems have been reported in other SSA countries leading to calls for strengthening these malaria laboratories to improve standardisation, validation protocols, personnel training, and quality assurance (Dini and Frean 2003).

Additional concerns facing malaria control efforts include the rising costs of antimalarials particularly for residents in low-income communities and the side effects associated with long-term use of these therapies in endemic regions (Margai and Minah 2007). Also problematic is the growing public distrust of drug efficacy due to the increasing presence of counterfeit antimalarials (Greenwood 2010). These are compounded further by the inability of governments to continue these programs. Most of the efforts are intermittent and short-lived due to the fiscal challenges facing these countries. Following below is a case study illustrating the kinds of challenges associated with the disease intervention efforts in resource poor settings. We start with a contextual background for the case study and then proceed to discuss the research objectives, methods, data analysis and findings.

## A Case Study to Reduce Malaria Burden in a Distressed Community

*National Context for the Study*

With funding from a British non-profit agency, a pilot intervention program for malaria was developed and implemented in Freetown, the capital city of Sierra Leone (Margai and Minah 2007). The rationale for conducting this study was based on both historical and current contextual factors: perennially high rates of malaria, extreme poverty, civil war, and poor access to health resources. Sierra Leone has had a long-standing reputation as one of the most malarious regions in West Africa. As early as the 1800s, the British had dubbed this region a 'white man's grave' due to high malaria fatality counts among their colonial officers. These dire conditions had prompted two British scientific expeditions to investigate the mosquito-malaria relationship, and develop preventive measures. Sadly enough, one of the preventive measures suggested was racial segregation, recommending that the homes of the Europeans be built on elevated areas, far removed from the indigenous people in the low-lying areas of Freetown (Frenkel and Western 1988).

At the time of our study, malaria accounted for roughly 40 per cent of the outpatient morbidity in Sierra Leone. The disease was endemic in the country with an annual average of one malaria episode per person. The health risks associated with malaria were exacerbated further by a brutal 11-year civil war (1991–2002) that had disrupted all societal institutions, killing and maiming thousands of people, internally displacing about 250,000, while forcing others to flee to neighbouring countries.

In the post-war period, development and economic progress in Sierra Leone has been painfully slow. To date, approximately 66.4 per cent of the population lives below the national poverty line. When placed within a global context, the percentage of people living below $2.00 a day is 76.1 per cent. Evidence of the intensity of national poverty can be further discerned by the Multidimensional Poverty Index (MPI) produced recently by Alkire et al. (2011) using data from the 2008 Demographic and Health Survey (DHS). The MPI shows that 43.9 per cent of the population is multi-dimensionally poor, implying significant deprivation in multiple indicators such as education, living standards, and health.

With high rates of poverty, most residents cannot afford the conventional drugs used to prevent or treat the malaria. As shown in Table 2.1, a comparison of the costs and side effects associated with the commonly available drug therapies points to an urgent need for alternative and sustainable therapies. Choloroquine, the cheapest drug in the market, is no longer efficacious in Sierra Leone with a confirmed failure rate of about 39 per cent. The other conventional drugs shown to be effective, such as Lariam or Malarone are expensive with potential side effects associated with prolonged use. The latter are used primarily by foreigners or other visitors from the developed world who could afford these therapies and are only likely to spend a short duration in these endemic areas, thus minimising the side effects.

**Table 2.1    Comparison of AntiMalarials (therapies and prophylaxes) by costs, efficacy and potential side effects**

| Drug | Cost per treatment (Estimated Dollars) | Efficacy | Potential side Effects |
|------|----------------------------------------|----------|------------------------|
| *Resochin (Chloroquine)* | 2 | Poor | Hearing Impairment |
| *Pyrimenthamin +Sulfadoxine(Fansidar)* | 6 | Poor | Allergic reactions |
| *Mefloquine/Lariam* | 60 | High | Cardiac failure, Psychosis |
| *Atovaquon + Proguanil (Malarone)* | 60 | Limited data | Abdominal problems |

*Source:* Minah and Margai, 2008.

Another challenge facing the country is the limited availability of health resources (medical staff, equipment, laboratories) required to mount an effective campaign against malaria. There are inadequate health facilities and few health practitioners due to high levels of 'brain drain'. Despite the reputable academic and health training institutions that once existed in the country, many of these professionals have emigrated in search of more lucrative job opportunities and better living conditions elsewhere.

For the study at hand, it was important to assess the national risk profiles of the disease based on the physical environment, treatment seeking patterns, and the spatial extent of bednet coverage. We utilised maps generated from MARA-ARMA models showing the seasonal dimensions of malaria, and geographic risk profiles based on vegetation, elevation, temperature and precipitation (MARA-ARMA 1998). We also assessed the spatial coverage of bednets using the 2008 DHS dataset. The data was collected from 350 spatially representative population clusters. The variables were brought into a GIS for geostatistical interpolation. The derived map shows the locational disparities in the distribution of bednets across the country (Figure 2.3). The results show that bednet coverage is still below the global and national target rate of 80 per cent. The maximum coverage is about 60 per cent observed in selected parts of the country such as the Bo, Koinadugu and Moyamba districts. All other regions including the western province (where Freetown is located) are performing under par in terms of meeting the target rates for bednet coverage.

Overall, addressing the economic, social and political challenges noted above while striving to meet the malaria targets set by the WHO are an uphill challenge for this

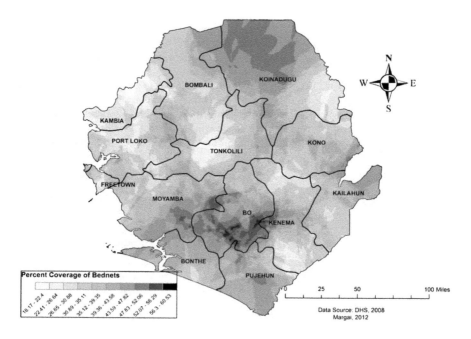

**Figure 2.3      Spatial coverage of bednets in districts across Sierra Leone**

The key goal of the intervention study was to explore the use of sustainable, affordable and efficacious therapies to reduce the burden of *P.falciparum* among the residents in this community. Emphasis was placed on Complementary and Alternative Medicine (CAM) with various modalities that are often used alongside conventional therapies. The study relied specifically on *Tropica nosode* as a promising and safe naturopathic therapy for malaria. *Tropica nosode* is a prophylaxis developed exclusively for P. *falciparum*. It belongs to the realm of homeopathic remedies for malaria that have been recognised in the literature for more than 200 years since Hahnemann's discovery (Hahnemann 2003; Golden 2007). Unfortunately, few studies have fully documented the efficacy of these remedies in Africa. In the absence of formally established clinical trials, the reports have been anecdotal, and some studies plagued with methodological problems such as poor or limited sampling, short-term testing, and data quality assurance issues (Wilcox and Bodeker 2004). Our goal in the current study was to overcome these limitations by developing a rigorous data driven approach that relied on a double blind randomised control method to guide the intervention study.

**Research Design and Methods**

The study was carried out in four phases. The first phase, initiated in June 2006, entailed the preparation and review of the research protocols, purchasing of medical equipment and project staff recruitment. The project team consisted of the lead principal investigator, a practicing paediatrician and homeopath with decades of experience in administering both conventional and homeopathic drugs in children; the Co-principal Investigator with decades of experience in environmental health risk assessment and spatial data analysis; an epidemiologist, a local health coordinator, two community organisers, four lab technicians and four nurses. Following intense staff training, and several meetings with the community leaders, we embarked on subject recruitment through community meetings, and door to door campaigns. The goal was to recruit approximately 780 permanent residents living within a radius of 10 km of the Kroo Bay Health Center (KBHC), a centrally located clinic in the community. This sample size was determined based on the estimated outpatient morbidity rate of 40 per cent for malaria, and an anticipated 20 per cent attrition rate during the follow-up periods. Eligibility guidelines for the study were based solely on adults aged 18 years and older with no evidence of severe illness. Children and pregnant women were excluded. Overall, 731 residents agreed to participate in the project.

Following the standard research protocols, participants were asked to first complete an informed consent form followed by a detailed questionnaire documenting their personal case histories, use of exposure prevention measures such as mosquito bed nets, frequency of malaria diagnoses, the kinds of treatments used in the past, and knowledge of alternative treatment therapies. Other variables such as age, height, weight, gender, occupation and socio-economic attributes were collected. Under supervision and care of the physician, participants underwent a comprehensive physical exam including the collection of blood samples to test for malaria. The blood slides were sent to the lab for microscopic examination and diagnosis. For positive cases, the parasitic density was assessed by the lab technicians. To further assess the level of accuracy in diagnosis, 10 per cent of the interpreted blood slides were sent to an independent lab for cross validation.

Based on the medical exams and lab tests, all individuals exhibiting clinical symptoms of malaria (high temperature >37.5° C, and high levels of asexual forms of P *falciparum* in the blood) were treated promptly using Quinine and Paracetamol, the state recommended therapy. Of the 731 registrants, 534 had very low or negligible parasitic burden. These 534 subjects were formally enrolled in the study. These subjects were randomised into two groups, with the first group of 289 subjects receiving five pellets of *Tropica nosode*. The second group of 245 subjects received five placebo pellets that were similar in form to the homeopathic therapy. All drugs were administered on site and patients were advised to report any potential health problems, specifically malaria symptoms, to the nursing staff at the health centre. Subjects were assigned unique numbers, and given identification cards with their name, age, gender, address. These identifiers were entered in the computerised database and a medical ledger for use in subsequent phases. Community health workers were required to visit these neighbourhoods regularly over the course of the year to check on the health status of these registrants.

Overall, the project lasted for four phases, and the procedures established in Phase 1 were replicated four months later in Phase II, and thereafter in Phase III, and Phase IV. In each phase, patients completed a follow-up survey, a health exam, and submitted a blood sample. Patients with negative test results were re-enrolled in phases, II (404 persons), III (347 persons) and IV (297 persons). During each phase, participants who tested positive with clinical signs of high temperatures and high levels of parasitemia were treated. As shown in Table 2.2, the overall distribution of patients was fairly consistent across the phases with 55 per cent of the participants receiving homeopathic prophylaxis and 45 per cent receiving inactive pellets. At the completion of the pilot study all of the data was compiled and analysed.

**Table 2.2       Distribution of eligible participants across treatment groups in Phases I, II, III and IV**

| Eligible Participants | Baseline Phase I | Follow-up Phase II | Follow-up Phase III | Follow-up Phase IV |
|---|---|---|---|---|
| *Malaria Prophylaxis* | 54% (n1=289) | 57% (n1=237) | 55% n1=194) | 55% (n1=167) |
| *Placebo* | 45% (n2=245) | 40% (n2=167) | 43% n2=153) | 43% (n2=130) |

**Statistical Data Analysis and Results**

Of the 731 participants who registered for the project, the average age was 38.6 years, and 73 per cent were females. The average length of stay in the community was 18.5 years. Literacy levels were very low with more than half of the subjects having no formal education (55 per cent). Employment levels were equally low with only a third (34 per cent) of the residents working in the informal sector selling small goods and vegetables.

   *a. Malaria Symptoms and Treatment Seeking Patterns*: The participants were asked several questions about symptoms of fever and malaria, frequency of malaria episodes, the source of and type of treatment received during the past year. Nearly three quarters (74 per cent) of the participants reported frequent episodes of fever. About 81 per cent reported that they had experienced at least one episode of fever within the past month. When asked about the frequency of malaria episodes, the average number of malaria episodes reported by patients was 3.24. These statistics were fairly representative of this community, which, as noted earlier, was highly vulnerable due to the confluence of risks. When asked about where they sought treatment for malaria, the three most common sources of treatment cited were the government hospital (23.8 per cent), local pharmacies (29.8 per cent) and itinerant drug vendors (19.2). The latter are locally untrained and illegal vendors who have stalls, or conduct door-to door visitations in the community sometimes offering counterfeit drugs and other therapies for a host of diseases. For the drugs frequently used to treat malaria, surprisingly, more than half of the residents cited Chloroquine (56.9 per cent) despite the documented resistance of P. *falciparum* parasites to this drug. Quinine, which was the state recommended therapy at the time, was cited by only 10 per cent of the respondents and some noted allergic reactions. Others mentioned Fansidar (17.5 per cent) and Native/Tribal Medicines (11.6 per cent).

   *b. Use of bednets and other preventive approaches*: Participants were asked about the use of bed nets and other devices that assist in malaria prevention. Only 16 per cent had bednets and when asked whether, it had been used the night before, only about 12 per cent indicated that they had used it the night before. The individuals with bednets had received these only about a month ago following a local NGO sponsored project that had given away bednets to lactating mothers. Other than bednets, the most common devices cited for warding off mosquitoes were mosquito coils and sprays. Due to the expenses involved, most residents in this community do not use these preventive devices on a regular basis.

*c. The Effectiveness of the Malaria Prophylaxis*: The efficacy of the malaria prophylaxis among these registrants was assessed using two kinds of statistical analysis. The first set of analysis involved a phase-by-phase evaluation of the data comparing the risks of malaria diagnosis among the homeopathic and placebo groups. The results generated from the medical examinations completed during Phase I confirmed that malaria was prevalent in the community. Evidence from the blood test results showed that nearly 29 per cent tested positive for malaria with a mean parasitic density of 401/*ul*. A total of eight clinical cases were identified based on the diagnostic criteria established in the study. In analysing the data in subsequent phases, only 3 clinical cases were observed in phase II, 0 in Phase III, and 3 in Phase IV. Overall, the most significant effect of the homeopathic therapy was evident in Phase II. In this second phase, the risk of getting malaria was 3.6 times higher in the placebo group than the homeopathic group. Unfortunately, the protective effect of the homeopathic therapy observed in Phase II was not sustained in Phases II and IV. The results in Phases III and IV were marginal and no statistically significant differences were observed between the two groups.

The second set of analyses was completed at the end of the pilot project during which a data subset was compiled. The latter consisted of only the participants for whom we had complete data across all four phases. This second analysis was necessary since the study followed a longitudinal approach in which the attrition rates from phase to phase was about 20 per cent and subjects were likely to drop out for a variety of reasons. Focusing solely on those for whom we had complete data across the board, the analytical findings were more hopeful, suggesting potential benefits of the Tropica nosodes in maintaining a low parasitic count of the parasites within the community. Within the one year period, the mean density of malaria parasites declined from 76.35/*ul* to 7.74/*ul* among all patients (see Table 2.3). A statistical comparison of the pre- and post-intervention phase confirmed that the observed reduction in malaria parasitic density was significant.

**Table 2.3**　　**Mean parasitic densities among valid subjects participating in all phases**

| Phases | Clinical Cases of Malaria | Mean Parasitic Density | Standard Error | Confidence Interval | |
|--------|---------------------------|------------------------|----------------|-------------|-------------|
| | | | | Lower Bound | Upper Bound |
| I | 8 | 76.335 | 19.790 | 37.309 | 115.402 |
| II | 3 | 23.099 | 6.786 | 9.710 | 36.488 |
| III | 0 | 18.508 | 3.432 | 11.737 | 25.279 |
| IV | 3 | 7.740 | 2.143 | 3.511 | 11.969 |

*Note:* Valid N=195; Difference in parasitic density between Phase I and IV t=4.125 p<0.001***.

**Research Challenges and Lessons Learned**

Overall, the results of this malaria intervention study were promising on several counts. First, when analysing the data on a phase by phase basis, the *Tropica nosode* therapy was found to be most effective during the first four months, immediately after the initial dosage was administered to subjects. Thereafter, the protective effects were significantly less evident in the study population. For those who took the therapy year round however, the results were more compelling with the overall parasitic burden significantly lower in the treatment group than the placebo group. Using the comprehensive data compiled across the four seasons, the results offered a positive indication of the long term benefits of homeopathic prophylaxis in reducing the overall parasitic burden of the disease among residents in the community. Since this was a pilot intervention study, a subsequent study to validate the long term and protective effects of this therapy is warranted.

The challenges encountered during this study also provided valuable lessons that underscored the interconnectedness between development and health in general, and revealed new insights for tackling these complexities in resource poor settings. As once noted by Desai and Potter (2009), doing development research and intervention projects entails many practicalities and realities on the ground that may often lead to a complex, professionally demanding, and nuanced experience. This intervention study, in particular, was demanding and wrought with challenges that required a high level of adaptability, prompt decision-making, and re-adjustment of research procedures to make changes as needed. For example, we encountered a large number of participants with similar names and addresses. Also, during the rainy season, many subjects lost their ID cards due to repetitive flooding of their homes. To address these challenges, we developed multiple identifiers, along with digital and manual health records to enable the cross-referencing of participant information during the follow-up phases. Another problem was that the lab technicians, especially in the independent lab had trouble interpreting some of the slides obtained during the recruitment phase. We needed to take immediate action to maintain the quality of the slides in subsequent phases. Lab technicians were instructed to use only pre-filtered stains, extend the normal staining times, and ensure proper storage conditions prior to transferring the slides to the independent lab for validation. These steps were critical in maintaining the overall quality of the stains, hence, a better accuracy of the blood test results in the subsequent phases.

A third and perhaps most formidable challenge was the scheduling conflict during Phase II with the religious month of Ramadan (which is difficult to anticipate ahead of time because it based on the lunar calendar). Since nearly 80 per cent of the residents in this community were Muslims, the project team quickly realised that some adjustments had to be made to cope with the situation. Specifically, there were two areas of concern: i) many of the patients were fasting and could not take their medication on site (the most reliable means of drug administration to ensure patient compliance); ii) Among those who were strict adherents of the Islamic faith, they indicated that it was against the religious codes to have their blood samples taken during the month of Ramadan; those subjects refused to complete their blood tests. To cope with the situation, the research team schedule was modified to include evening work hours to enable subjects to visit the KBHC after breaking fast. Other subjects were given the opportunity to take their medication home, and given instructions on when and how to take the medication. Due to concerns about patient compliance, a separate data code was created in the database denoting patients who took their medication on site versus those who opted to take it home. This variable was later analysed and no significant impacts were observed as a result of these adjustments.

Finally, this study illustrated the importance of community buy-in and engagement to promote disease prevention and control initiatives. Given the low literacy rates, this study required intense educational campaigns to sensitise the community about the dangers and symptoms of malaria, and our efforts to address these challenges. A two-hour radio program led by the lead investigators and community leaders was broadcast nationally to discuss the objectives of the study. Several meetings were also held, first with the elected political leaders and community representatives, all of whom later became very instrumental in communicating the project objectives to their constituents. This participatory approach enabled us to move forward with our efforts to address the malaria risks in this community.

## Conclusions

The global burden of malaria remains unacceptably high particularly within SSA where the majority of deaths and disabilities attributable to the disease occur. Our review of the literature revealed that the disease is complexly intertwined with low economic development and poverty thus demanding the integration of economic and health reform policies to simultaneously address these problems. We also presented a number of global programs aimed at curbing malaria morbidity through treatment approaches, and exposure prevention strategies such as the distribution of ITNs, larviciding and IRS. Unfortunately, the success of these approaches so far has been rather limited due to a range of environmental, political, socio-behavioural, and economic barriers, notwithstanding the changing climate and growing parasitic resistance to the existing therapies.

The case study in Sierra Leone was presented to illustrate these inherent challenges in disease intervention by utilising a sample of 731 residents in a low-income community using a naturopathic prophylaxis. The findings from the pilot study also offered a glimpse of the hurdles that are typically encountered when undertaking these development and health projects, and the need for research adaptability, fluidity, public awareness, and community engagement to ensure greater success in these efforts. Overall, as the global quest for malaria control programs continues, it is important to raise public awareness about these efforts and to continue to explore the promising qualities of complementary therapies as safe, cost-effective, and sustainable strategies for reducing the disease burden in endemic regions.

## References

Alkire, S., Roche, J.M., Santos, M.E. and Suman, S. 2011. *Sierra Leone Country Briefing*. Oxford Poverty & Human Development Initiative (OPHI) Multidimensional Poverty Index Country Briefing Series. [Online]. Available at: www.ophi.org.uk/policy/multidimensional-poverty-index/mpi-country-briefings/ [accessed: 22 August 2012].

Batisso, E., Habte, T., Tesfaye, G. et al. 2012. A stitch in time: a cross-sectional survey looking at long lasting insecticide-treated bed net ownership, utilization and attrition in SNNPR, Ethiopia. *Malaria Journal*, 11, 183.

Castro, M.C. and Fisher, M.G. 2012. Is malaria illness among young children a cause or a consequence of low socioeconomic status? Evidence from the United Republic of Tanzania. *Malaria Journal*, 11, 161. Available at: doi:10.1186/1475-2875-11-161.

Cropper, M.L., Hailec, M., Lampiettib, J. et al. 2004. The demand for a malaria vaccine: evidence from Ethiopia. *Journal of Development Economics*, 75, 303–18.

Demographic and Health Surveys. 2008. Sierra Leone. MEASURE DHS. Calverton, MD: ICF Macro.

Desai, V. and Potter, R.B. 2009. *Doing Development Research*. Thousand Oaks, CA: Sage Publications.

Dini, L. and Frean, J. 2003. Quality Assessment of malaria laboratory diagnosis in South Africa. *Transactions of the Royal Society of Tropical Medicine and Hygiene*, 97(6), 675–7.

Dongus, S., Nyika, D., Kannady, K. et al. 2007. Participatory mapping of target areas to enable operational larval source management to suppress malaria vector mosquitoes in Dar es Salaam, Tanzania. *International Journal of Health Geographics*, 6, 37.

Eng, J.L., Thwing, J., Wolkon, A. et al. 2010. Assessing bed net use and non-use after long-lasting insecticidal net distribution: a simple framework to guide programmatic strategies. *Malaria Journal*, 9, 133.

Frenkel, S., and Western, J. 1988. Pretext or prophylaxis? Racial Segregation and Malarial Mosquitoes in a British Tropical Colony: Sierra Leone. *Annals of the Association of American Geographers*, 78(2), 211–28.

Gallup, J. and Sachs, J. 2001. The economic burden of malaria. *American Journal of Tropical Medicine and Hygiene*, 64(1,2)S, 85–96.

Golden, I. 2007. *Vaccination & Homeoprophylaxis? A Review of Risks and Alternatives.* Isaac Golden Publications: Gisborne, Australia.

Greenwood, B. 2010. Anti-malarial drugs and the prevention of malaria in the population of malaria endemic areas. *Malaria Journal*, 9(Suppl 3): S2.

Guyatt, H.L. and Snow, R.W. 2001. The epidemiology and burden of Plasmodium falciparum-related anemia among pregnant women in sub-Saharan Africa. *American Journal of Tropical Medicine and Hygiene*, 64, 36–44.

Hahnemann, S.C.F. 2003. *Organon of Medicine.* London: Orion Publishing Group.

Holding, P.A. and Kitsao-Wekulo, P.K. 2004. Describing the burden of malaria on child development: What should we be measuring and how should we be measuring it? *Am J Trop Med Hyg*, 71(Suppl. 2), 71–9.

Lengler C. 2004. *Insecticide-Treated Bednets and Curtains for Preventing Malaria.* Cochrane Database of Systematic Reviews.

MARA/ARMA. 1998. Towards an Atlas of Malaria Risk. First Technical Report of the MARA/ARMA Collabouration, Mapping Malaria Risk in Africa/Atlas du Risque de la Malaria en Afrique (MARA/ARMA). Durban, South Africa, 31pp.

Margai, F.M. 2010. *Environmental Health Hazards and Social Justice: Geographical Perspectives on Race and Class Disparities.* London: Taylor and Francis, UK; Earthscan.

Margai, F.M. and Minah, J. 2007. *The Use of Homeopathic Treatment Approaches to Reduce the Prevalence of Malaria in Depressed Communities.* Protocol Registration System. Available at: Clinical Trials.gov NLM identifier NCT00351013.

Malaney, P., Spielman, A. and Sachs, J. 2004. The malaria gap. *American Journal of Tropical Medicine and Hygiene*, 71, 141–6.

Mathanga, D.P. and Bowie, C. 2007. Malaria control in Malawi: are the poor being served? *International Journal for Equity in Health*, 6, 22. Available at: doi:10.1186/1475-9276-6-22 .

Minah, J. and Margai, F.M. 2008. The Use of Malaria Nosodes to reduce the Prevalence of Malaria in Depressed Communities. *International Coethener Exchange*, 7, 25–9.

Omran, A.R. 1971. The Epidemiological Transition: A theory of the Epidemiology of Population Change. *The Milbank Memorial Fund Quarterly*, 49(4), 509–38.

Sachs, J. and Malaney, P. 2002. The economic and social burden of malaria. *Nature*, 415, 680–85.

Samba, E.M. 2004. Bridging the Gap: Linking Research, Training, and Service delivery to reduce the Malaria burden in Africa. *American Journal of Tropical Medicine and Hygiene*, 71(Suppl. 2), 71–9.

Stratton, L., O'Neill, M.S., Kruk, M.E. and Bell, M.L. 2008. The Persistent problem of malaria: Addressing the fundamental causes of a global killer. *Social Science and Medicine*, 67, 854–62.

Wilcox , M.L. and Bodeker, G. 2004. Traditional herbal Medicines for malaria. *British Medical Journal* Volume, 329, 1156–9.

Worrall, E., Basu, S. and Hanson, K. 2005. Is malaria a disease of poverty? A review of the literature. *Tropical Medicine and International Health*, 10(10), 1047–59.

World Health Organization (WHO). 1996. *Larviciding: Introduction, definition, Objectives and Scope*. [Online]. Available at: http://whqlibdoc.who.int/hq/1996/WHO_CTD_VBC_96.1000_Rev1_(chp6–11).pdf [accessed: 27 August 2012].

World Health Organization(WHO). 2011. *World Malaria Report 2011*. Geneva. [Online]. Available at: http://www.who.int/malaria/world_malaria_report_2011/en/ [accessed: 27 August 2012].

# Chapter 3

# The Geography of Maternal Mortality in Nigeria

Joseph R. Oppong and Jane Ebeniro

## Introduction

Maternal mortality, the death of a woman while pregnant or within one year after termination of pregnancy (Koonin et al. 1988; Lindroos 2010), is a serious problem in Nigeria and other developing countries. In 2005, 533,000 of the 536,000 global maternal deaths (99 per cent) occurred in developing countries (WHO 2007). While having only 2 per cent of the world's total population, Nigeria accounted for 10 per cent of the world's total maternal deaths in 2010 (Zozulya 2010). In 2008, the United States and Britain had an estimated 24 and 12 maternal deaths per 100,000 live births, respectively, but Nigeria had 840 deaths, about 35 and 70 times more, respectively (UNICEF 2010). However, the spatial variation of Nigeria's maternal mortality and the explanatory factors remain unclear.

This chapter examines the geography of maternal mortality in Nigeria. It uses a vulnerability theoretical framework and argues that adverse life situations such as maternal death do not affect populations uniformly, but vary with social and economic factors in place of residence (Chambers 1989; Oppong 1998; Ghosh and Kalipeni 2005). Examining these vulnerabilities spatially is crucial to the prevention and control of these risks, in our context, maternal mortality in Nigeria.

## Understanding Vulnerable Populations and Maternal Mortality in Nigeria

The status of a woman in society is a critical determinant of maternal mortality. In Nigeria's patriarchal society, where decisions about reproduction, family finances and education are made by men and early marriage and childbirth are encouraged, maternal mortality is high (Hodges 2001). Education, critically important for women's status in society (Ghosh and Olson 2007; Chakrapani et al. 2010), is low among Nigerian women, leaving many women dependent or with limited ability for self-support. Moreover, increased time spent in formal education extends a woman's age at first marriage and childbirth, and increases lifetime wages significantly (Psacharopoulos and Patrinos 2002), but poverty limits access to healthcare services, transportation and adequate nutrition (Hodges 2001). The cost of healthcare, coming from a tight household budget, is proportionally much higher for the poor, regardless of the quality of service they receive (Filippi et al. 2006), and poor women are less likely to seek prompt medical attention (Harrison 1997; Graham et al. 2004; Prata et al. 2009).

Poverty is a major determinant of birth outcomes in Nigeria. Demographic and Health Survey data on place of delivery shows that poor women are less likely to give birth in a healthcare facility with skilled healthcare providers (NPC 2008). In addition, 30 per cent of Nigerian women identified lack of money to pay for health care as a major obstacle to accessing health care. Distance to a healthcare facility and the cost of transportation were considered as significant obstacles (NPC 2008). Moreover, Nigerian women tend to have low levels of education. About 41.6 per cent of Nigerian women have no education at all, 21.4 per cent have primary education, and 31.1 per cent have secondary education, while only 5.9 per cent have a college degree. There is a strong negative correlation between level of education and access to financial resources or the wealth quintile. Because the lowest wealth quintile for women was 68.7 per cent and the highest was 5.8 per cent (NPC 2003), unless these disadvantaged populations are targeted as high risk populations, progress in safe delivery efforts will remain unsuccessful.

**Prenatal Care and Maternal Mortality**

Prenatal care is critically important for healthy pregnancy outcomes, but not readily available for those who need it most in Nigeria. Prenatal care provides women with the knowledge about what to do if complications arise during pregnancy, childbirth, or the period immediately after childbirth when maternal death is most likely. It also provides education on proper maternal nutrition, treatment for infections (e.g., malaria, syphilis, and tetanus), and testing for HIV/AIDS. An important component of prenatal care visits is counselling on safe sex practices and contraceptive use to prevent unwanted pregnancies and sexually transmitted diseases. Good prenatal care can detect high risk pregnancies and prevent most major pregnancy complications that require emergency obstetrical care. The World Health Organisation recommends that pregnant women should have at least three prenatal care hospital visits to ensure a normal pregnancy (Lindroos 2010). According to the Nigerian Population Commission (1999), while 64 per cent of Nigerian women received some form of prenatal care or health care services during pregnancy, access is much lower in rural areas.

Poor quality emergency care, resulting from shortage of medical personnel, drugs and supplies, is the norm in most rural health facilities in Nigeria. Thus, arriving at a healthcare facility may not necessarily lead to immediate commencement of treatment (Hodges 2001), because the nearest or most accessible healthcare facility may not be sufficiently equipped to address the emergency. Typically transportation to access a better equipped healthcare facility is lacking, thereby compounding and complicating further the pregnancy (Thaddeaus and Maine 1994).

**Cultural Practices, Religion and Maternal Mortality**

Gender inequality that is rooted in cultural and religious norms is a huge factor in maternal mortality; it controls access to food and medical care for pregnant women. Specifically, some Islamic religious practices keep reproduction under strict male supervision and control, and encourage early marriages and pregnancies often before pelvic maturity (Wall 1998). For example, *purdah* (wife seclusion), limits access to medical care for women, and produces high rates of female illiteracy. Generally, maternal mortality occurs more frequently among women who have babies at high and low extremes of maternal age (women younger than 20 and above 40 years of age) (UNFPA 2004; WHO 2006). This is because for those younger than 20 years, their reproductive organs are not mature enough to carry a pregnancy.

Cultural values and perceptions are also important factors in maternal mortality. For example, some pregnant women's perception of blood loss may determine how they act and whether or not they seek prompt medical attention during an emergency (Thaddeus and Nangalia 2004). While some women believe that bleeding during pregnancy is healthy and necessary because it eliminates impurities in a woman (i.e. pain, swelling and poison) (Sargent 1982), others fear that excessive bleeding can drain the life out of a new mother (Obermeyer 2000). Thus, the belief that excess bleeding is necessary for the cleansing process contributes to the late recognition of excessive bleeding, postpartum haemorrhage or other symptoms of risky pregnancies.

In some societies, the church building is a preferred place for childbirth due to the belief that the 'holy environment' of the church would protect both mother and child from evil spirits and witchcraft. Also, certain religions, such as Jehovah Witnesses, do not allow blood transfusions under any circumstances. This clearly endangers the life of the mother after childbirth (Chukuezi 2010).

Moreover unsafe abortion is a huge problem. Globally, 72 per cent of all deaths in women under age 19 are attributed to complications of unsafe abortions including cervical tearing, haemorrhage, pelvic infection, infertility and death (Zabin and Kiragu 1998).

Access to healthcare services, which includes prenatal care, childbirth and postnatal care, is largely determined by geographical location and cost. Proximity, affordability of healthcare services, and quality of service are important determinants of access to maternal healthcare. The Federal Ministry of Health (2011) states that approximately 71 per cent of Nigerians have a primary healthcare facility within a 5 km radius to their homes but many of these facilities are not functional due to a lack of equipment, essential supplies and qualified staff. The few healthcare facilities located in rural areas are often poorly equipped, under- and poorly-staffed and inaccessible due to distance, bad roads, and high cost of transportation. Consequently, rural and urban differences in distance to health care facilities translate into significantly higher rural mortality rates – 828 per 100,000 live births versus an urban rate of 531 (Federal Ministry of Health 2011). Moreover, as is the case with many health outcomes, mothers in the poor rural areas and impoverished urban areas have a higher risk of developing illnesses and complicated pregnancies, have poorer nutrition, and face more challenges in accessing timely healthcare.

In summary, the percentage living in poverty, educational attainment, religious affiliation, access and quality of health care, and age at marriage and childbirth are expected to explain maternal mortality variations in Nigeria. Understanding the variations of maternal mortality in Nigeria, especially at the state level will assist local authorities in determining specific vulnerable people and places to target in order to reduce maternal mortality as envisaged by Millennium Development Goal 5.

## Hypothesis and Research Questions

Four main hypotheses are tested in this research;

*Hypothesis 1:* Maternal mortality rates are influenced by access to health care. Areas with a higher number of women with no postnatal care and low percentage of women who delivered in a healthcare facility will have a higher maternal mortality rate.

*Hypothesis 2:* Low socioeconomic status, defined by the percentage of women living in poverty (living on less than USD$1.25 a day), and the percentage of women with less than secondary school education, will have a positive relationship with maternal mortality.

*Hypothesis 3:* Age at first marriage and childbirth is related to maternal mortality. Women younger than 20 years at first marriage and women who fall within the age extremes at first childbirth will have a higher risk of pregnancy-related complications resulting in death.

*Hypothesis 4:* Religious beliefs are a predictor of maternal mortality. Areas that are predominantly Muslim will have a higher mortality rate than areas that are predominantly Christian.

## Methodology and Data Sources

Data on maternal mortality rates were obtained from the Federal Ministry of Health, Port Harcourt for the year ending 2010 since that was the only accessible and most current data available. All the explanatory variables were obtained from the Nigerian Demographic and Health Survey (DHS) 2008, a nationally representative sample survey of 36,800 women aged 15–49 drawn from all 37 Nigerian states, with a minimum of 950 completed interviews in each state (NPC 2008). A correlation matrix was developed using the Factor Analysis tool to examine the relationships among all the 17 tested variables and maternal mortality. The goal was to determine which factors had the strongest relationships and second, which factors had the strongest influence on maternal mortality rates in Nigeria.

## Results

Maternal mortality in Nigeria is highly concentrated in the North West and North Eastern regions of the country, although, smaller pockets of high maternal deaths occur in the rural south as well as in some major urban areas such as Lagos and Rivers State (Figure 3.1). Generally, the further north, the higher the maternal mortality rates and the more concentrated the spatial patterns relative to the southern region of the country. As Table 3.1 shows, more than 80 per cent of the states have rates exceeding the national average of 545 maternal deaths per 100,000 live births. Kano State, a predominantly Muslim state with a large urban population, records the highest mortality rate at 2,200 maternal deaths per 100,000 live births. Lagos State, the largest metropolitan area of Nigeria, has the second highest mortality rate at 2,100 deaths per 100,000 live births. These high rates may be attributed to a large urban impoverished population, in the case of Lagos State and early child marriages and child birth due to religious beliefs in the case of Kano State.

In Table 3.2, component 1 accounts for 46.4 per cent of the total variation in maternal mortality, component 2 accounts for 27.6 per cent of the total variation, and component 3 accounts for 7.7 per cent of the total variation in maternal mortality in Nigeria. These three components alone account for a cumulative percentage of approximately 82 per cent of maternal mortality in Nigeria and can be used to give a better understanding of the spatial pattern of maternal death rates in the country.

Component 1 in table 3.3 correlates highly with low access to healthcare, characterised by a high percentage of early childbirth (women aged 15–19 at first childbirth), no postnatal care, and a low percentage of women who had skilled birth assistance or delivered at a healthcare facility. It also correlates highly with a low percentage of women who had postnatal care administered by a skilled provider, a high Muslim and

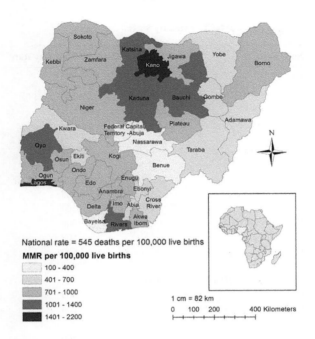

National rate = 545 deaths per 100,000 live births

**MMR per 100,000 live births**
- 100 - 400
- 401 - 700
- 701 - 1000
- 1001 - 1400
- 1401 - 2200

1 cm = 82 km

0    100    200         400 Kilometers

**Figure 3.1      Map showing maternal mortality rates (MMR) by state**

rural population, low educational attainment, difficulty accessing drugs, a percentage of women who required male permission to seek medical assistance, no health insurance, and early marriage. Component 2 captures the percentage of the Christian and rural population with limited access to drugs and no health insurance. The final component seems to capture healthcare services and correlates highly with the percentage of women who did not receive postnatal care, had difficulty accessing drugs and required male permission to seek medical attention.

*Access to Healthcare*

The percentage of women delivering in a health care facility and women with access to postnatal care are presented in Figures 3.2 and 3.3. The southern states of Lagos, Osun, Ekiti, Edo, Imo, Abia and Anambra had the highest rates of women who delivered in a healthcare facility (67–94 per cent) while northern states such as Sokoto, Kebbi and Zamfara had between 4–21 per cent. Similarly, Kebbi, Sokoto, Niger, Zamfara, Katsina, Kano, Bauchi and Adamawa states in the northeast and northwest have the highest rates of women who had no postnatal care visits.

*Socioeconomic Status*

The second hypothesis proposed that socioeconomic status, defined by poverty and educational attainment, would determine mortality rates in Nigeria. Thus, women who

**Table 3.1      Maternal mortality rates by state**

| No. | State | Maternal Mortality Rate |
|-----|-------|-------------------------|
| 1 | Abia | 700 |
| 2 | Adamawa | 700 |
| 3 | Akwa-Ibom | 900 |
| 4 | Anambra | 1,000 |
| 5 | Bauchi | 1,100 |
| 6 | Bayelsa | 400 |
| 7 | Benue | 1,00 |
| 8 | Borno | 1,000 |
| 9 | Cross River | 700 |
| 10 | Delta | 1,000 |
| 11 | Ebonyi | 500 |
| 12 | Edo | 800 |
| 13 | Ekiti | 600 |
| 14 | Enugu | 800 |
| 15 | Federal Capital Territory – Abuja | 300 |
| 16 | Gombe | 600 |
| 17 | Imo | 900 |
| 18 | Jigawa | 1,000 |
| 19 | Kaduna | 1,400 |
| 20 | Kano | 2,200 |
| 21 | Katsina | 1,400 |
| 22 | Kebbi | 800 |
| 23 | Kogi | 800 |
| 24 | Kwara | 600 |
| 25 | Lagos | 2,100 |
| 26 | Nassarawa | 400 |
| 27 | Niger | 1,000 |
| 28 | Ogun | 900 |
| 29 | Ondo | 800 |
| 30 | Osun | 800 |
| 31 | Oyo | 1,300 |
| 32 | Plateau | 800 |
| 33 | Rivers | 1,200 |
| 34 | Sokoto | 900 |
| 35 | Taraba | 500 |
| 36 | Yobe | 500 |
| 37 | Zamfara | 800 |
|   | *National Average* | *545* |

**Table 3.2    Total Variance Explained**

| Component | Rotation Sum of Squares | | |
|---|---|---|---|
| | Total | % of Variance | Cumulative % |
| 1 | 7.896 | 46.446 | 46.446 |
| 2 | 4.691 | 27.596 | 74.043 |
| 3 | 1.307 | 7.688 | 81.731 |

*Note:* Extraction Method: Principal Component Analysis.

**Table 3.3    Component matrix**

| | Component | | |
|---|---|---|---|
| | 1 | 2 | 3 |
| | Access to healthcare | Place of residence and religion | Healthcare quality |
| 15–19 at 1st childbirth | 0.919 | -0.233 | -0.133 |
| 25–49 at 1st childbirth | -0.938 | 0.070 | 0.091 |
| No postnatal care | 0.834 | 0.042 | 0.333 |
| Delivered through a skilled provider | -0.944 | 0.012 | 0.057 |
| Delivered at a healthcare facility | -0.910 | 0.014 | 0.123 |
| Postnatal care through a provider | -0.915 | 0.034 | 0.125 |
| Urban | -0.716 | -0.603 | 0.050 |
| Rural | 0.716 | 0.603 | -0.050 |
| Christian | -0.792 | 0.536 | 0.052 |
| Muslim | 0.784 | -0.543 | -0.074 |
| Less than secondary education | 0.957 | 0.025 | 0.031 |
| Access to drugs (medication) | 0.611 | 0.247 | 0.505 |
| Required male permission | 0.607 | -0.020 | 0.494 |
| No health insurance | 0.422 | 0.367 | 0.134 |
| Less than 20 at 1st marriage | 0.964 | -0.124 | -0.096 |
| Less than 20 at 1st sexual intercourse | 0.266 | 0.335 | -0.724 |
| Living in Poverty | 0.938 | 0.000 | -0.033 |

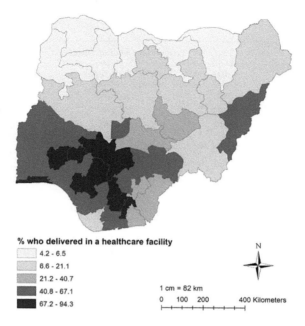

**Figure 3.2      Map showing women who gave birth in a healthcare facility**

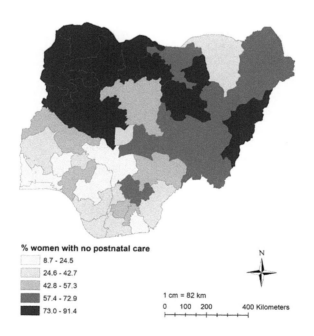

**Figure 3.3      Map showing women with no access to postnatal care**

reside in the predominantly poor, rural areas and who have less than secondary school education would be at a higher risk of developing pregnancy-related complications resulting in death. Access to health care services varies geographically in the rural/urban areas in Nigeria as prenatal care is more accessible in the urban areas relative to the rural areas. The largest urban areas are concentrated in the Southwestern part of the country with a smaller pocket in the Northeastern state of Borno.

The Federal Capital Territory of Abuja, Osun, Lagos and Anambra States have the highest urban populations in the country. Rural areas are highly concentrated in the northern part of Nigeria with Sokoto, Zamfara, Jigawa, Taraba and Benue having the largest rural populations in the country.

Figure 3.5 shows the percentage of women living in below $1.25 a day. Sokoto, Zamfara, Katsina, Jigawa, Yobe and Bauchi states in the north and Ebonyi state in the southeast record the highest rates of female poverty in Nigeria at 42–92 per cent of the female population living in poverty. The percentage of women who have less than a secondary school education is illustrated in Figure 3.4. This population would have a higher risk for early age pregnancies and would therefore develop complications during pregnancy. The northern region of Nigeria has the highest concentration of populations with the least educational attainment. Northern border states, which are predominantly Muslim, such as Sokoto, Zamfara, Jigawa, Katsina, Borno and Yobe have some of the largest low educational attainment populations with 91–96 per cent of the population having less than secondary school education. The southern states of Rivers, Imo, Anambra and Abia record lower populations with less than secondary education (37–56 per cent). In other words, the southern region records a higher educational attainment relative to the northern region.

*Maternal Age*

The third hypothesis proposes that age at first marriage and age at first childbirth influences maternal death rates in Nigeria. Areas with a high percentage of women who were married before 20 years and areas with a high percentage of women who had their first childbirth between the ages of 15–19 are at a higher risk of developing pregnancy-related complications resulting in death.

Figure 3.6 shows the percentage distribution of women who had their first marriage before age 20. All the northeastern and northwestern states recorded the highest percentage of females who were married before 20. In fact, about 86–93 per cent of the population had their first marriage before age 20. Lagos, Imo and Abia states in the southern region recorded the lowest percentage of the population with 32–37 per cent of the female population having their first marriage before they were 20 years of age.

Sokoto, Zamfara, Katsina, Jigawa, and Borno states in the northern region had the highest population with 42–65 per cent of women who had their first childbirth between 15–19 years (Figure 3.7). On the other hand, Lagos, Anambra, Imo and Enugu states in the southern region had a low population with only 2–6 per cent of women who had their first childbirth in the same age range.

*Religious Beliefs*

The fourth hypothesis proposes that maternal mortality rates will vary among the different religions and due to early marriages and childbirth, Muslims are at a higher risk to developing pregnancy-related complications and dying as a result of those complications. Figure 3.8

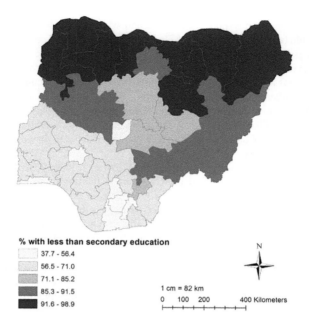

**Figure 3.4     Map showing women with less than secondary education**

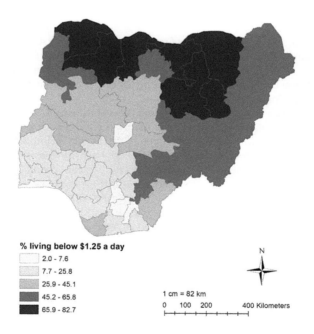

**Figure 3.5     Map showing women living below $1.25 a day**

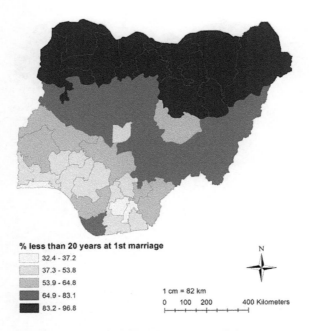

**Figure 3.6     Map showing women less than 20 years at first marriage**

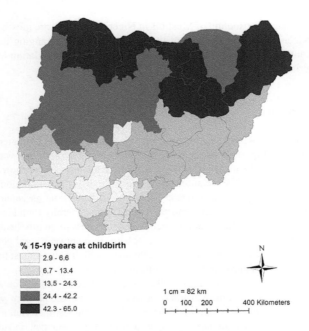

**Figure 3.7     Map showing women 15–19 years at first childbirth**

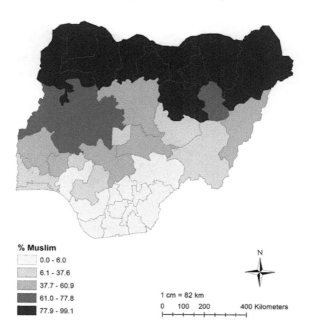

**Figure 3.8      Map showing female Muslim distribution**

shows the percentage distribution of Muslims in Nigeria. Muslims are mostly concentrated in northern Nigeria with a percentage of the Muslim population ranging between 78–99 per cent. In contrast, Christians comprise 86–99 per cent of the population in the southern states of Nigeria.

## Discussion of Results

The objective of this research was to examine the spatial patterns of maternal mortality in Nigeria and the important explanatory factors. Maternal mortality was higher and concentrated in the northern region of Nigeria where Muslims are the more predominant residents. There was a positive relationship between the Muslim population and poverty, difficulty accessing drugs at healthcare facilities, skilled birth assistance, and rural populations. In contrast, low maternal mortality rates were generally found in mostly urban areas with skilled birth assistance and women who had access to quality healthcare. These areas were usually occupied by Christians. The relationship between rural populations and high maternal mortality has been extensively examined, which may suggest the importance of residential location and proximity to a healthcare facility.

The percentage of women who had less than a secondary school education was positively correlated with the per cent of the Muslim population. Also, female poverty was high in the predominantly rural northern region of Nigeria where the highest maternal mortality rates also exist. Nevertheless, it is important to note that poverty also exists in rural as well as some major urban areas in the southern region of Nigeria. For instance, Lagos state, a major urban area and the economic core of Nigeria, had the second highest maternal mortality rate of 2,100 deaths per 100,000 live births while the predominantly rural Benue State had only 100 deaths per 100,000 live births but had over 80 per cent female poverty.

It was also hypothesised that as early marriage and early childbirth increases, maternal mortality would also increase. Results showed positive correlation between early marriage and early childbirth showing that they are higher in the northern states with the highest maternal mortality rates. This suggests that women who had their first childbirth between 15–19 years have a higher risk of developing pregnancy-related complications resulting in deaths.

## Conclusion

A factor analysis revealed the importance of three major components characterised by access to healthcare, religion/place of residence and quality of healthcare. These three components suggested that areas with a higher risk of vulnerability to developing pregnancy-related complications resulting in death would be predominantly Muslim, rural, and would have a high percentage of poverty. It also suggests that low educational attainment, early childbirth, early marriage and no health insurance would be characteristics of these vulnerable populations. The three extracted components labelled as access to healthcare, religion/place of residence and quality of healthcare, accounted for about 82 per cent explanation of the spatial pattern of maternal mortality in Nigeria. Therefore, mothers aged 15–19 at first childbirth residing in the predominantly rural areas, especially in the rural northern regions and impoverished urban southern regions of Nigeria should be targeted as a vulnerable population for intervention programmes such as accessible and better quality healthcare facilities, free prenatal and postnatal care. Although educating these vulnerable populations on the importance of prenatal care visits in order to prevent and monitor complicated pregnancies is an important step in the reduction of maternal mortality in Nigeria, empowerment of these women is paramount to reaching this goal especially in societies where women are totally dependent on male supervision and control, including obtaining permission before seeing a physician, which has been shown to limit timely access to healthcare.

### Future Research

The maternal mortality data used for this research was collected at the state-level and may be suspect for inaccuracy. Future research should seek data at a finer scale, perhaps at the district level, to illuminate intra-state level maternal mortality rates. Future research should also look at the proximity to and distribution of hospitals as well as the total number of physicians and mid-wives in each state, as another measure examining if readily accessible healthcare services and skilled birth assistance has an impact of maternal mortality in Nigeria.

## References

Chakrapani, V., Newman, P.A., Shunmugan, M. and Dubrow, R. 2010. Prevalence and Contexts of Inconsistent Condom Use among Heterosexual Men and Women Living in India: Implications for Prevention. *AIDS Patient Care and STDS*, 24(1): 49–58.

Chambers, R. 1989. Vulnerability, Coping and Policy. *IDS Bulletin*, 20(2), 23–32.

Chukuezi, C. 2010. Socio-Cultural Factors Associated with Maternal Mortality in Nigeria. *Journal of Social Sciences*, 1(5), 22–6.

Federal Ministry of Health, Port Harcourt. 2011. *State-Level Statistics on Neonatal Mortality Figures in Nigeria*. Port Harcourt: Federal Ministry of Health.

Filippi, V., Ronsmans, C., Campbell, O. et al. 2006. Maternal Health in Poor Countries: The Broader Context and a Call for Action. *Lancet*, 368(9546), 1535–41.

Ghosh, J. and Kalipeni, E. 2005. Women in Chinsapo, Malawi: Vulnerability and Risk to HIV/AIDS. *Journal of Social Aspects of HIV/AIDS*, 2(2), 320–32.

Ghosh, J. and Olson, B. 2007. HIV/AIDS in South Africa and India: Understanding the Vulnerability Factors, in *Geographic Perspectives on Cities, Regions and Society*, edited by G. Pomeroy, C. Cusak and B. Thakur. New Delhi: Concept Publishing Co.

Graham, W., Fitzmaurice, A., Bell, J. and Cairns, J. 2004. The Familial Technique for Linking Maternal Death and Poverty. *Lancet*, 363, 23–7.

Harrison, K. 1997. Maternal mortality in Nigeria: The Real Issues. *African Journal of Reproductive Health*, 1, 7–13.

Hodges, A. 2001. *Children's and Women's Rights in Nigeria: A Wake-Up Call, Situation, Assessment and Analysis*. UNICEF/National Planning Commission, Nigeria.

Koonin, L., Atrash, H., Rochat, R. and Smith, J. 1988. *Maternal Mortality Surveillance, United States 1980–1985*. [Online]. Available at: http://www.cdc.gov/mmwR/preview/mmwrhtml/00001754.htm.

Lindroos, A. 2010. *Antenatal Care and Maternal Mortality in Nigeria*. A Report Written for the Public Health Program – Exchange to Nigeria. [Online]. Available at: http://www.uku.fi/kansy/eng/antenal_care_nigeria.pdf [accessed: March 2012].

Nigerian Population Commission (NPC) [Nigeria]. 1999. *Nigerian Demographic and Health Survey 1999*. Abuja, Nigeria: National Population Commission and ICF Macro.

Nigerian Population Commission (NPC) [Nigeria]. 2003. *Nigerian Demographic and Health Survey 2003*. Abuja, Nigeria: National Population Commission and ICF Macro.

National Population Commission (NPC) [Nigeria]. 2008. *Nigeria Demographic and Health Survey 2008*. Abuja, Nigeria: National Population Commission and ICF Macro.

Obermeyer, C. 2000. Pluralism and pragmatism: Knowledge and Practice of Birth in Morocco. *Medical Anthropology*, 14, 180–201.

Oppong, J.R. 1998. A Vulnerability Interpretation of the Geography of HIV/AIDS in Ghana, 1986–1995. *Professional Geographer*, 50(4), 437–49.

Prata, N., Sreenivas, A., Vahidnia, F. and Potts, M. 2009. Saving Maternal Lives in Resource-Poor Settings: Facing Reality. *Health Policy*, 89(2), 131–48.

Psacharopoulos, G. and Patrinos, H. 2002. Returns to Investment in Education: A Further Update. *Policy Research Working Paper 2881*. Washington, DC: World Bank. [Online]. Available at: http://wwwwds.worldbank.org/external/default/WDSContentServer/IW3P/IB/2002/09/27/000094946_02091705491654/Rendered/PDF/multi0page.pdf.

Sargent, C. 1982. Solitary Confinement: Birth Practices among the Bariba of the People's Republic of Benin, in *Anthropology of Human Birth*, edited by M.A. Kay. Philadelphia: F.A. Davis Company.

Thaddeus, S. and Maine, D. 1994. Too Far To Walk: Maternal Mortality in Context. *Social Science and Medicine*, 38(8), 1091–110.

Thaddeus, S. and Nangalia, R. 2004. Perceptions Matter: Barriers to Treatment of Postpartum Hemorrhage. *Journal of Midwifery and Women's Health*, 49(4), 293–7.

UNFPA. 2004. *State of World Population, 2004*. Available at: http://www.unfpa.org/swp/2004/english/ch9/page5.html.

UNICEF. 2010. *State of the World's Children*. New York, UNICEF.

Wall, L. 1998. Dead Mothers and Injured Wives: The Social Context of Maternal Morbidity and Mortality among the Hausa of Northern Nigeria. *Studies Family Planning*, 29(4), 341–59.

World Health Organisation. 2006. UNFPA. *Pregnant Adolescents*. Geneva: World Health Organization.

World Health Organisation. 2007. *Maternal mortality in 2005*. Maternal Mortality Estimates Developed by WHO, UNICEF and UNFPA. Geneva: World Health Organisation.

Zabin, L. and Kiragu, K. 1998. The Health Consequences of Adolescent Sexual and Fertility Behavior in Sub-Saharan Africa. *Studies in Family Planning*, 29, 210–32.

Zozulya, M. 2010. *Maternal Mortality in Nigeria: An Indicator of Women's Status.* [Online]. Available at: http://www.consultancyafrica.com/index.php?option=com_content&view=article&id=358:maternal-mortality-in-nigeria-an-indicator-of-womens-status&catid=59:gender-issues-discussion-papers&Itemid=267.

Chapter 4

# Sex [Work] and [Structural] Violence: A Study of Commercial Sex Workers in Budhwar Peth, Pune, India

Jacqueline P. Hellen and Vandana Wadhwa

## Introduction

Adult prevalence rate of HIV/AIDS in India is low, approximately 0.3 per cent (Mozumder and Nora 2009; National AIDS Control Organisation [NACO] 2010), but in terms of absolute numbers, India ranks third in the world with an estimated 2–3.1 million adult people living with HIV/AIDS (PLHA) (Gutierrez et al. 2010). To adequately address prevention efforts, the Indian government established the nodal agency NACO, and the National Aids Control Programme (NACP), now in its third phase (NACO 2010). Additionally, under the national free Anti-Retroviral Therapy (ART) program launched in 2004, the Indian government has worked in tandem with several non-governmental Organisations (NGOs), establishing several HIV centres and hospitals for free treatment of PLHA (John, Rajagopalan and Madhuri 2006; NACO 2010).

NACP Phases II and III have emphasised strategies such as Greater Involvement of People with HIV/AIDS (GIPA) and working with NGOs as stakeholders and partners (NACO 2010). However, despite these increased interventions and efforts, HIV control measures in India are often hindered by lack of information and awareness, stigma and taboo associated with sex and HIV/AIDS, and hegemonic social structures (Steinbrook 2007; Ghosh, Wadhwa and Kalipeni 2009; Mozumder and Nora 2009; Wadhwa 2012; Wadhwa, Ghosh and Kalipeni 2012), all of which are also evidenced by this study.

Since the first case of AIDS was diagnosed in India in 1986, female sex workers (FSWs) have been targeted and blamed for the spread of the epidemic (Wadhwa 2012). Over the past two decades, men who have sex with men (MSMs) have also been similarly stigmatised; the marginalisation and criminalisation of these groups has served to drive their activities underground, further isolating them from educational, counselling, testing and treatment services (Steinbrook 2007). As a result, national rates of HIV prevalence are high for these groups; about 5 per cent and 7.3 per cent among FSWs and MSMs, respectively. HIV prevalence rates as high as 30 per cent have also been found in some sex worker populations in several districts of the state of Maharashtra where the study area is located, particularly in Pune, Mumbai, and Thane (Mozumder and Nora 2009; NACO 2010).

At the time this study was conducted in 2009, HIV prevalence rates at Budhwar Peth's ante-natal clinics were just above 40 per cent (Mascarenhas 2011), making this red light district of Pune a prime candidate for studying the reasons behind risk to HIV exposure among sex-workers and the efficacy of programmatic interventions being conducted by several NGOs operating in the area. Ironically, according to the most recent release of data (Mascarenhas 2011), HIV prevalence rates in Budhwar Peth have fallen steeply since the study was conducted. Increased rates of HIV-related knowledge, condom use, voluntary counselling, testing, and treatment of sexually transmitted infections (STIs) and opportunistic infections among sex workers in Budhwar Peth are largely attributable to two community-led NGOs that operate here: Vanchit Vikas and Udaan Trust.

The qualitative field-study conducted by the first author attempted to uncover the impact of the work of Vanchit Vikas and Udaan Trust on sexual health awareness and practices of commercial sex workers (CSWs) in Budhwar Peth. In the process, however, the study also uncovered power dynamics that are embedded in socio-cultural expressions of structural violence, such as the stigmatisation of sex-workers, homophobia, and marginalisation of transgender (TG) people. A gender-based hierarchy was also revealed within the red-light area, wherein male sex workers (MSWs) and transgender sex workers (TGSWs) possessed better levels of sexual health knowledge, practices, outcomes and autonomy as compared to FSWs. Further, a paradox was revealed, wherein the work of Vanchit Vikas and Udaan Trust seemed to mitigate such gender differentials, but at the same time also amplify them in other ways. This chapter seeks to present such inequities in sexual health and rights within a conceptual framework built upon themes emerging from survey-type structured interviews of 30 sex workers, supplemented by in-depth interviews of a subset of six participants.

## Study Context

### Commercial Sex Work in India and Implications on HIV/STI incidence

It is estimated that there are about three million CSWs in India, of whom 40 per cent are children (Ministry of Woman and Child Development 2008). More specific estimates are difficult due to the stigmatisation and the clandestine nature of sex work in India; approximate estimates for CSWs vary from 800,000 to two million for FSWs and over 200,000 for MSWs, although the sexual practices, sometimes for gifts and money, of over two million MSMs complicates estimates further (Khan 1999; Steinbrook 2007).

Commercial sex work in India is often a consequence of social, cultural, and economic vulnerabilities. For women and girls, predominant factors associated with engaging in commercial sex work are linked to low socio-economic status and/or disempowerment, such as widowhood, abandonment by family/husbands, rape/incest and exploitation, illiteracy, and economic pressures by family and larger society; for example, the inability of lower castes to find any mode of survival outside of sex work. To a small degree, the appeal of 'fast money' and sexual curiosity have also been cited as factors (Chattopadhyay, Bandyopadhyay and Duttagupta 1994; Thappa, Singh and Kaimal 2007; Sahni, Shankar and Apte 2008). Additionally, despite its illegality throughout India, the '*Devadasi*' (God's handmaiden) system is still practiced in some Hindu temples, where young girls from impoverished families are married to and thus dedicated to different gods and goddesses for various temple tasks, but primarily provide sexual services to priests and temple patrons (O'Neil et al. 2004; Thappa, Singh and Kaimal 2007; Blanchard et al. 2005).

Many of the same reasons for entering commercial sex work as given above also apply to male and transgender sex workers, such as abandonment by family or weak family ties, rape/exploitation, economic need, as well as sexual curiosity/need and easy access to money. However, marginalisation and stigmatisation of non-normative sexual and gender expressions is also a large factor; sex work is sometimes the only way such individuals might claim their sexual or gender identity – such 'self-realisation' can also often be prompted by conscious choice, regardless of stigma, either due to sexual desire or need for interaction with peers (Khan 1999; Bhaskaran 2004; Lorway et al. 2009).

Same-sex relations in South Asia, including India, do not always follow the neat categorisations often found in Western discourses of sexuality and gender, which makes it difficult to generalise the nature of male sex work as well. Complex interplays of sexual and gender performativities exist: for example, in the case of sex workers, identities encompass '*Kothis*' (self-identified, typically feminised males who follow social gender roles by preferring to be penetrated) and '*hijras*' (transgender or 'third sex' people, some of whom are ritually castrated, who also usually have a '*kothi*' sexual performity; they dress according to female gender norms, and although historically considered 'auspicious' in Hindu mythology and thus even in contemporary society, in reality they often hold a social status below that of FSWs). However, not all '*kothis*' or '*hijras*' are sex workers. 'Gay' identities as defined in western discourse are also becoming more visible in urban upper and middle-class India, as is the concept of '*gigolo*'. There are many more complex sexual performativities, such as the concept of '*masti*' where men and adolescents engage in sexual acts but do not deem it as 'having sex'; it is viewed more as 'play'. Any of these identities may be engaged in for paid sex, although '*Panthis/giriyas*' are typically the clients and/ or pimps, and are *kothi*-identified 'real men'; they are almost always the penetrators, also engage in heterosexual behaviour, and are or will be married (Khan 1999; 2004; Bhaskaran 2004; Steinbrook 2007).

CSWs in India often face discrimination, violence and abuse, marginalisation, manipulation and/or rape, with little opportunity for justice. Additionally, most CSWs report that they either do not practice safe sex (use of condoms and lubricants, for example), or lack the agency to negotiate it. These factors have contributed to high rates of HIV/STIs in these groups (Khan 2004; Chakrapani et al. 2007; Steinbrook 2007; Sahni, Shankar and Apte 2008; Betron and Gonzales-Figueroa 2009; Karandikar and Próspero 2010). Evidence from various empirical studies bears this out: for example, the prevalence of HIV and STIs in MSWs is 17 and 58 per cent respectively and is 41 and 61 per cent respectively in TGs in Mumbai (Shinde et al. 2009). There is a HIV prevalence of 54 per cent in Pune (Brahme et al. 2006) and an average of 14.5 per cent across South India (Ramesh et al. 2008).

More than 80 per cent of HIV infections in India are transmitted during unprotected heterosexual sex (Mozumder and Nora 2009; NACO 2010), and much of it can be attributed to men's utilisation of FSW services. Nationally, an estimated 4 per cent or 8.5 million men aged 15–49 years were clients of FSWs in a given year, of whom slightly over half were married, and many of whom had highly mobile lifestyles. Consistent condom use is low, thus, these clients act as 'bridge populations' who aid in the diffusion of HIV/STIs into the general population and back into high-risk groups (Subramanian et al. 2008; Gaffey et al. 2011).

*Study Site and the work of Vanchit Vikas and Udaan Trust*

The city of Pune is situated in the west-central part of the Western state of Maharashtra, India, and is known as the state's 'cultural capital' (Encyclopaedia Britannica 2012). Budhwar Peth ('Wednesday market') is a densely populated *bazaar* area in inner Pune. The red-light district is estimated to be the third largest in the country, with a population of over 5,000 sex workers. Living conditions are often unsanitary, with basic amenities frequently lacking (Raveendhran 2009).

Vanchit Vikas ('Upbringing/uplifting the Deprived') has established two facilities in Budhwar Peth under the Mukta Project, which operates in partnership with Pathfinder International ('Mukta Project: India'). It provides a plethora of free services to prevent transmission and reduce the burden of HIV/AIDS and STIs among CSWs and PLHA, and to increase their utilisation of health services. The Mukta Project also works with regular partners and clients of male, female and TG sex workers. It operates two facilities within Budhwar Peth: (i) the Spruha treatment centre, which provides free or inexpensive treatment and health care for HIV, STIs and opportunistic infections, and lab facilities for faster diagnoses of HIV and Tuberculosis, and (ii) a free, voluntary counselling and treatment STI clinic that predominantly targets brothel and non brothel-based CSWs. This clinic also offers services to MSMs and the general population, including free government-provided condoms for patients in a confidential and safe setting.

A facility of the Udaan Trust is also located in Budhwar Peth and is committed to empowering and supporting MSMs, TGs, MSWs, and TGSWs, who have faced sexual assault, physical abuse, neglect, or discrimination through providing them legal and health services. The latter includes free HIV/AIDS and STI education and counselling, building behavioral skills to prevent transmission, and providing social support.

## Research Design and Ethics

This study is based upon qualitative field research done by the first author from September through December 2009, under the aegis of The Alliance for Global Education, which partners with Fergusson College and the College of Military Engineering, Pune. Faculty from the latter two and the Directors of Vanchit Vikas acted in advisory capacity through the duration of protocol design and fieldwork. All research ethics conformed to the Ethical Guidelines for Social Science Research in Health as laid down by the National Committee for Social Science Research in Health (NCESSRH 2000).

Since a primary purpose of the study was to assess the quality of Vanchit Vikas and Udaan Trust services, male/female/transgender CSWs were required to have some length of exposure to interventions by the two agencies. Therefore, a qualitative study design was used to obtain in-depth understanding of their sexual health awareness, outcomes and rights; a purposive sample of 30 participants (14 FSWs, 14 MSWs, and two TGSWs) who were consumers of Vanchit Vikas and Udaan Trust services was obtained for survey-type structured interviews, keeping research parameters and adequate gender representation in mind. A subset of six participants (two FSWs, two MSWs, and two TGSWs) provided in-depth interviews, and an additional three female participants from the larger pool also voluntarily added information beyond the structured interviews. Two mock structured interviews were conducted in order to ensure their feasibility and flow; one female participant and one male participant were interviewed.

*Eligibility Criteria*

Participants were eligible to participate in the study if they were over the age of 18 and were regular attendees of either the Vanchit Vikas or Udaan Trust facilities. Therefore, all female participants had to have visited either the Vanchit Vikas clinic or the Vanchit Vikas Spruha treatment centre in any capacity at least once before their current visit, and all male participants were required have attended the Udaan Trust facility in Budhwar Peth at least twice in the past week. All participants conducted their business within the Budhwar Peth red-light district; female participants were solely brothel-based sex workers, while male participants were non-brothel based, reflecting the general pattern of sex work in this area. The male participants were either MSWs or TGSWs; any MSM not receiving financial compensation for sexual acts were excluded from the study. Participants received no incentives for participation.

*Interview Administration and Consent Procedures*

Participants were either recruited while waiting for health services in the Vanchit Vikas clinic or during their time to socialise with peers. Male sex workers were either interviewed at the Vanchit Vikas clinic or Udaan Trust while female sex workers were interviewed solely at the Vanchit Vikas clinic, since Udaan Trust only supports MSWs and TGSWs. The research team obtained the informed consent of each participant after a professional female translator read a statement in either Hindi or Marathi (depending on the native language of the participant), describing the purpose, objectives, methodology, risks and benefits of the study, and the sensitive content of the interviews (see 'Data and Analysis'). Before the structured interview began, each participant was asked if they would also consent to participate in a more in-depth interview after the completion of the former, and were apprised of its content (see 'Data and Analysis'), after which consent was obtained again. Participants were also informed that participation was entirely voluntary, and that they could choose not to answer any question or to terminate the interview at any time for any reason. They were also assured of complete anonymity. No names were associated with any of the structured or in-depth interviews.

All interviews were conducted in a private room including only the translator, the participant, and the lead author. All interviews were conducted uniformly by the same female translator in Hindi or Marathi. Both types of interviews were translated from English to Hindi or Marathi by the translator before the interviews began, and read out loud to each participant by the same female translator, since many of the participants were illiterate. Each structured interview lasted between 30 and 60 minutes, and each in-depth interview took an average of an additional half-hour. Detailed field notes were taken by hand, then transcribed by the professional female translator, and later translated from either Hindi or Marathi into English by the same translator after the interviews completion.

*Data and Analysis*

The structured interviews comprised questions on individual knowledge of HIV/STIs, participants' sexual practices, access to and use of HIV/STI testing, and treatment history. In-depth interviews were semi-structured, and utilised the life-history method to gain insights on participants' personal stories as CSWs in Budhwar Peth, including when and why they first engaged in sex work, motivations for continuing in sex work, earnings and income, experiences with discrimination/abuse, and general sexual health and rights. Additionally, field observations of the operations of Vanchit Vikas and Udaan Trust were also conducted.

Transcripts from the interviews, and observations from the field were analysed and coded, then grouped into emergent themes within the qualitative research framework of 'grounded theory', which allows for the findings to be linked with the existing or new theoretical frames (Miles et al. 1994; Strauss et al. 1998). Since the transcriptions were not verbatim, 'thick descriptions' have largely been eschewed except in the rare cases these were available from the transcriptions.

## Findings and Analysis

Combining evidence from both types of interviews and field observation, key findings were thematically grouped and are discussed below. In the structured interviews, data from MSWs and TGSWs were combined, since the practices and life-experiences of the two groups were similar in many ways. This is consistent with similar clubbing of these categories in other research (Khan 2004; Shinde et al. 2009).

### Commonalities of Exploitation and Marginalisation

This theme emerged primarily from the in-depth interviews, manifest in participant's accounts of marginalisation from society, exploitation, discrimination, stigma, oppression, and violence/abuse. All except one of the in-depth interview participants mentioned that they had entered the trade due to coercion or exploitation; all of them began sex work before age 20, on average at age 12, and one of them below the age of 10. Their stories regarding first engagement in sex work spoke to economic and sexual exploitation and trauma, such as being kidnapped from their village and sold to a brothel owner, or as recounted by one of the MSWs: 'When I was in the 5th standard, I was raped by my teacher and [soon after] became a sex worker.'

Marginalisation was also cited as a reason for engaging in sex work; some MSWs entered the trade since they saw it as the only way of being able to express their sexuality and being accepted by a group of peers. In India, sex and related issues, such as sex work or HIV/AIDS, is considered taboo, and is stigmatised. Sex workers are often segregated from general society, and CSWs and PLHA are often shunned and ostracised. Additionally, individuals not considered 'mainstream' to normative gender/sexual expression are also stigmatised, and often subjected to harassment and abuse, frequently in violent ways (Chakrapani et al. 2007; Steinbrook 2007; Betron and Gonzales-Figueroa 2009; Ghosh, Wadhwa and Kalipeni 2009; Wadhwa, Ghosh and Kalipeni 2012). The above participants also spoke of similar stigma and discrimination perpetrated by general society, as well as incidents of rape and violence/abuse, sometimes at the hands of authority figures such as police officers. One MSW mentioned that his family rejected him since he tested positive for HIV, while a TGSW recounted having sustained severe injuries on multiple occasions due to rape.

The exception to these narratives was of a woman who was a '*devadasi*' – she was married at age 12 and encouraged by her husband to begin her 'duty' at age 13, according to the custom prevalent in her village. While any researcher/reader from outside the communities where this custom is practiced might find this tradition no less than exploitation, the participant herself felt no such victimhood. She was the only female participant who reported no sense of dissatisfaction towards her work, or discrimination or stigma, since her work was seen by her and her community as performance of religious duty. She also mentioned never having to face any abuse or rape from patrons or others, possibly due to her status as the 'the Lord's servant' (Blanchard et al. 2005). As reported in other studies on the topic, such customs when sanctioned by society have provided a way for women to enjoy a certain status while saving them from likely penury (O'Neil et al. 2004; Blanchard et al. 2005).

*Gender-based Differentials and Disparities*

This theme was manifest in four key yet overlapping findings from the study, namely, gender differentials in: (i) knowledge about HIV/STIs; (ii) sexual health practices; (iii) sexual health outcomes, and related and perhaps causative of the previous three; and (iv) empowerment/agency. Male and transgender sex workers had superior levels of almost all four aspects as compared to their female counterparts. The work of Vanchit Vikas and Udaan Trust in Budhwar Peth should be borne in mind as a context for these findings.

*Knowledge/Awareness about HIV/STIs*

According to the third National [Indian] Family Health Survey (IIPS and Macro International 2007), national awareness levels regarding HIV/STIs are generally higher amongst men than women; the low levels of awareness among women are typically attributable to lower literacy levels, higher taboo and lower agency regarding access to sexual knowledge and information (Wadhwa 2012; Wadhwa, Ghosh and Kalipeni 2012). The survey-type structured interviews revealed that regarding general awareness of HIV/AIDS and STIs, all MSWs including TGSWs reported awareness of both, with the exception of one who did not know about HIV; in contrast, more than half (57 per cent) of the FSWs were unaware of STIs and 36 per cent were unaware of HIV/AIDS. When tested on specific knowledge of STI symptoms, all male and transgender participants could name at least one, and were at least four times more likely to know five or more symptoms than female participants.

Regarding knowledge about the nature, spread, prevention and treatment of HIV/AIDS, a majority of FSWs were either unable to provide any information about HIV/AIDS or at most reported unprotected sex as a transmission mode, although 29 per cent did not think unprotected sex could result in transmission. In fact, condom use and health reasons for their use were completely foreign to several of the female respondents; one-fifth of FSWs claimed that condoms do not prevent the spread of STIs or HIV/AIDS. In contrast, all MSWs/TGSWs knew that unprotected sex is a possible mode of HIV transmission and that condoms are a preventive factor. They often reported a more comprehensive understanding of HIV transmission, choosing several correct answers from all given options, including that HIV/AIDS is incurable (38 per cent) and that HIV attacks the body's ability to fight disease (31 per cent). About half of the MSWs/TGSWs reported other correct information about HIV/AIDS, including several if not all modes of transmission and specific STI symptoms.

While a majority of FSWs reported that they had been given information regarding STIs (64 per cent) and all but one had been taught about the use of condoms, rates of access to such information were universal among the MSWs/TGSWs. Additionally, knowledge of safe sexual practices was also disparate; 2 FSWs incorrectly stated that a condom could be reused after sexual intercourse, in contrast to all 16 MSWs who answered this question correctly. This has direct bearing on the following sub-section.

*Sexual Health Practices*

While all CSWs showed a higher rate of condom usage than studies of other areas have shown, particularly where safe-sex interventions are not intensive (Khan 2004; Subramanian et al. 2008; Shinde et al. 2009; Gutierrez et al. 2010), it should to be noted that actual incidence of condom use was higher among FSWs. All FSWs reported easy access to free condoms, and 86 per cent of them said they used condoms with all clients. A much lower 69 per cent of MSWs/TGSWs reported that they use condoms with all clients, with 93 per cent saying they had convenient access to free condoms when needed. Additionally, 88 per cent of MSWs/TGSWs but almost all FSWs claimed they always replace a damaged condom. The relatively low condom usage by MSWs/TGSWs is consistent with findings from other studies (Khan 2004; Shinde et al. 2009), and the higher usage rates among FSWs likely speak to the success of safe-sex interventions in Pune and Budhwar Peth (Brahme et al. 2006).

Despite lower condom usage, 81 per cent of MSWs/TGSWs said that they always refuse service if a client refuses to use a condom, while only 64 per cent of FSWs answered similarly. Of the MSWs/TGSWs who reported having an STI, all said they refused to provide service if the client did not want to use a condom, while 30 per cent of FSWs said they still provide services in that situation. The majority of CSWs who reported having unprotected sex claimed to do so with a regular partner, since it denoted greater emotional intimacy. Other predominant reasons given for not using condoms included financial incentives for unprotected sex, and lack of enjoyment from the client (thus potential loss of clientele). For example, according to one MSW: 'I agree to not use a condom if my client promises me more money and removes before ejaculating. I do not refuse sex without a condom when I really need the money because I can get 1,000 to 2,000 Rupees extra.'

About 69 per cent of MSWs/TGSWs claimed they used lubricants during sex to prevent tears that could facilitate infections, but none of the FSWs did so, placing themselves and 'bridge populations' at higher risks of infections. Moreover, while all MSWs/TGSWs reported the practice of washing their genitals between clients, a small percentage of FSWs (14%) did not do so.

*Sexual Health Outcomes and Healthcare Access*

Possibly related to greater knowledge of health risks, the MSWs/TGSWs accessed healthcare facilities more frequently and reported fewer STI-related symptoms. Many initial symptoms of HIV and particularly other STIs can be attributed to benign causes, but symptoms such as genital sores and blisters, odorous discharge, and painful or bloody urination, are probable signs of STIs. While both male and female participants had similar rates of ever having been diagnosed with an STI (just above a third), 71 per cent of FSWs reported such symptoms at the time of the study, while a much lower 31 per cent of MSWs/TGSWs reported experiencing them.

Access to treatment and related information were also often disparate; although all participants mentioned they had received STI testing services at some point of time, only 78 per cent of FSWs mentioned receiving related counselling regarding condom use, while this was universal for MSWs/TGSWs. Of the 15 CSWs who experienced STI symptoms, three FSWs reported issues accessing testing services or receiving free medications, but none of the MSWs/TGSWs in this subset reported any such issues.

*Levels of Empowerment/Agency*

Empowerment and agency have been defined in various ways; the definition used here is from Watts and Bohle (1993) who have ascribed to it multiple contextual processes, including those of decision-making and negotiation, and access to monetary and other resources. Agency is simply defined here as the translation of these processes and assets into the ability to take action.

Financial autonomy is usually an integral component of empowerment; from the in-depth interviews, it was evident that the MSWs/TGSWs were able to command more monetary resources than their female counterparts. MSWs/TGSWs reported fewer clients (between one to a maximum of four) but earned more per day than FSWs, with daily earnings ranging between Rs. 2,000–3,000 depending on number of clients and condom use. FSWs earned much less, about Rs. 500–600 on average per day, if they serviced multiple clients (only about two-thirds of the FSWs reported one to four clients every day, with the rest reporting 5–10 or more). Additionally, FSW's earnings were all affected by age, perceived beauty and condom use. FSWs made much less money per client than MSWs/TGSWs because the FSW population in Pune is much larger, increasing competition. They also often have multiple children for whom they are financially responsible, further driving them into poverty and financial desperation (Raveendhran 2009). In addition, FSWs' net income is reduced since they often have to provide a share of their income to the brothel owner.

The very fact that the majority of FSWs were brothel-based and the MSWs/TGSWs were not belies the fact that the latter have a greater degree of autonomy. Affiliation with a brothel seemed to affect not just the financial aspect of empowerment, but various other themes touched on in previous sub-sections. For example, the FSWs interviewed reported that brothel owners frequently block access to treatment and care, either because they view it as unnecessary drain of time and therefore money, or due to the stigma that is attached to attending an HIV/STI related clinic, which then affects potential draw of clientele. Also, since a third party (the pimp/madam/brothel owner) often arranges for, or is involved in each sexual transaction between an FSW and her client, FSWs have less power than non-brothel based MSWs/TGSWs to negotiate condom use and/or to deny sexual relations. Since they receive higher payment for unprotected sex with a client, the mediator's incentive is to discourage such behaviour. Thus, FSWs often lack the knowledge, confidence, financial security, and/or independence to refuse service. In fact, one FSW proffered: 'New, younger girls are forbidden to negotiate for condom use or go to the clinic for education by their madams or pimps to get the highest possible pay-cut per client.'

*Paradoxical Role of Vanchit Vikas and Udaan Trust*

Field observation revealed that Vanchit Vikas and Udaan Trust were both performing essential roles in alleviating many of the issues highlighted above, from creating networks of safety and inclusion for these marginalised groups, to providing essential education, counselling, testing and treatment services. Due to these efforts, Vanchit Vikas and Udaan Trust were able to mitigate some of the differentials in health and power dynamics; for example, findings above showed that Vanchit Vikas was able to boost condom use amongst the FSWs, which should be able to impact health outcomes in the long run – in fact, some effect of this is already visible (Mascarenhas 2011). Additionally, Udaan Trust's approach of keeping empowerment issues of MSWs/TGSWs central to their focus was successful in removing some of the stigma and marginalisation experienced by them.

However, the different approaches and roles of the two NGOs, as well as the slightly different consumer base they served also had the reverse effect of amplifying some differentials. Udaan Trust has been particularly successful by incorporating the social milieu of MSWs/TGSWs into its efforts, and providing an inclusive and safe haven for social interaction, while also promoting the use of health and education services provided by Vanchit Vikas. Further, Udaan Trust practiced an egalitarian peer-outreach approach to influence healthy behaviours and effect self-efficacy and empowerment, in contrast to Vanchit Vikas, where outreach to FSWs was performed mainly by a few experienced outreach workers who were well known in the community and regularly interacted with FSWs and their madams/pimps, and mostly focused on education and health services. Although Vanchit Vikas increased accessibility, availability, and affordability to health services for the FSW population, it failed to incorporate service utilisation barriers into input strategies, not investing as much in addressing social and structural barriers to healthcare access and behavioural change through FSW empowerment. For example, since madams/pimps/brothel owners collect about half of the monthly earnings of their 'wards', FSWs have very little autonomy to negotiate for condom use or deviate from the brothel and work to utilise Mukta Project services. As a result, gender differentials in health and empowerment between FSWs and MSWs/TGSWs was sometimes exacerbated, while hegemonic structures that affected FSWs in Budhwar Peth were allowed to remain largely unaddressed.

Thus, while both NGOs had a decidedly positive impact on their client populations, Udaan Trust's model of incorporating empowerment and giving a voice to MSWs/TGs in combination with services provided at Vanchit Vikas, addressed their needs more holistically. For FSW's, the benefit from Vanchit Vikas was evident, but the missing component of empowerment meant that the differentials that exist in patriarchal society continue to exist.

## Conceptual Framework: 'Othering' and 'Hegemonic Masculinities' as Indicators of Structural Violence

Amongst the emergent findings, it is impossible not to note the differential power dynamics that exist at various levels. Structural violence has been used in the context of HIV/AIDS in the field of health geography to signify how socio-economic constructs and institutions can inflict further harm upon already marginalised and disempowered groups (Kalipeni, Oppong and Zerai 2007; White, Pope and Malow 2009). Within the context of HIV/AIDS in India, Wadhwa (2012) elucidates how socio-cultural factors such as stigma/taboo and patriarchal structures are symptomatic of power differentials and cause harm and suffering to vulnerable populations or persons.

For a more nuanced appreciation of structural violence in the present context, it is essential to understand two other conceptual frames. The first concept is that of 'Othering/ Otherness', which also describes the first level of power differentials visible in the context of the study. 'Othering' has been extensively used in radical and critical studies to describe marginalisation of individuals or groups on the basis of race, gender, class, disability, and various other social axes (for a review of the concept, see Canales 2000; Johnson et al. 2004; Gregory et al. 2009). It has also been used to describe the stigmatisation of persons with perceived or actual HIV-positive status (Dear et al. 1997; Petros et al. 2006). Within this study, one of the levels of differential power dynamics is indicated in such displays of 'othering', through mechanisms such as the 'marking' of CSWs from society as the 'immoral Other', and the perceptible 'othering' also faced by those who do not adhere to heteronormative ways and the binary gender norm of larger society.

The second level of differential power dynamics overlaps with the first, in that a gender/ sexuality hierarchy is clearly apparent within the larger social context, and within the world of commercial sex work in Budhwar Peth. This is explainable through the concept of 'hegemonic masculinities' (Connell 1987). On its face, 'hegemonic masculinities' implies male power and domination as found in patriarchal systems. This is the case in the study area, where regardless of various similar structural barriers faced by MSWs, TGSWs, and FSWs, the former still had greater levels of awareness about HIV/STIs, better health and access to healthcare, and higher levels of autonomy as compared to FSWs, largely because FSWs have limited agency regarding some decisions. This is in itself a function of the hierarchical structure within the red-light district, which still follows a patriarchal framework where male clients and their interests are paramount, and the FSWs are economically and socially disempowered.

However, this does not imply that MSWs and TGSWs always have agency, or are not at a disadvantage in the same social and/or economic terms. For example, one MSW said that he is occasionally unable to demand condom use, and as substantiated by another, this is more often the case when clients are forceful or abusive. This is where the richer complexities of 'hegemonic masculinities' come into play. Since various social axes intersect that of gender, intra-gender power tensions are created; subordinated 'marginalised masculinities' exist along the axes of caste, class, age, sexuality, and other such interstices (Connell and Messerschmidt 2005). Thus, hegemonic masculinities work to create vulnerabilities for men as well as women, as is the case for the MSWs/ TGSWs in this study, where they face ridicule, violence, and marginalisation. According to Gaffney and Beverley (2001: 133), '... like women, for male sex workers, hegemonic and heterosexist constructs ensure that they also occupy a subordinated position within society'.

Thus, the two theoretical frames of 'othering' and 'hegemonic masculinities' are 'grounded' by the themes of exploitation/marginalisation and gender differentials that emanate from the field study. These two in turn support the larger conceptual frame of structural violence, as apparent from the words of Parker et al. (2000, S23):

> ... the interactive or synergistic effects of social factors such as poverty and economic exploitation, gender power, sexual oppression ... [create] what can be described as forms of "structural violence," which directly determine the social vulnerability of groups and individuals.

## Conclusion

Based on the survey and interview responses, we found that despite similar structural barriers of severe discrimination and social marginalisation faced by the sex workers, MSWs and TGSWs displayed better sexual health knowledge and practices on average, and higher levels of autonomy as compared to the FSWs, who faced additional structural barriers of a hierarchical work environment. Udaan Trust was able to facilitate better outcomes largely due to their dual focus on health as well as empowerment by providing a safe environment and using positive peer models. Modelled behaviour is capable of altering personalised perceptions of detriments or benefits associated with particular behaviour, in turn influencing an individual's actions and health behaviours (McAlister, Perry and Parcel 2008). Thus, Udaan Trust has captured the concept of observational learning to motivate MSWs/TGSWs towards self-regulation, personal accountability and responsibility for actions, and adopting healthier behaviours.

At the time of the study, observations and findings suggested that the Mukta Project has not been as successful in reduced risks among FSWs because Vanchit Vikas failed to establish a similar environment for observational learning and empowerment. Prevention efforts and objectives of the Mukta Project were muted by inability to address structural barriers such as deterrents to clinic or treatment centre attendance placed by brothel owners/ madams/pimps and also the stigma and anxiety faced by FSWs that utilising such services will expose or implies STI status. Whereas Udaan Trust has worked to provide a safe social atmosphere for the male sex workers to proactively receive education and care, female sex workers only attended the Vanchit Vikas clinic for testing, education, and medications after they experienced STI symptoms.

Previous studies have shown that community-based HIV interventions that incorporate lowering contextual structural barriers and tackling local aspects of structural violence are more successful at reducing HIV risk among sex workers (Argento et al. 2011; Ghose, Swendeman and George 2011). It is important and interesting to note that at the time of writing, a news release about Budhwar Peth reported statistics supporting evidence of the immense success of the Mukta Project. According to the release (Mascarenhas 2011) prevalence rates of HIV at antenatal clinics in Budhwar Peth had declined from the astounding high of 41.2 per cent in 2008 to 13 per cent in 2011. Apart from the provided health services, this decline is primarily being accredited to a sense of empowerment created by the setting up of a community-learning centre as part of Mukta Project interventions in 2009. The centre is run by a 'core committee' of 12 members, all drawn from the resident community of FSWs. It functions as a 'learning site' for life and vocational skills and also as a forum for airing and resolving issues related to their work and everyday lives, which fosters greater autonomy among the FSWs (Mascarenhas 2011).

While welcome news of an extraordinary degree, 13 per cent is still a high prevalence rate that requires that due vigilance be maintained in the operation of the projects that offer services in Budhwar Peth. Towards this end, some weaknesses noted in Vanchit Vikas' operations should be addressed by incorporating peer-outreach models (Argento et al. 2011; Ghose, Swendeman and George 2011), instituting structural interventions such as raising awareness and facilitating attitudinal changes regarding MSWs/TGSWs and FSWs among local police, brothel owners, and society (Laga et al. 2010), and maximisation of Vanchit Vikas' existing facilities that cater to FSWs' child care needs. These would greatly help in reducing the inequities characteristic of structural violence in the study area.

Future research directions could include in-depth examination of the opportunities and barriers faced by Vanchit Vikas and Udaan Trust, and strengthening the activities that are resulting in enabling FSWs to find greater agency over their health and lives. Long-term policy implications that need to be seriously considered after examining the structural barriers existing in the study area include outreach to client populations regarding health behaviours and social attitudes, decriminalisation and possible legalisation of sex work; the latter has been put forward for consideration to the government of India by judges of the Indian Supreme Court (Subramanian et al. 2008; BBC News 2009; Karandikar and Próspero 2010).

In concluding, it is evident from the study observations and literature that the greatest impact occurs from community led interventions; it is difficult not to see the truth in the following words:

> ... local "spaces of marginality" are much more than a "space of deprivation" [but] also a site of radical possibility, a space of resistance. (bell hooks 1990, 342 in Herod 2010, xiii)

## References

Argento, E., Reza-Paul, S., Lorway, R. et al. 2011. Confronting structural violence in sex work: lessons from a community-led HIV prevention project in Mysore, India. *AIDS Care*, 23(1), 69–74.

Betron, M. and Gonzalez-Figueroa, E. 2009. *Gender Identity, Violence, and HIV among MSM and TG: A Literature Review and a Call for Screening*. Washington, DC: Futures Group International, USAID Health Policy Initiative, Task Order 1.

Bhaskaran, S. 2004. *Made in India: Decolonizations, Queer Sexualities, Trans/national Projects*. New York, NY and Basingstoke, England: Palgrave Macmillan.

Blanchard, J., O'Neil, J., Ramesh, B. et al. 2005. Understanding the social and cultural contexts of female sex workers in Karnataka, India: Implications for prevention of HIV infection. *The Journal of Infectious Diseases*, 191(S1), S139–46.

Brahme, R., Mehta, S., Sahay, S. et al. 2006. Correlates and trend of HIV prevalence among female sex workers attending sexually transmitted disease clinics in Pune, India (1993–2002). *Journal of Acquired Immune Deficiency Syndromes*, 41(1), 107–13. [Online]. Available at: http://journals.lww.com/jaids/Fulltext/2006/01010/Correlates_and_Trend_of_HIV_Prevalence_Among.17.aspx [accessed: 5 February 2012].

Canales, M.K. 2000. Othering: Toward an understanding of difference. *Advances in Nursing Science*, 22(4), 16–31.

Chakrapani, V., Newman, P., Shunmugam, M. et al. 2007. Structural violence against *kothi*-identified men who have sex with men in Chennai, India: a qualitative investigation. *AIDS Education and Prevention*, 19(4), 346–64.

Chattopadhyay, M., Bandyopadhyay, S. and Duttagupta, C. 1994. Biosocial factors influencing women to become prostitutes in India. *Biodemography and Social Biology*, 41(3–4), 252–9.

Connell, R.W. 1987. *Gender and Power: Society, the Person and Sexual Politics*. Stanford, CA: Stanford University Press.

Connell, R.W. and Messerschmidt, J.W. 2005. Hegemonic masculinity: Rethinking the concept. *Gender and Society*, 19(6), 829–59.

Dear, M., Wilton, R., Gaber, S.L. and Takahashi, L. 1997. Seeing people differently: The sociospatial construction of disability. *Society and Space*, 15(4), 455–80.

Encyclopædia Britannica. 2012. *Pune*. [Online]. Available at: http://www.britannica.com/EBchecked/topic/483487/Pune [accessed: 31 January 2012].

Gaffey, M.F., Venkatesh, S., Dhingra, N. et al. 2011. Male use of female sex work in India: A nationally representative behavioural survey. *PLoS ONE*, 6(7), e22704. Available at: doi:10.1371/journal.pone.0022704.

Gaffney, J. and Beverley, K. 2001. Contextualizing the construction and social organization of the commercial male sex industry in London at the beginning of the twenty-first century. *Feminist Review*, 67, 133–41. Available at: doi:10.1080/01417780150514556.

Ghose, T., Swendeman, D.T. and George, S.M. 2011. The role of brothels in reducing HIV risk in Sonagachi, India. *Qualitative Health Research*, 21(5), 587–600.

Ghosh, J., Wadhwa, V. and Kalipeni, E. 2009. Vulnerability to HIV/AIDS among women of reproductive age in the slums of Delhi and Hyderabad. *Social Science and Medicine*, 68(4), 638–42. [Online]. Available at: http://www.ncbi.nlm.nih.gov/pubmed/19070950 [accessed: 25 January 2012].

Gregory, D., Johnston, R., Pratt, G., Watts, M. and Whatmore, S. 2009. *The Dictionary of Human Geography*. 5th edition. Chichester, UK: Wiley-Blackwell.

Gutierrez, J., McPherson, S., Fakoya, A., Matheou, A. and Bertozzi, S.M. 2010. Community-based prevention leads to an increase in condom use and a reduction in sexually transmitted infections (STIs) among men who have sex with men (MSM) and female sex workers (FSW): The Frontiers Prevention Project (FPP) evaluation results. *BMC Public Health*, 10(1), 497. [Online]. Available at: http://www.biomedcentral.com/1471–2458/10/497 [accessed: 26 January 2012].

Herod, A. 2010. *Scale*. New York, NY: Routledge.

IIPS and Macro International. 2007. *National Family Health Survey 2005–2006 – India (NFHS-3), 2005–06: India: Volume I*. Mumbai, India: International Institute for Population Sciences. [Online]. Available at: http://www.nfhsindia.org/NFHS-3%20Data/VOL-1/India_volume_I_corrected_17oct08.pdf [accessed: January 20, 2012.]

John, K., Rajagopalan, N. and Madhuri, N. 2006. Brief Communication: Economic comparison of opportunistic infection management with antiretroviral treatment in people living with HIV/AIDS presenting at an NGO clinic in Bangalore, India. *Journal of the International AIDS Society*, 8(4), 24.

Johnson, J., Bottorf, J. and Browne, A. 2004. Othering and being othered in the context of health care services. *Health Communication*, 16(2), 253–71.

Kalipeni, E., Oppong J.R. and Zerai, A. (Guest Editors). 2007. HIV/AIDS in Africa: Gender, agency and empowerment. Special Issue of *Social Science and Medicine* 64(5), 1015–50.

Karandikar, S. and Próspero, M. 2010. From client to pimp: Male violence against female sex workers. *Journal of Interpersonal Violence*, 25(2), 257–73.

Khan, S. 1999. Through a window darkly: Men who sell sex to men in Bangladesh and India, in *Men Who Sell Sex: International Perspective on Male Prostitution and HIV/AIDS*, edited by P. Aggleton. Philadelphia: Temple University Press, 195–212.

Khan, S. 2004. *MSM and HIV/AIDS in India: A Briefing Summary*. London: Naz Foundation International.

Laga, M., Galavotti, C., Sundaramon, S. and Moodie, R. 2010. Editorial: The importance of sex-worker interventions: the case of Avahan in India. *Sexually Transmitted Infections*, 86(S1). Available at: http://sti.bmj.com/content/86/Suppl_1/i6.full.pdf, doi:10.1136/sti.2009.039255 [accessed: 9 February 2012].

Lorway, R., Reza-Paul, S. and Pasha A. 2009. On becoming a male sex worker in Mysore: Sexual subjectivity, 'empowerment', and community-based HIV prevention research. *Medical Anthropology Quarterly*, 23(2), 142–60.

Mascarenhas, A. 2011. Budhwar Peth: HIV prevalence down from 41% to 13% in 3 years. *The Indian Express*, 13 December. [Online]. Available at: http://www.indianexpress.

com/news/budhwar-peth-hiv-prevalence-down-from-41-to-13-in-3-yrs/887226/ [accessed: 25 January 2012].

McAlister, A., Perry, C. and Parcel, G. 2008. How individuals, environments, and health behaviors interact: Social cognitive theory, in *Health Behavior and Health Education: Theory, Research, and Practice*, edited by K. Glanz, B. Rimer and K. Viswanath. San Francisco: Jossey-Bass.

Miles, M.B. and Huberman, M.A. 1994. *Qualitative Data Analysis*. 2nd edition. Beverly Hills, CA: Sage Publications.

Ministry of Women and Child Development. 2008. *India country report-2008*. New Delhi: Ministry of Women and Child Development and the United Nations Office on Drugs and Crime.

Mozumder, S. and Nora, E. 2009. *HIV/AIDS in India*. [Online]. Available at: http://siteresources. worldbank.org/SOUTHASIAEXT/Resources/223546–1192413140459/4281804– 1231540815570/5730961–1235157256443/HIVAIDSbriefIN.pdf [accessed: 25 January 2012].

Mukta Project: India. [Online]. Available at: http://www.pathfind.org/site/PageServer? pagename=Programs_India_Projects_Mukta [accessed: 29 January 2012].

NACO. 2010. *Annual Report 2009–10*. New Delhi: Ministry of Health and Family Welfare [Online]. Available at: http://www.nacoonline.org/upload/AR%202009–10/NACO_ AR_English%20corrected.pdf [accessed: 1 August 2011].

NCESSRH. 2000. *Ethical Guidelines for Social Science Research in Health*. Mumbai: National Committee for Ethics in Social Science Research in Health, Centre for Enquiry into Health and Allied Themes. [Online]. Available at: http://www.cehat.org/ publications/ethical2.html [accessed: 22 August 2009].

O'Neil, J.O., Orchard, T., Swarankar, R.C. et al. 2004. Dhandha, dharma, and disease: Traditional sex work and HIV/AIDS in rural India. *Social Science and Medicine*, 59(4), 851–60.

Parker, R.G., Easton, D. and Klein, C.H. 2000. Structural barriers and facilitators in HIV prevention: A review of international research. *AIDS*, 14, S22/S32.

Petros, G., Airhihenbuwa, C.O., Simbayi, L. et al. 2006. HIV/AIDS and 'Othering' in South Africa: The blame goes on. *Culture, Health and Sexuality*, 8(1): 67–77.

Ramesh, B.M., Moses, S., Washington, R. et al. 2008. Determinants of HIV prevalence among female sex workers in four south Indian states: Analysis of cross-sectional surveys in twenty-three districts. *AIDS*, 22(S5), S35–44.

Raveendhran, R. 2009. Business shrinking, Budhwar Peth sex workers turn to part-time jobs. *The Indian Express*, 25 June. [Online]. Available at: http://www.indianexpress. com/news/business-shrinking-budhwar-peth-sex-workers/481067/ [accessed: 25 January 2012].

Sahni, R., Shankar, V.K. and Apte, H. 2008. *Prostitution and Beyond: An Analysis of Sex Work in India*. Los Angeles, CA: Sage Publications.

Shinde, S., Setia, M.S., Row-Kavi, A., Anand, V. and Jerajani H. 2009. Male sex workers: Are we ignoring a risk group in Mumbai, India?. *Indian Journal Dermatology, Venereology and Leprology*, 75: 41–6. [Online]. Available at: http://www.ijdvl.com/ text.asp?2009/75/1/41/45219 [accessed: 9 February 2012].

Steinbrook, R. 2007. Perspective: HIV in India – A complex epidemic. *New England Journal of Medicine*, 356(11), 1089–93.

Strauss, A.L. and Corbin, J.M. 1998. *Basics of Qualitative Research: Techniques and Procedures for Developing Grounded Theory*. Thousand Oaks, CA: Sage Publications.

Subramanian, T., Gupte M.D., Paranjape, R.S. et al. 2008. HIV, sexually transmitted infections and sexual behaviour of male clients of female sex workers in Andhra Pradesh, Tamil Nadu and Maharashtra, India: results of a cross-sectional survey. *AIDS*, 22(S5), S69–79.

Thappa, D.M., Singh, N. and Kaimal, S. 2007. Prostitution in India and its role in the spread of HIV infection. *Indian Journal of Sexually Transmitted Diseases*, 28(2). [Online]. Available at: http://medind.nic.in/ibo/t07/i2/ibot07i2p69.pdf [accessed: 25 January 2012].

Wadhwa, V. 2012. Structural violence and women's vulnerability to HIV/AIDS in India: understanding through a 'Grief Model' framework. *Annals of the Association of American Geographers*, 102(5).

Wadhwa, V., Ghosh, J. and Kalipeni, E. 2012. Factors Affecting the Vulnerability of female slum youth to HIV/AIDS in Delhi and Hyderabad, India. *GeoJournal.* 77(4), 475–88.

Watts, M. and Bohle, H. 1993. The space of vulnerability: The causal structure of hunger and famine. *Progress in Human Geography*, 17(1), 43–67.

White, R.T., Pope, C. and Malow, R. 2009. HIV, public health, and social justice: Reflections on the ethics and politics of health care, in *HIV/AIDS: Global Frontiers In Prevention/Intervention*, edited by C. Pope, R. White and R. Malow. London and New York: Routledge.

# Chapter 5
# Aboriginal Health and Development: Two Steps Forward and One Step Back?

Kathi Wilson, Mark. W. Rosenberg and Ashley Ning

## Introduction

In 2006, more than one million individuals in Canada identified themselves as an Aboriginal person.[1] The Aboriginal population accounted for 3.8 per cent of the total Canadian population in 2006, which is an increase from 2.8 per cent in 1996 (Statistics Canada 2006). In comparison, Indigenous people make up 15 per cent of the total population in New Zealand whereas in the United States and Australia they account for just 2 per cent of the population. As a group, the Aboriginal population in Canada is much younger and growing at a much faster rate than the general Canadian population. Between 1996 and 2006, the Aboriginal population increased by 45 per cent, which is much higher than the 8 per cent increase for the non-Aboriginal population (Statistics Canada 2006). In 2006, the median age of the Aboriginal population was 27 years in comparison with 40 years among the non-Aboriginal population (Statistics Canada 2010). Approximately 30 per cent of the Aboriginal population is less than 15 years of age compared with only 17 per cent in the non-Aboriginal population (Statistics Canada 2008).

Like Indigenous peoples in other countries, the Aboriginal population in Canada has experienced a history of oppression and marginalisation as a direct result of colonial policies that aimed to erase Aboriginal culture and assimilate Aboriginal people into the dominant (i.e., colonising) population. Such policies, and their ongoing legacy, have resulted in numerous health disparities that continue to exist today. While it is beyond the scope of this chapter to provide a detailed overview of this colonial legacy, a few significant examples deserve mention.

Beginning with the arrival of European settlers in the fifteenth century, Aboriginal people were physically displaced from traditional territories and this culminated with the creation of the reserve system in the late nineteenth century. Originally reserves were areas of land that were set aside for the use of First Nations with the legal title to the land held by the Crown (Canada 2004). Reserve land was often marginal (i.e., did not support either

---

1    The term Aboriginal is used in this paper to refer to the three broad indigenous groups in Canada – the First Nations, Inuit and Métis populations. Each of these groups has a unique history and distinct relationships to the federal government as it pertains to health and health care. The term First Nations was introduced around the 1970s to replace the term 'Indian', which many Aboriginal people deemed to be politically incorrect (Canada 2004). The Inuit are Aboriginal peoples who live in Canada's most northern regions. Originally, the term Métis was used to describe the children of Cree women and French fur traders living in the prairie region of Canada. In the contemporary context, 'Métis means a person who self-identifies as Métis, is of historic Métis Nation Ancestry, is distinct from other Aboriginal Peoples and is accepted by the Métis Nation Council' (MNC 2010).

traditional hunting, fishing and gathering or economic activities such as farming) and situated in isolated locations (i.e., removed from the non-Aboriginal population). In addition to physical displacement from traditional territories, the Aboriginal population in Canada was displaced socially and culturally through policies that sought to erase their cultural values and customs (Canada 1996). Such policies had significant impacts on health and healing. For example, amendments to the *Indian Act* banned specific traditional ceremonies and gatherings, which resulted in many being pushed underground and some practices being lost for generations (Canada 1996; Waldram et al. 2006). Perhaps the most aggressive step the government took towards assimilation was the creation of the government-church run residential schools. The goal of the schools was to replace the Aboriginal cultural system with a European one (Canada 1996). The first residential schools opened in the late 1800s, reaching a total of 80 schools across the country by the 1930s with the last school closing in the mid-1990s (AFN 2009). Aboriginal children were forcibly removed from their homes to become educated and 'civilised' in the schools. However, it is only within the last 30 years that survivors of the residential school system began disclosing the physical, mental, and sexual abuse they suffered as students in the residential school system (Canada 1996, Castellano et al. 2008). As a result of the residential schools system and other government policies aimed at assimilation, Aboriginal communities experienced a significant loss of cultural knowledge in general and healing knowledge in particular (Waldram et al. 2006).

The estimated number of Aboriginal children who attended residential schools over the period they existed is estimated at approximately 150,000 (CBC News 2008). The direct and indirect impacts on their physical and mental health cannot be estimated but it is safe to say that the lasting legacy of the negative impacts of the residential school system manifests itself in the health and social problems faced by today's Aboriginal population and the wide gaps in health and social problems when compared to the non-Aboriginal population. In this chapter we argue that while some of the gaps in health status between Aboriginal and non-Aboriginal populations have narrowed in terms of health status and social and economic development, the improvements have been uneven and new inequalities in health and well-being have emerged, particularly among Aboriginal youth. We seek to explain these gaps through both historical and current lenses of racism and racist strategies that hold back widespread improvements in health and the development of Aboriginal Peoples.

## Biomedical Understandings of Aboriginal Health

It is well documented that Aboriginal peoples in Canada suffer from much higher levels of morbidity and mortality than the non-Aboriginal population (Enarson and Grzybowski 1986; Hammond et al. 1988; Young 1991; MacMillian, Offord and Dingle 1996; Trovato 2001; Allard, Wilkins and Berthelot 2004; Smylie et al. 2010). However, it is important to note that we have witnessed some specific improvements in Aboriginal health over time. For example, the gap in life expectancy between 'status Indians' and the general Canadian population declined from approximately 11 years in 1980 to less than seven years in 2001. In addition, recent projections suggest that the gap in life expectancy will be further reduced by 2017 (Statistics Canada 2010). Disparities in both infant and overall mortality rates also appear to be decreasing. For example, research has shown that among Status Indians in British Columbia, rates of infant mortality have dropped since the 1950s from 100 per 1,000 births to 4.0 deaths per 1,000, almost equal to the non-Aboriginal infant mortality rate of 3.7 deaths per 1,000 births (BC Ministry Health Office Planning 2001). Beyond mortality, the Aboriginal population in Canada has also experienced some improvements with respect to certain health conditions, specifically infectious diseases. For example, death rates from tuberculosis have been estimated to have been as high as 700 per 100,000 during the early twentieth century (Clark, Riben and Nowgesic 2002). However, tuberculosis rates have rapidly declined over recent decades. During the early 1980s the incidence of tuberculosis dropped to 148 per 100,000 (Smeja and Brassard 2000) and by 1996 this was further reduced to 35.8 per 100,000 among Status First Nations (FitzGerald, Wang and Elwood 2000). Despite these improvements, rates of tuberculosis still remain disproportionately high compared to the non-Aboriginal population (2 per 100,000) (FitzGerald et al. 2000).

Overall, improvements in life expectancy and infectious diseases are reflective of the Aboriginal population undergoing an epidemiologic transition, characterised by a decline in the incidence of infectious diseases and a rise in the incidence of chronic, non-communicable diseases (specifically cancer, diabetes and cardiovascular diseases). For example, First Nations have experienced significantly lower incidences of both cancer and cancer related mortalities compared to the non-Aboriginal population (Elias et al. 2011). Between 1984–1988 the cancer mortality rate of First Nations was 40 per cent below that of the non-Aboriginal population (Elias et al. 2011). However, rates have been steadily rising such that by 2001 cancer was the third leading cause of death among First Nations males and second leading cause of death among First Nations females (Tjepkema et al. 2009). There are a number of factors that may be contributing to the increased occurrence of cancer within the Aboriginal population including genetics and the environment (Moore et al. 2006, Dong et al. 2008; Esteller 2008). In addition, the change in lifestyle among Aboriginal population brought on by colonialism is linked to a number of health risks, which may be associated with the rise in cancer incidence. For example, the higher rates of smoking among Aboriginal populations may be linked with an increased risk of cancer (Elias et al. 2011). Furthermore, diabetes mellitus and obesity, which affect Aboriginal peoples at a greater rate than non-Aboriginals, have been linked to various cancers (Everhart and Wright 1995; Calle et al. 2003; Coughlin et al. 2004). Rates of diabetes are estimated to be 2 to 5 times higher for First Nations compared to non-Aboriginals (Oster and Toth 2009). In addition, Aboriginal peoples experience obesity rates that are more than double that of the non-Aboriginal population and without intervention it is expected that the prevalence of obesity will only continue to increase among Aboriginal populations (Ng, Corey and Young 2012). Not only do diabetes and obesity increase one's risk of cancer, both are also known risk factors for cardiovascular disease (CVD). Despite an overall decline in the incidence of CVD and associated deaths in North America, rates continue to rise for the Aboriginal populations in Canada (Retnatkaran et al. 2005). While these measures of health and well-being are important, we argue that it essential to broaden the definition of health and well-being beyond that represented in the epidemiologic and biomedical perspectives found in much Aboriginal health research (presented above) to encompass both health and social issues, the latter we argue represents a new health gap particularly between the younger Aboriginal population and the non-Aboriginal population.

## Socioeconomic Inequalities and Emerging New Health Inequalities

Youth represent a significant proportion of the Aboriginal population with nearly half (48 per cent) of all Aboriginal peoples currently under the age of 24 (Statistics Canada 2006).

However, despite their youthfulness, Aboriginal peoples remain disproportionately burdened by social and health disparities with much higher levels of poverty, unemployment, abuse, addiction, obesity and suicide (Disant et al. 2008).

Health statistics and research examining the health of Aboriginal youth are lacking in comparison to the data available for the Aboriginal population as a whole. Yet, from the limited information to which we do have access a grim and often dark portrait is painted depicting the health of Aboriginal youth. There is a growing awareness of both the historical and social inequalities suffered by many Aboriginal peoples, but the intergenerational impacts of these are still being uncovered. It is acknowledged that the factors shaping the health of Aboriginal youth are intertwined between both historical injustices and current inequities (Standing Senate Committee on Aboriginal Peoples 2003).

The socioeconomic inequalities experienced by Aboriginal youth are immense and unfortunately many Aboriginal youth are born into a life of disadvantage. Living below the low-income-cut-off is a reality for many Aboriginal peoples. In 2005, approximately 28 per cent of Aboriginal children 15 years of age and younger lived in low-income households (Collin and Jensen 2009). In the same year, almost 20 per cent of Aboriginal youth between the ages of 16 and 24 lived in low-income families as compared with only 9.8 per cent of non-Aboriginal youth. Rates of poverty are 63 per cent higher among Aboriginal youth who are living alone or living with individuals to whom they are not related by blood, marriage or adoption (Collin and Jensen 2009). This statistic is particularly worrisome given that Aboriginal youth are three times more likely than non-Aboriginal youth to be estranged from their families due to placement in foster care or adoption (Disant et al. 2008).

Undoubtedly, a life of poverty can severely impact one's health and development. Research has shown that very early on an individual's social economic status (SES) can have direct impacts upon health and well-being and that poverty in childhood can have long-lasting effects into adulthood (Hill and Sandfort 1999). Among the Aboriginal population, the rippling health effects of poverty begin with its destructive forces upon the most basic elements essential to human life, food and shelter.

While Canada ranks sixth on the UN Human Development Index (Human Development Report 2011) many First Nations reserves can be best described as deplorable; substandard housing, lack of potable water and proper sanitation continue to shape the lives and health of reserve residents and those living in the far North. Aboriginal peoples are four times more likely to experience crowding and one out of every four Aboriginal people live in houses which are in need of major repair (McIntyre, Connor and Warren 2000). Such conditions can increase the risk for infectious diseases such as tuberculosis (Clark, Riben and Nowgesic 2002) and gastrointestinal viruses (Rosenberg et al. 1997). For example, Inuit infants and children have the highest rates of lower respiratory tract infections in the world, which have been directly linked to their living conditions (Kovesi et al. 2007). Furthermore, high incidences of Otitis Media (Ayukawa et al. 2004) and bacterial and viral infections such as pneumonia, gastroenteritis, and bacterial meningitis underlie the majority of early childhood morbidity and mortality of Inuit children (Jenkins 2002) and are linked to substandard living conditions.

As we have seen from the income disparities described earlier it is no surprise that Aboriginal families are over-represented among those individuals experiencing hunger (McIntrye et al. 2000). Nutritional deficiencies amongst Aboriginal peoples remain a persistent problem, especially for those families living in poverty. Such deficiencies can manifest themselves as larger health problems (e.g., nutritional rickets) and may greatly affect physical and intellectual development (Moffatt 1994). Tied to nutrition is food security, which for many Aboriginal communities is a continual struggle. Aboriginal peoples experience numerous barriers to access to nutritious foods. For example, among Aboriginal peoples living in remote areas where healthy, fresh food items are not readily available. In remote areas food is transported by air from southern locations, making those heavier often nutritious foods a high cost commodity and more likely to be replaced by lighter weight, non-perishable foods, such as 'junk' food. Essentially, lighter is cheaper and unhealthier, but it is these lighter food options that are most accessible to Aboriginal households. The high cost of milk has been linked to the severity of dental caries present in Inuit children (Zammit et al. 1994) and as milk is replaced with high fructose drinks such as carbonated soft drinks the risk of obesity and diabetes has been shown to increase for many Aboriginal youth (Croucher Todd 2010). In addition, many Aboriginal peoples live in communities with contaminated food and water sources. Knowing that traditional food sources are environmentally contaminated limits the mix of healthy foods available for consumption.

In addition to the barriers listed above, dramatic changes to Aboriginal cultures and lifestyles observed over the past 50 years, specifically those related to diet and the adoption of sedentary lifestyles, have given way to major health concerns for Aboriginal youth. At one time non-existent in Aboriginal communities, today both obesity and Type II diabetes (T2D) are affecting Aboriginal youth at alarming rates. Findings from the First Nations Regional Longitudinal Health Survey revealed that of those First Nations on reserve, 14 per cent of youth and 36.2 per cent of children were considered obese (Collin and Jensen 2009). The high prevalence of obesity has been linked with a corresponding rise in frequency of T2D and is particularly worrisome given both are risk factors for CVD (Zorzi et al. 2009).

More than 50 per cent of Aboriginal youth reside in urban areas (Statistics Canada 2006). For some the city is the only home they have ever known while for others the city is a place to go in search of opportunities unavailable to them in their home communities. Although the city can be a success for some, for others the urban promise of a better future does not always become a reality. The urban landscape can pose numerous barriers to Aboriginal youth in search of housing, employment and education.

The links between education, employment and income are well known. It is clear that education leads to greater income opportunities and as such education can be considered a significant determinant of health (Hull 2005). Although the education gap is narrowing, the high school completion rate for Aboriginal youth remains low and a large gap persists between those Aboriginal and non-Aboriginal university graduates at rates of 8 per cent compared to 23 per cent respectively (Statistics Canada 2006). Unfortunately, the low percentage of Aboriginal university graduates indicates the barriers they experience are overwhelming for most.

The link between SES and education is double-barrelled. Education can very well be a means of improving one's SES, but this glimmer of hope is undermined by the dark reality that for those individuals from families of low SES achieving higher education is unlikely (Mendelson 2006). As those individuals living with scarce resources may be required to allocate their time to fulfill immediate needs to survive such as housing and food this negative link may be stronger than one would predict. Many Aboriginal youth are placed in positions requiring greater responsibilities beyond that of education and commonly leave school to seek employment, to care for siblings or simply due to problems within the home that may interfere with their learning (Standing Senate Committee on Aboriginal Peoples 2003). It should be noted that overall Aboriginal peoples tend to pursue post-secondary education at later stages in their lives, perhaps demonstrating those challenges and barriers to education are mainly tied to childhood and youth experiences. One experience specific to Aboriginal youth are the high rates of teen pregnancy with 20 per cent of all First Nations births involving a teen mom compared to 5.6 per cent for the general Canadian population (Disant et al. 2008). The responsibilities of young mothers often result in their school absence contributing to the high drop-out rates witnessed for Aboriginal youth.

Aboriginal peoples living in cities are twice as likely to live in poverty compared to the non-Aboriginal population (Disant et al. 2008). The unemployment rate for Aboriginal youth between the ages of 15 and 24 is triple the rate of non-Aboriginal youth. Often times those youth migrating to the city soon realise they are lacking the basic skills and experience required to obtain even the most basic employment for which the city had initially enticed them (Standing Senate Committee on Aboriginal Peoples 2003).

As visible minorities, discrimination arises in both the job and housing markets leaving many Aboriginal youth defeated and forced to occupy marginal and often dangerous spaces. Despite a decrease in the overall number of Aboriginal peoples living in crowded homes, the numbers remain high with Aboriginal peoples four times more likely to live in crowded dwellings compared to non-Aboriginals (Statistics Canada 2006). Additionally, a link has been drawn between crowding and health outcomes related to violence, stress and injury (Lauster and Tester 2010), thus only exacerbating the poor health conditions of many Aboriginal peoples.

Among Aboriginal youth, mortality rates are three times greater than that of non-Aboriginal youth. Furthermore, Aboriginal youth are four times more likely to suffer an injury, the most prevalent being suicide with rates 5–6 times higher than non-Aboriginal youth (Coleman et al. 2001). Suicide is the leading cause of death of those First Nations and Inuit between the ages of 10 and 24 (Disant et al. 2008). The risk of suicide increases with several factors including history of physical and sexual abuse, alcohol and substance abuse, relative poverty, low education, poor parenting, social isolation, and feelings of hopelessness (Fraser 2009). The list of risk factors here are not exhaustive, but each of these factors represent conditions that Aboriginal peoples experience at a much higher rate than non-Aboriginals. Suicide rates are, however, not experienced evenly across Aboriginal communities. There has been a link shown between those communities with greater cultural continuity and local control and lower rates of suicide (Chandler and Lalonde 2008). Additionally, increased family and community connectedness, community involvement, school success, and spirituality have been observed to serve as protective factors to suicide prevention (Fraser 2009). Although suicide accounts for a large portion of injuries among Aboriginal youth, injuries related to motor vehicle collisions, violence, abuse, falls and exposure (frostbite/hypothermia) also exist as major health concerns affecting Aboriginal youth (Health Canada 2001).

Substance abuse including marijuana, inhalants and stimulants are all too familiar amongst Aboriginal youth and for many can become a problem at a very early age. For example, the highest risk period for inhalant initiation is between the ages of 10–13 and on average first use occurs at 11.5 years of age (Coleman et al. 2001). Aboriginal youth are three times more likely to be victims of abuse or violence (Disant et al. 2008) and this risk increases for those youth whose access to employment and a steady source of income are limited. It has been argued that economic marginalisation may push Aboriginal youth to pursue illegal enterprises as a primary source of income (Standing Senate Committee on Aboriginal Peoples 2003). Aboriginal incarceration rates have been steadily increasing and this is particularly true for Aboriginal youth. In 1998, 13 per cent of those youth admitted to correctional services self-identified as Aboriginal, 10 years later this number rose to

17.9 per cent (Perreault 2009). Overall, Aboriginal peoples comprise 20 per cent of those behind bars despite comprising only 3 per cent of the national population (Perreault 2009). In a study completed with Aboriginal ex-gang members themes of discrimination, racism, structural inequalities and lack of opportunity were frequently reported as causal factors to gang involvement (Grekul and LaBoucane-Benson 2008). Many revealed poverty and family dysfunction as precursors to their recruitment. Lacking a sense of identity and belonging, youth often turn to the welcoming arms of gangs for a sense of purpose and family (Grekul and LaBoucane-Benson 2008). It has been found that those youth without a high school diploma or employment are at greater risk of committing crimes that will lead to incarceration (Perreault 2009), again emphasising the importance of access to education and meaningful employment for youth.

For young Aboriginal females, illegal activities often take shape in the form of prostitution, not only subjecting them to significant risk of violence and injury, but as well jeopardising their health and well-being. Finding oneself in a position of despair and poverty can lead to engagement in risky behaviour such as trading sex for shelter, food or drugs. Aboriginal peoples are over-represented amongst those living with both HIV and AIDS. Once primarily transmitted sexually, HIV has grown to an epidemic occurring amongst intravenous drug users, accounting for 17 per cent of new infections in 2006 (Duncan et al. 2011). This fact is of concern given Aboriginal peoples comprise a significant proportion of those suffering drug addictions (McCormick 2000; Coleman, Charles and Collins 2001). Prior to 1993, 1.3 per cent of reported AIDS cases were found in the Aboriginal population; however, this number jumped to an astonishing 13.4 per cent in a matter of ten years and, of those, 25 per cent are under the age of 30 (Health Canada 2004). In the last decade, infections of HIV have rapidly increased among Aboriginal populations whom accounted for 27.3 per cent of new infections in 2006 (Public Health Agency of Canada 2007). Thirty per cent of all Aboriginal HIV cases occur among those aged 20 and 29 years of age in comparison to 20 per cent of non-Aboriginal cases (Centre for Infectious Disease Prevention and Control 2003). Research indicates Aboriginal youth are at high risk for HIV infection and become infected at a younger age than non-Aboriginals (Canadian Aboriginal AIDS Network 2003). Seventy per cent of Aboriginal youth become sexually active before the age of 15 and less than 20 per cent practice safe sex (i.e., consistent condom use) (Myers et al. 1993). The frequency of Aboriginal youth engaging in risky sexual behavior is confirmed by their significantly higher rates of sexually transmitted infections with reported rates of Chlamydia seven times that of the non-Aboriginal population (Disant et al. 2008), in addition to high rates of pregnancy both which have been found to be predictors for HIV infection (Canadian Aboriginal AIDS Network 2003).

## Conclusions

It is evident that Aboriginal peoples experience profound health inequalities that are exacerbated by greater social inequalities. Furthermore, the inequalities experienced by young Aboriginal peoples can be understood as manifestations of the disturbing legacy left behind from colonisation and the residential school system. The effects of colonisation have been perpetuated across generations and communities of Aboriginal peoples and have compounded racism, poverty and violence making them commonplace in the lives of too many Aboriginal youth. Reacting to these hardships places the health and lives of Aboriginal youth at risk as they attempt to escape them through various means such as urban migration, street involvement and drug use (Canadian Aboriginal AIDS Network 2003). The feedback loops among racism, poverty and violence, urban migration, street involvement and drug use are contributing to an emergence of new health inequalities including prevalent alcohol and substance abuse, injury, suicide, incarceration rates, and most shockingly the recent and rapidly growing cases of HIV and AIDS seen among Aboriginal youth. Unfortunately, such experiences shed light on only darker realities and present tragedies that extend far beyond the lives of Aboriginal youth as they threaten future generations of Aboriginal Peoples. The social and economic costs of not addressing the health needs of Aboriginal peoples today will be far greater in the future. This speaks to the need for further research and policy committed to improving the lives of Aboriginal youth to ensure a sustainable future for Aboriginal peoples across the country.

## References

Allard, Y., Wilkins, R. and Berthelot, J. 2004. Premature mortality in health regions with high Aboriginal populations. *Health Reports, 15*(1). 51–60.

Assembly of First Nations (ANF). 2009. *History of residential schools.* Ottawa. [Online]. Available at: http://www.afn.ca/residentialschools/history.html.

Ayukawa, H., Bruneau, S., Proulx, J. et al. 2004. Otitis media and hearing loss among 12–16 year old Inuit of Inukjuak, Quebec, Canada. *International Journal of Circumpolar Health, 64*, 312–14.

BC Ministry Health Office Planning. 2001. *BC's provincial health officer's annual report 2001: the health and well-being of Aboriginal peoples in British Columbia.* [Online]. Available at: http://www.health.gov.bc.ca/pho/pdf/phoannual2001.pdf.

Calle, E., Rodriguez, C., Walker-Thurmond, K. et al. 2003. Overweight, obesity, and mortality from cancer in a prospectively studied cohort of U.S. adults. *The New England Journal of Medicine, 348*, 1625–38.

Canada. 1996. Royal commission on Aboriginal peoples. In Looking forward, looking back, Vol. 1. Ottawa: Department of Indian and Northern Affairs. [Online]. Available at: http://www.collectionscanada.gc.ca/webarchives/20071124125216/http://www.ainc-inac.gc.ca/ch/rcap/sg/sg1_e.html.

Canada. 2004. *Words First: An Evolving Terminology Relating to Aboriginal Peoples in Canada.* Ottawa: Communications Branch Indian and Northern Affairs Canada.

Canadian Aboriginal AIDS Network. 2003. Strengthening Ties – Strengthening Communities: An Aboriginal Strategy on HIV/AIDS in Canada. Ottawa, ON: Canadian Aboriginal AIDS Network.

Castellano, M.B., Archibald, L. and DeGagné, M. 2008. *From Truth to Reconciliation: Transforming the Legacy of Residential Schools.* Ottawa: Aboriginal Healing Foundation.

CBC News. 2008. *Residential schools: a history of residential schools in Canada.* [Online]. Available at: http://www.cbc.ca/news/canada/story/2008/05/16/f-faqs-residential-schools.html.

Centre for Infectious Disease Prevention and Control (CIDPC). 2003. HIV/AIDS Among Aboriginal Persons in Canada: A Continuing Concern. HIV/AIDS Epi Updates. Ottawa, Ontario: Health Canada, 35–40.

Chandler, M., and Lalonde, C. 2008. Cultural continuity as a moderator of suicide risk among Canada's First Nations, in and Healing Traditions: The Mental Health of

Aboriginal Peoples in Canada, edited by L.J. Kirmayer and G. Valaskakis. Vancouver: University of British Columbia Press, 221–48.

Clark, M., Riben, P. and Nowgesic, E. 2002. The association of housing density, isolation and tuberculosis in Canadian First Nations communities. *International Journal of Epidemiology, 31*(5), 940–45.

Coleman, H., Charles, G., and Collins, J. 2001. Inhalant use by Canadian Aboriginal youth. *Journal of Child and Adolescent Substance Abuse*, 10(3). 1–20.

Collin, C. and Jensen, H. 2009. A statistical profile of poverty in Canada. (Report # PRB 09–17E). [Online: Library of Parliament]. Available at: http://www.parl.gc.ca/Content/ LOP/ResearchPublications/prb0917-e.pdf.

Coughlin, S., Calle, E., Teras, L. et al. 2004. Diabetes Mellitus as a predictor for cancer mortality in a large cohort of US adults. *American Journal of Epidemiology, 159*(12), 1160–67.

Croucher, Todd, S. 2010. Food security in Paulatuk, NT: opportunities and challenges of a changing community economy. Master's Thesis. Edmonton: University of Alberta.

Disant, M., Hebert, C., Bergeron, O. et al. 2008. Aboriginal youth and social inequalities in health. [Online: Quebec Population Health Research]. Available at: http://www. santepop.qc.ca/bulletin.php?l=en&id=68.

Dong, L., Potter, J., White, E. et al. 2008. Genetic susceptibility to cancer. *The Journal of the American Medical Association, 307*(14), 1480–542.

Duncan, K., Reading, C., Borwein, A. et al. 2011. HIV incidence and prevalence among Aboriginal peoples in Canada. *AIDS Behaviour, 15*, 214–27.

Elias, B., Kliewer, E., Hall, M. et al. 2011. The burden of cancer risk in Canada's Indigenous population: a comparative study of known risks in a Canadian region. *International Journal of General Medicine, 4*, 699–709.

Enarson, D.A. and Grzybowski, S. 1986. Incidence of active tuberculosis in the native population of Canada. *Canadian Medical Association Journal*, 134(10), 1149–52.

Esteller, M. 2008. Epigenetics in cancer. *The New England Journal of Medicine, 358*, 1148–59.

Everhart, J. and Wright, D. 1995. Diabetes Mellitus as a risk factor for pancreatic cancer. *The Journal of the American Medical Association, 273*(20), 1605–9.

FitzGerald, J., Wang, L. and Elwood, R. 2000. Tuberculosis: 13. control of the disease among Aboriginal people in Canada. *CMAJ, 162*(3), 351–5.

Fraser, S. 2009. Current approaches to Aboriginal youth suicide prevention. Canada: Institute of Community & Family Psychiatry Jewish General Hospital: Culture & Mental Health Research Unit, 1–156.

Grekul, J. and LaBoucane-Benson, P. 2008. Aboriginal gangs and their (dis)placement: contextualizing recruitment, membership and status. *Canadian Journal of Criminology and Criminal Justice*, 50(1), 59–82.

Hammond, G.W., Rutherford, B.E., Malazdrewicz, R. and MacFarlane, N. 1988. Haemophilus Influenzae Meningitis in Manitoba and the Keewatin District, NWT: Potential for mass vaccination. *Canadian Medical Association Journal*, 139, 743–7.

Health Canada. 2001. *Unintentional and intentional injury profile for Aboriginal People in Canada: 1990–1999*. Ottawa, ON: Minister of Public Works and Government Services Canada.

Health Canada. 2004. *Understanding the HIV/AIDS epidemic among Aboriginal peoples in Canada: the community at a glance*. Ottawa: Health Canada.

Hill, M. and Sandfort, J. 1999. Effects of childhood poverty on productivity later in life: Implications for public policy. *Children and Youth Services Review*, *17*(1), 91–126.

Hull, J. 2005. Post-secondary education and labour market outcomes Canada, 2001. Winnipeg: Prologica Research Inc.

Human Development Report. 2011. *Sustainability and Equity: A Better Future for All*. New York: United Nations Development Programme.

Jenkins, A. 2002. Factors influencing the health of Canadian Inuit infants Canada. Master's Thesis. Montreal: McGill University, 101.

Kovesi, T., Gilbert, N., Stocco, C. et al. 2007. Indoor air quality and the risk of lower respiratory tract infections in young Canadian Inuit children. *CMAJ*, 177(2). 155–60.

Lauster, N. and Tester, F. 2010. Culture as a problem linking material inequality to health: On residential crowding in the Arctic. *Health and Place*, *16*, 523–30.

MacMillan, H., MacMillan, A., Offord, D. and Dingle, J. 1996. Aboriginal health. *Canadian Medical Association Journal*, *155*(11), 1569–626.

McCormick. R. 2000. Aboriginal traditions in the treatment of substance abuse. *Journal of Counseling and Psychotherapy*, 34(1), 25–32.

McIntrye, L., Connor, S., Warren, J. 2000. Child hunger in Canada: results of the 1994 national longitudinal survey of children and youth. *CMAJ*, *163*(8), 961–5.

Mendelson, M. 2006. Aboriginal peoples and post-secondary education in Canada. [Online: Caledon Institute of Social Policy]. Available at: www.caledoninst.org/Publications/PDF/595ENG.pdf.

Métis Nation Council (MNC). 2010. Citizenship. Métis Nation Council. [Online]. Available at: http://www.metisnation.ca/index.php/who-are-the-metis/citizenship.

Moffatt, M. 1994. Current status of nutritional deficiencies in Canadian Aboriginal people. *Canadian Journal of Physiology and Pharmacology*, 73, 754–8.

Moore, L., Huang, W. and Hayes, R. 2006. Epidemiologic consideration to assess DNA methylation from environmental exposures to cancer. *Annals of the New York Academy of Science*, *983*, 181–6.

Myers, T., Calzavara, L., Cockerill, R. et al. 1993. *Ontario First Nations AIDS and Health Lifestyle Survey*. Ottawa, Ontario: National AIDS Clearinghouse, Canadian Public Health Association.

Ng, C., Corey, P. and Young, T. 2012. Divergent body mass index trajectories between Aboriginal and non-Aboriginal Canadians 1994–2009 – an exploration of age, period and cohort effects. *American Journal of Human Biology*, *24*, 170–76.

Oster, R. and Toth, E. 2009. Differences in the prevalence of diabetes risk-factors among First Nation, Métis and non-Aboriginal adults attending screening clinics in rural Alberta, Canada. *Rural and Remote Health*, *9*(2), 1170.

Perreault, S. 2009. The incarceration of Aboriginal peoples in adult correctional services. (Report No. 85–002-X). [Online: Statistics Canada]. Available at: http://www.statcan.gc.ca/pub/85–002-x/2009003/article/10903-eng.pdf.

Public Health Agency of Canada. 2007. HIV/AIDS epi updates, November 2007. Ottawa: Public Health Agency of Canada.

Retnakaran, R., Hanley, A., Connelly, P. et al. 2005. Cigarette smoking and cardiovascular risk factors among Aboriginal Canadian youths. *CMAJ*, *173(*8), 885–9.

Rosenberg, T., Kendall, O., Blanchard, J. et al. 1997. Shigellosis on Indian reserves in Manitoba, Canada: its relationship to crowded housing, lack of running water, and inadequate sewage disposal. *American Journal of Public Health*, *87*(9), 1547–51.

Smeja, C. and Brassard, P. 2000. Tuberculosis infection in an Aboriginal (First Nations) population in Canada. *The International Journal of Tuberculosis and Lung Disease*, *4*(10), 925–30.

Smylie, J., Fell, D., Ohlsson, A. and the Joint Working Group on First Nations, Indian, Inuit, and Métis Infant Mortality of the Canadian Perinatal Surveillance System. 2010. A Review of Aboriginal Infant Mortality Rates in Canada: Striking and Persistent Aboriginal/Non-Aboriginal Inequities. *Canadian Journal of Public Health*, *101*(2), 143–8.

Statistics Canada. 2006. Aboriginal peoples in Canada 2006: Inuit, Métis and First Nations, 2006 Census. (Report No. 97 -558 -X I.E.). Available at: http://www12.statcan.ca/census-recensement/2006/as-sa/97–558/p6-eng.cfm.

Statistics Canada. 2008. *Educational Portrait of Canada, Census 2006*. (Report No. 97–560-X2006001). Available at: http://www12.statcan.gc.ca/english/census06/analysis/education/pdf/97–560-XIE2006001.pdf.

Statistics Canada. 2010. *Projections of the Aboriginal Populations, Canada, Provinces and Territories, 2001 to 2017* (Report No. 91–547-XIE). Available at: http://www.statcan.gc.ca/pub/89–645-x/2010001/c-g/c-g013-eng.htm.

Standing Senate Committee on Aboriginal Peoples. 2003. *Urban Aboriginal youth: an action plan for change*. Available at: publications.gc.ca/collections/collection.../YC28–0–372–6-eng.pdf.

Tjepkema, M., Wilkins, R., Senecal, S. et al. 2009. Mortality of Metis and registered Indian adults in Canada: an 11-year follow-up study. *Health Reports*, *20*, 31–51.

Trovato, J. 2001. Aboriginal mortality in Canada, the United States and New Zealand. *Journal of Biosocial Science*, *33*(1), 67–86.

Waldram, J.B., Herring, A.D. and Young, K.T. 2006. *Aboriginal Health in Canada: Historical, Cultural and Epidemiological Paerspectives* (2nd ed.). Toronto: University of Toronto Press.

Young, T.K. 1991. Prevalence and correlates of Hypertension in a Subarctic Indian population. *Preventive Medicine*, 20, 474–85.

Zammit, M., Torres, A., Johnsen, D. and Hans, M. 1994. The prevalence and patterns of dental caries in Labrador Inuit youth. *Journal of Public Health Dentistry*, *54*(3), 132–8.

Zorzi, A., Wabi, G., Macnab, A. and Panagiotopoulos, C. 2009. Prevalence of impaired glucose tolerance and the components of metabolic syndrome in Canadian Tsimshian First Nations youth. *Canadian Journal of Rural Medicine*, *14*(2), 61–7.

# PART II
# Health Access and Utilisation in Developing Countries

Chapter 6

# The Place of 'Health' in Social Health Insurance in Developing Countries: A Study in Ghana's Upper West Region

Jenna Dixon and Paul Mkandawire

## Financing Health Care in Developing Countries

Around the turn of the new millennium, in part fuelled by the global initiatives of the millennium development goals, a noticeable uptick in attention began to be paid to the role of health care systems in improving the wellbeing of peoples in developing countries. Indeed many international organisations including the WHO, the World Bank, and the German Agency for Technical Cooperation have been urging poor country governments to enact policy to allow the establishment of health insurance schemes so that poor people could afford to obtain health care (Hsiao and Shaw 2007). It is not surprising then, that Hsiao and Shaw (2007, 1) point to 'a wave of Social Health Insurance initiatives' that has swept across Africa, Asia, and Latin America.

This comes against a backdrop of decades of Structural Adjustment Programmes (SAPs), which were supported by some of the very institutions now calling for reform, such as the World Bank and International Monetary Fund. The SAPs, though diverse in consequences, had for the most part led to a drastic reduction in public expenditure and public investment in national health care sectors across the developing world. The fallout of these policies has been well documented by many, and at the very least is recognised to have disproportionately impacted society's most vulnerable populations – women, children, the poor, and those in rural areas (Konadu-Agyemang 2000). As health care required out-of-pocket payments at the time of service, most people enacted the 'wait and see' strategy, delaying contact with the formal health system as long as possible, while others went into great debt to finance their health care needs. The 1990s can therefore be understood as a period of regression in the overall health for the people of developing countries. The contemporary shift away from the health policies found during the era of SAPs and the relatively recent institutional advocacy for a reform in health financing towards health insurance schemes raises an intriguing, but often not asked, question – *can these institutions which are rooted in the ideology of free markets and private property rights genuinely support health reforms that are founded on the ethic of collective wellbeing and social inclusion?*

## What is Health Insurance?

Health insurance is a concept whereby people pre-pay for coverage, and together pool the risks associated with the costs of falling ill. By paying into their coverage, individuals avoid the potential for extreme out of pocket payments that could come from a serious illness, and thus health insurance helps protect people from catastrophic financial loss. As well, the plans ensure that people are covered for basic care and thus can help control illness with medical attention before it becomes more serious. In this sense, health insurance has been recognised as an important resource for breaking the downward spiral of poverty and ill-health (Xu et al. 2003). Further, since the cost is spread over a very large group of people and often subsidised by the government, health insurance represents an effective tool for expanding coverage to the poor.

Amongst others, Ghana, Rwanda and Thailand have adopted forms of Social Health Insurance (SHI) to finance their health care systems, and still more governments such as the Kingdom of Lesotho have begun investigating the feasibility of starting these programmes in their countries. These programmes have undoubtedly been met with both success and challenges. This mixed success has prompted studies which increasingly focus on evaluating the true extant of accomplishments and failures associated with the SHI schemes. However, the goal of this chapter is different in that it instead seeks to shift attention to examining the true nature of these programmes, the range of activities that constitute them, and how they are rolled out in practice. This chapter is structured around the argument that in its current formulation, the SHI model while avoiding the designation of a private health insurance model, shares fundamental similarities with the private health insurance arrangement. We reveal this connection by interrogating some of the key assumptions on which these insurance programmes are founded and making the links between these assumptions and the substantive contents of these schemes in terms of the portfolio of activities and practices that constitute SHI schemes. We also draw on empirical data from Ghana – one of the countries which has been successfully operating a SHI – to demonstrate that the reductionist manner in which health has been conceptualised within the scheme is not only irreconcilable with local understandings of health, but also serves to mask broader social and political contexts that shape community health.

## Types of Health Insurance Schemes

Health insurance can generally be divided into four different types (Hsaio and Shaw 2007). The first is *Private Insurance*, which requires individuals to pay premiums out of pocket, though private schemes are voluntary. Usually this type of insurance transaction is made directly with an insurance company, which likely makes a notable profit off of these insurance plans. The second type is *Community Based Insurance*. Like private insurance, this is voluntary and premium payments are made out of pocket by the individual participating. However the pool of participants for CBI's is usually much smaller and based within a geographically defined locality. CBI schemes are also usually not geared towards making a profit, but to cover the health care needs of the community. The third type of health insurance to be considered is a *National Insurance* plan. National Insurance plans are funded primarily through tax revenues and organised via national governments as benefits automatically extend to all citizens. National Insurance is common in more developed economies, such as Europe and North America, with populations that can handle higher tax levels.

Finally, and of primary focus here, is the *Social Health Insurance* (SHI) model. SHI plans draw from a variety of sources for funding, including employer/employee contributions, government (tax-based) contributions, and private out of pocket contributions. SHI is mandatory for employees of formal sector organisations that pay into them, and often made technically mandatory for entire populations including the informal sector of the economy. However, as our case study of Ghana will demonstrate, mandatory participation (and the premium payments that come with them) is a policy not easily or readily enforced. The SHI model has a long history since it was first implemented in Germany in 1883 (Saltman and Dubois 2004). Currently, more than 30 countries worldwide have instituted a form of social health insurance coverage, though most of these are higher income countries such as Belgium, Austria and Luxemburg. Individuals become members not necessarily by virtue of citizenship, but rather because they must pay a contribution which can take the form of a payroll tax for those formally employed or a subsidy by the government in the case of those who are extremely poor.

All models of health insurance rest on the notion that illness is largely accidental, characterised by a high degree of uncertainty. The SHI model further assumes that although a relatively small number of people will suffer from serious illness in a society at any given point in time, the resulting debility can lead to permanent injury, disability and even loss of life. According to SHI theory, individuals act as rational and risk-averse economic agents. Based on this assumption it is expected that it would be in their best interest to seek protection against accidental insults to health and wellbeing that would result in disability.

Ideally, the SHI model works by pooling high and low risk people into one integrated health insurance system whose primary aim is to circumvent the problem of adverse selection. Adverse selection is a serious problem in health insurance because the poor in society – who are the most likely to need coverage – may actually fail to enrol in the insurance scheme on economic grounds, while young healthy individuals may be reluctant to enrol in a scheme that also includes high risk groups. These circumstances justify a mandatory SHI system operated by the state and backed by appropriate legislation in order to compel the well-off members who usually have the option to sign up in private health insurance scheme to be part of the SHI system as well.

Notwithstanding the foregoing virtues, the SHI model suffers from fundamental theoretical and practical flaws. In this next section we introduce the conceptual framework of the 'social determinants of health' and our understanding of the large scale social, structural and economic influences in which people are deeply embedded and how that has been proven to influence health. Given this, we then outline four main areas where the assumptions underlying SHI, and the rhetoric surrounding the policymaking of SHI, can be found to be in conflict with the basic tenets of the social determinants of health.

## The Social Determinants of Health

Around the same time that the popularity was rising of alternative health care financing models, there was also renewed attention within public health circles towards the critical mass of evidence acknowledging the importance of the economic and social factors that contribute to health (Dixon 2000). In light of this, the WHO compiled 10 distilled messages for policy makers and the public on the evidence of the social determinants of health (SDH), later expanded into a book (Marmot and Wilkinson 1999). The 10 messages are as follows: health follows a social gradient; stress damages health; the health impacts of early development and education last a lifetime; poverty and social exclusion cost lives; stress in the work place increases risk of disease; job security improves health; unemployment causes illness and premature death; social supports and supportive networks improve health; alcohol, drug and tobacco use are influenced by the social setting; healthy food is a political issue; healthy transport means walking and cycling and good public transport. For our discussion here it is not one particular message that is important but the thrust of the entire argument – namely that health is in large part determined far beyond the individual level and that any discussion on health must recognise the social, economic, political and other structural elements that feed an individual's health status.

The SDH perspective has become a basic part of our underlying approach to research in many fields of study related to health, including serving as an important marker in the cultural turn from medical to health geography. Certainly there is ample evidence of the theory's power. Both on an international scale and at a more local scale, inequities in health arise out of broader inequities in society. The foremost example of this is to compare gross national product (GNP) per capita and life expectancy, as the overall direction of the relationship is the same across the globe – (national) wealth equals (national) health. But this difference is not just between the developed and developing world. Notable in demonstrating that health inequalities are powerful even within nations and even within relatively close socioeconomic standards has been the Whitehall study. The Whitehall study (Marmot and Shipley 1996) followed British civil servants for three decades, all of whom were living in a relatively affluent life with steady office-based employment. Divided into a hierarchy of employment grades the participants showed that over time there was strong correlation with this hierarchy and mortality risk. This relationship held not only for overall mortality but for the major causes of death as well (Marmot et al. 1984). Thus, the problems of inequality in health are not restricted to grand material differences in living standards, but primarily in our identities within our own social contexts.

While an important move forward, admittedly Marmot and Wilkinson compilation of evidence is based almost exclusively on data from richer (developed) countries and targeted at European policy makers. Does the relevance of this framework translate to poorer or developing contexts? Indeed it does, just not rigidly into the 10 messages described above. The Commission on Social Determinants of Health (CSDH) was set up by the WHO in 2005 to address these questions on a more global scale. Their work is rooted in the understanding that global inequities in health are socially determined:

> These inequities in health, avoidable health inequalities, arise because of the circumstances in which people grow, live, work, and age, and the systems put in place to deal with illness. The conditions in which people live and die are, in turn, shaped by political, social, and economic forces. (CSDH 2008, ii)

Given this, the CSDH outlined three overarching recommendations to 'close the gap' in health inequalities. The commission's first call is to improve the daily living conditions of people in developing countries. This addresses issues such as education, environmental and housing conditions, land rights, fair employment, social protection and universal access to health care. Second, tackle the inequitable distribution of power, money and resources. This would often include the basic components on which society is organised, such as gendered divisions of power, as well as wrestling with large scale issues in the global financial system. Finally, continue to measure, evaluate and take action on these problems.

We draw on the SDH framework for this chapter in order to buttress our argument that the rhetoric around health insurance fails to account for the broader social forces that actually contribute to health. While the CSDH (2008) actually does endorse health insurance schemes for developing countries, we note that they have carefully wedged it in as part of the larger effort to improve living conditions and fight power inequities. In the following section we compare the assumptions of SHI to the SDH framework.

## The Social Health Insurance Model *versus* the Social Determinants of Health?

By establishing an arena where the indemnified pay a stipulated premium in exchange for an agreed package of health services, SHI essentially operates on a similar principle as the private health insurance while avoiding the nomenclature of the private sphere. In setting a clearly defined set of commodities and services to be provided to a given group of people on *quid pro quo* basis, the SHI, like the private insurance, establishes a service market where premiums and benefits are traded between two parties. On the one side of exchange are enrollees or prospective patients and on the other is the insurance scheme, the supplier of those services aimed at restoration of health. The resultant social contract gives rise to the expectation that enrollees agree to monetary payments in return for health care for all who are a part of the scheme. Those who cannot enrol are excluded from benefitting from its services. While polices are put in place to subsidise the extreme poor, this does not cover every citizen with a tight financial budget. Though health is often considered to be a public good and a right for all, the manner in which it is packaged for health insurance effectively transforms it into a private good where consumption is contingent on the ability to pay and therefore excludes those who lack purchasing power. While the SHI certainly theoretically avoids some of the pitfalls of the private insurance model, such as excluding the extreme poor on economic grounds and having more affordable pricing in practice, the model does not operate in a manner that is entirely different from the private model.

One of the most important points of incongruity between the SDH perspective and the SHI model relates to the manner in which the very notion of health has been operationalised. By packaging insurance coverage as a distinct set of services, the SHI model essentially suggests that wellbeing can be reduced to discrete set of experiences, amenities and commodities. When seen from this perspective, it is easy to understand that in its current formulation the SHI model conceives the attainment of health as predicated on availability of a prescribed range of drugs, treatments, procedures, supplies, and services to be dispensed by the health worker at a given time. The SHI's categorical conceptualisation of health does not resonate with the real life experience of health a process, where an individual's health is seen as the ability to rally from insults and continually adapt to the changing environment rather that a set of individual practices and commodities employed to deal with sporadic disease episodes (Earikson and Meade 2010). For instance, Avotri and Walters (1999) have found Ghanaian women's health to be very much a product of years of labour, pains, and psychological stress, as opposed to one acute medical problem.

Further, this apparent static conception of health artificially fixes health in time, allowing little or no scope for understanding the role of historical factors in shaping the contemporary experience of health. Notwithstanding, the role of agency, vulnerability to disease emerges from interconnecting global, national, regional, and local factors. Power imbalances systemic to the process of globalisation deserve scrutiny in the understanding and spread of diseases (Turshen 1999). Similarly, the legacy of colonialism still holds a strong influence over the broader social forces that shape ill-health in many developing countries (Coovadia et al. 2009).Such a reductionist approach to health is however understandable. It is consistent with other positivist assumptions on which the SHI is premised. For instance, even though the SHI bears the nomenclature of *social*, the framework is for the most part founded on the assumption of individualism where health insurance clients are assumed to be self-interested.

Furthermore, SHI's incorporates the assumption of rational choice – that clients in health insurance are rational economic actors who are self-interested and therefore will seek to maximise the health benefits that correspond to their premiums or prescribed insurance coverage. This assumption is inseparable from a related axiom of individualism, where personal independence and self-regard should take precedence over interdependence and communal interest. The assumption ignores the reality that people are socially embedded. Gender relations, for example, are an important form of social relation which is central in shaping health and vulnerability to disease (Bezner Kerr and Mkandawire 2010).

By implicitly invoking the assumption of individualism, the SHI model also fails to account for other social considerations such as cultural values or moral concerns. These hedonistic suppositions are especially problematic when examined in light of the fact that individuals also derive satisfaction from improved health and wellbeing of others (Sen and Willams 1982). Throughout much of the world people's sense of self is intertwined with that of others, a social relation that allows scope for a conception of health as a collective good rather than an individual or private property which can be procured from the market (Kalipeni et al. 2004).

Lastly, the notion that health is a commodity that can be transacted on the market may actually come in conflict with cultural understanding of health – where health is a sacred entity, comprising wellbeing and a virtue that transcends the nominal value of money. In such contexts, the notion of market exchange may be quite familiar and part of everyday life, but social norms may be such that exchanges are limited to other domains of society rather than health. Consequently, once 'health' is imported into the SHI model as a distinct commodity and a portfolio of activities and practices, it ignores and denigrates the social and cultural significance placed on life and deeper meanings attached to the notion of health and human existence.

Thus, although steering clear of the nomenclature and excesses associated with the private insurance model, the basic framework that would have legitimately placed these insurance schemes within the realm of the *social* is not reflected in the SHI model. From the foregoing, it is evident that the SHI closely approximates the private insurance scheme from which it purports to distance itself. Such is the character of the SHI model in that it sets a limit not only to the understanding of what constitutes health, but also to the understanding of the wider forces that impinge on it. Since these arguments in which the SHI model inadequately takes account of the SDH have so far been presented in abstract terms, we must now ground them in real, lived examples. Below, we present our case study of perceptions and experiences of health insurance in Ghana in order to illustrate all four of these themes in action.

## Study Context

### The Upper West Region of Ghana

The Upper West Region (UWR) spans an area of 18,476km² and accounts for 7.7% of the total land area in Ghana (Figure 6.1). The region has a total population of 618,730 people marking it with a relatively lower population density when compared to other regions in the country (Ghana Statistical Service 2008).

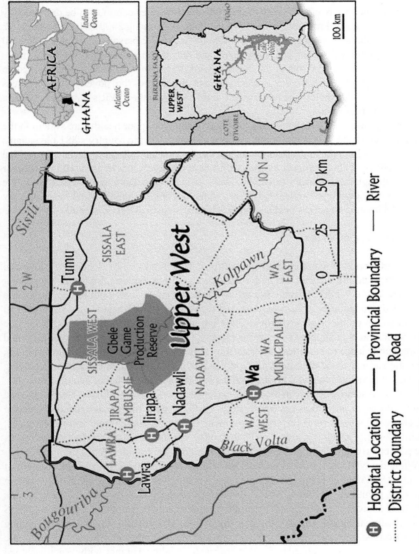

**Figure 6.1    Ghana's Upper West Region**

● Hospital Location    —— Provincial Boundary    —— River

...... District Boundary    —— Road

The UWR is one of the least-developed regions in Ghana, with only 17.5% of the total population characterised as urban. Only 5% of residents have attained any form of post-secondary education (Adjasi and Osei 2007). It is estimated that 69.8% of residents aged six years or older have never attended school, compared with the national average of 38.8%, and this has a cascading effect on the rate of unemployment in the region. Many decades of policy neglect partly explain why the region's literacy rates continue to be dramatically lower than the national rate (Anyinam 1994; Konadu-Agyemang 2000). The sex ratio is 92 males to 100 females, with an average household size of 7.2 persons. This has reinforced the already high levels of poverty with health and nutritional status being the worst in the country. For example, in terms of the upper poverty line of 90 Ghana *cedis* annual income (approximately $46 USD), 39.5% of Ghanaians live below the poverty line, whereas 79–96% in UWR live below the poverty line and 96–99% in the UWR's rural areas (Ghana Poverty Reduction Strategy 2005).

Spatially, uneven development has translated into a very poor health care system in the region. Presently, the UWR has six hospitals and only 17 of the country's 881 physicians. This represents both the lowest number of doctors in total as well as per population, with a ratio of 1:40,144. This is almost 8 times worse than Greater Accra Region with one doctor per 5,073 inhabitants (Ministry of Health Ghana 2011). Three quarters of households in the UWR live outside the recommended 8 km radius to a health facility, often meaning very long walks in order to access health services (Ghana Statistical Service 2008).

*Health Insurance in Ghana*

The Government of Ghana enacted the National Health Insurance Scheme (NHIS) into law in 2003, and the scheme was active nationwide within the next few years (Agyepong and Adjei 2008). While SHI schemes are still relatively rare in developing countries, the widespread unpopularity of the previous cost recovery model of health care, generated an arena in which politicians were provided the populace's support to create the NHIS. Due to the Structural Adjustment Programmes (SAPs), Ghana's focus on cost recovery resulted in poor maintenance of facilities, understaffing, reduction of pay and benefits, undermining of morale and increased absenteeism (Oppong 2001). Ghana, like many other developing countries in the same situation, implemented a pay-per-service model of health. There was, by result, a substantial decline in the use of mainstream medicine. Estimates have suggested regional drops in utilisation anywhere from 25–90%, with the greatest declines among the poor, women, and rural residents (Anyiman 1989; Waddington and Enimayew 1990; Hutchful 2002). During this era of SAPs the northern areas of Ghana, including the UWR, were particularly understaff and underfunded (Konadu-Agyemang 2000).

While the NHIS is technically mandatory for all citizens, there is little enforcement of this rule. Unlike other forms of insurance, only a small proportion of the NHIS' funding comes via premium payments. The vast majority of the NHIS revenue comes from the centralised sources of funding, and premium payments only accounting for 5% of all NHIS inflow (National Health Insurance Authority 2010). The centralised sources of funding (drawn from sources such as the 2.5% Value Added Tax and Social Security Funds) are channelled to the de-centralised nodes that operate the health insurance within each assigned district. Citizens may choose to purchase private insurance in addition to, or instead of, their local NHIS option, though private health insurance receives no additional funding from the government (Agyepong and Adjei 2008). While the insurance scheme is undeniably heavily subsidised by the government, in a context where the majority of the population lives below poverty line creates a situation where even modest premiums can constitute a major barrier to accessing health care for large sections of the population.

The evidence suggests that for those that are covered under the insurance programme, the NHIS has been found to be an effective tool for improving health outcomes (Mensah, Oppong and Schmidt 2010), and the NHIS has made impressive strides in enrolling Ghana's citizens. Official figures indicate that national enrolment started at 1.3 million people in 2005 and increased to 14.5 million people by 2009 (or 62% of the population) and a reported 18 million in 2010 (NHIA 2010; NHIA 2011). However, many studies indicate that Ghana is facing difficulties in enrolling poorer segments of society (Aikins and Dzikunu, 2006; Asante and Aikins, 2008; Dixon, Tenkorang and Luginaah, 2011; Jehu-Appiah, Aryeetey, Spaan, de Hoop, Agyepong and Baltussen, 2011; Witter and Garshong, 2009).

## Methods

This chapter forms part of the authors' larger study on a gender-based analysis of access and utilisation of the NHIS in the UWR. Research for the broader study was conducted in Ghana's UWR between May and December 2011 and consisted of a mixed-methods approach of more than 2,000 quantitative surveys, 17 focus group discussions (FGDs) and 26 in-depth interviews (IDIs). While evidence for this chapter is drawn from the qualitative phase of the research (the FGDs and the IDIs) the findings are guided by insights from the study as a whole.

To examine local perceptions and understandings of health vis-à-vis the NHIS, we adopted an interpretive approach conducted across the geographical space of the UWR. In many ways, the FGD serves as a microcosm of the processes underlying successful participant education (Kidd and Parshall 2000), as group members can ask one another questions, exchange anecdotes, and comment on one another's experiences and points of view. FGDs are particularly appropriate for facilitating the discussion of unfamiliar topics because the less inhibited members of the group often break the ice for shyer participants (Kitutilisationinger 1995). IDIs, on the other hand, compliment this method, by allowing for quieter participants to speak and assuring anonymity (Leavy and Hesse-Biber 2003).

To achieve maximum variation in diverse opinions, males and females of varying ages from 18 to 90+ years were recruited. Recruitment for the FGDs involved two steps. First, contact was made with village chiefs for preapproval and then contact with a local for broadcasting the time and purpose of the FGD. Participants were always made aware by the researcher of their right to choose participation. IDIs were similarly recruited but with individual contacts already established within villages, and with key informants such as village chiefs, community health workers and NHIS staff.

All FGDs were conducted outdoors under trees, were grouped into either male or female groups in order to provide social comfort to participants, and averaged approximately one to one and a half hours in length. The IDIs were conducted indoors in privacy and the participants were assured of their anonymity. IDIs varied greatly in length, between one half hour to three hours. All FGDs and IDIs were digitally recorded, with consent of the respondents. The FGDs and IDIs were led by the researcher and translated through a research assistant fluent in Dagaare or Waali (the language of the focus group informants). A checklist of topics (semistructured openended questions) guided the FGDs and IDIs. The checklist probed participants about several different topics related to their experiences with and opinions about the NHIS in the UWR. The checklist was designed to be flexible; new questions were added as necessary during the data collection process.

*Analysis*

After transcribing the audio recordings to digital copies a thematic analysis of the data was guided by our research. Following Strauss and Corbin (1998), we conducted line-by-line coding to produce textual elements that provides a means for organising explaining the data. The key categories under each theme were reviewed several times in order to ensure that concepts pertaining to the same phenomena were coded in the same category.

**Results**

The following results are organised around the four main themes: 1) health is actually an accumulation of experiences over the lifecourse and not a single incident in need of a single cure; 2) health is not necessarily a product of individual behaviour but shaped by wider community, social relationships and norms; 3) people take satisfaction for a collective wellbeing; and 4) health is sacred and valued beyond a market commodity. Direct quotations from the transcripts of the IDIs and FGDs are used to punctuate these themes and contextualise participants' responses. The participant's gender (M=Male, F=Female), the age of IDI participants and the type of discussion (FGD or IDI) are all provided at the end of each quotation.

*Wellbeing is not Discrete*

There was significant disjuncture between the SHI assumption of how illness occurs and how participants in our study described how they became ill. Participants stated over and over that their illness and pains came from the work they do day-in and day-out, not necessarily from any particular incident or disease:

> Us women, we wake up early in the morning go into the bush to look for foods, just to fend for the children. The morning the weather is always very cold so sometimes we get chills or get feverish. The men don't care, they just marry and bring you to the house and they make you give birth to children and they don't care about them. So every burden is on you, sometimes the psychology alone – thinking of the children and all those things – they make you fall sick most often. (F; FGD)

> [You see] that rice field? When it floods there is a lot of water so we stay in the water to harvest the crop or to cultivate the land. Because we stay in the water for a long period of time we mostly fall sick and sometimes we get mosquito bites and then malaria. So around September the land would be flooded but we have to stay in the water to continue work. (F, 59; IDI)

Further, many participants recognised that the health provided for within the health insurance 'does little to keep you healthy'. This view was particularly emphasised by our informants as they argued that paying for health insurance often competed with other household needs that are necessary in keeping people healthy:

Now the only thing we do here is subsistence farming and with this farming you have to feed your family, take care of their education, clothe them, and so many expenses! So you just end up selling the food that you would otherwise eat to register your health expenses. (Female, FGD)

If it doesn't rain properly and the lands are not fertile then we men are not able to afford fertiliser and then we can't produce enough. So when you get the money you either use it to buy food or decide whether to use it to pay for the health insurance. (F; FGD)

There is a lot of burden on us because when you get the money you are in a dilemma whether to pay children's [health insurance] fees, or to use it to buy food. Sometimes you are in a dilemma so when you use it for something and the rest left you just use it to also take care of yourself. We are asking you, if have some little money, would you use it to register the children or use it to go and buy some foodstuffs for the children to eat? Which one is better? (F, 29; IDI)

Further, when describing the nature of their illnesses many would draw on the concept of a 'cycle'. In doing so, they are challenging the assumption that their illness is one discrete problem and instead pointing to larger underlying causes. Both the man and woman below echo this sentiment:

When we are sick [we get treatment with] the health insurance. But when they give us the treatment and we come back, we won't recover fully. But we are forced to go and continue work ... Yeah, it's some kind of a cycle. (M, 40, IDI)

*[Demonstrating how to crack wood]* This is the labour we do to get money, but it really hurts our bodies. We go the hospital and they don't help us. You go to do the same kind of labour again and so you fall sick more often. (F, FGD)

By extension, when the health insurance coverage could not cure the underlying long-term problems, health care workers were likely just to prescribe pain killers. The paracetamol described below is an over-the-counter pain and fever reducer similar to Aspirin.

Now, if you are admitted to the hospital, you can rely on the fact that you don't have to pay for the bedding fees. But it doesn't matter if they don't give you any proper treatment. The only drug they give you is paracetamol, and it doesn't cure anything. (M;60; IDI)

A problem is that most of the time when you go to the hospital, there is only paracetamol that they give you instead of giving you other medication. You can't take it and recover, it will just kill the pains for now ... They give you paracetamol as pain killers, but they don't actually give us proper medication, so you come back, and it's like a cycle. (F, 23, IDI)

*Health Insurance is Influenced by Culture, Social Relationships and Community Morals*

Contrary to the assumptions underlying health insurance which tends to reduce health to a personal responsibility thereby artificially removing the individual from the social world around them, accounts of this study reveal that people's sense of self was intertwined with that of the wider community. In the UWR, social norms do not correspond with individualistic thinking. For instance, many participants noted a cultural obligation to take care of extended family:

> Sometimes in a family a brother can die so you have to take care of the children. So in that case all those children are yours, you count them as your own children. Some of these unfortunate things – you still are so young but you have so many children, when your brother dies you have to just take responsibility of all the children he has left behind and try to get them enrolled. (M, FGD)

As well, polygamous marriages which are common in the UWR, are embedded with responsibilities that seem to counter the individualised approach to enrolment:

> You know, here it is common that a man may have two wives. So if one wife decides to enroll with her own children then she may also enroll the children with the other woman. The husband will add the children and will just use one woman to enroll them. (F, FGD)

Gender roles have historically weighed strongly in decisions to pay for the health care of children in Ghana. In our study, many participants reflected these social norms around on who is responsible for paying for health insurance for the children:

> The insurance is important to both the husband and the wife. It's important because of the monetary problems – you have to register your wife and the children. If you register yourself leaving your wife and children and then if your wife falls sick … [Then people will] say you want her to die for you that is why you are registering yourself leaving her and the children. But if you register your wife and the children there will be peace in the family, (M, FGD)

> We women always end up paying to enroll the children and ourselves. You know, women are usually susceptible to sickness and other disease that are just only for women which are always common, especially here. [And then] if you have a child and the child is sick, it is actually you the woman who takes care of the child. They do everything with you so that is the more reason why women use the health insurance. (F, FGD)

Participants often reflected dissatisfaction with the individualised model of enrolment. In a social setting where everyone pitches in for everyone else, it seemed counterintuitive to have to pick and choose which individual people were going to be enrolled. This was especially so when a parent had limited income and could only enrol some of his or her own children:

> There are sometimes when you want to enroll all your children. But, maybe let's say, you have three children and you are only able to enroll two. The next time when the three are sick and you go [to the clinic] they will say they will not treat the person who is not registered. (F, 33, IDI)

*People Take Satisfaction in the Collective Wellbeing*

Further challenging the individualistic approach to health, participants in this study provided many examples of striving for a collective wellbeing. Primary amongst these examples were the numerous *susu* groups (informal collective in a community that members pay into in order to save money and give out loans to the group) set up to assist in paying for health insurance enrolment:

> Sometimes when the man cannot afford everything she just goes to some kind of *susu* group ... They contribute money together and put it down. So when your insurance expires and you don't have money, you just simply go there and take money and come and pay for the insurance and you will repay into the group fund eventually. Yes it is better this way, so everyone can keep their health insurance. (F, FGD)

> They get the money from the group and pay for all of them – they themselves, their husband and their children. Later on when they have money, their husband gives them money to go and pay back the loan they took from the group, or they themselves also can pay it back. So their husbands know about the group, the whole community actually works together like this. (F, FGD)

As the NHIS policy currents stands, children can only be enrolled under the membership of an already enrolled adult. Reflecting a commitment to the whole community, as opposed to self interest in one's own health, it was extremely common for adults to want to put all their money towards enrolling the children:

> You have to register the child for four Ghana *cedis*, so depending on the number of children you have you have ... and due to the large household sizes, most often our community has plenty children ... and it's expensive. So sometimes we find it hard to register all the children. We would even prefer to register the children and leave ourselves, because the children's health is more important. So those are the problems we are facing. (F, 46, IDI)

> You see, because we are adults we are very particular about the children. As an adult we maybe have lived most of our lives already and our health is not really important. But the 4 Ghana *cedis* charge for the children is a problem for us. We prefer, even if we can't register ourselves, we want to always register the children so that the children can enjoy health care. (M, 50, IDI)

Similarly, when participants talked about the benefits of the NHIS, it was rarely just as individuals. The discussion often reflected on prosperities to the community as a whole:

> [Meningitis] and measles were rampant here, it killed mainly children, but now with this health insurance when we notice those signs we rush to the hospital. (F, FGD)

> Most of us [adults] used to suffer from stomach pains, malaria and hernia. And you know all those who were suffering from hernia, we went the hospital for an operation and we are now free ... People used to die through some of those things. (M, FGD)

### Health is Not a Commodity

The people of the UWR were somewhat familiar with the idea that health was something to be bought, due to their previous experience with pay-per-service system. However, there was often an expression of discomfort that the health insurance model did not change this. There was a general assumption that the NHIS would remove the commodification of health:

> When the [NHIS] policy came they taught us that it was going to solve all of our health problems, because when you register you know that no matter how seriously you fall sick you are going to get treatment. But as it ends up, if you fall sick and you go to the hospital the personnel will tell you there are no drugs you have to go the market to buy it. That kind of behaviour is really hitting us. Because we save up all our money to go and register and they end up going to the hospital only to be told it's no good. (M, IDI, 31)

The problem was especially apparent when it came to pharmaceuticals. Participants often expressed a feeling that regaining health boiled down to the ability to pay for drugs:

> Some of the drugs are not being covered by the health insurance and when we fall sick and go to the hospital they will give us a form to go to the drugstore and buy the drugs. In that case you may not have money to buy the drugs so some of us suffer. How can that be? Why must we always just keep paying and paying? (F, FGD)

> I know a woman who went to the pharmacy to collect her drugs and they told her that her drugs are not covered by the health insurance. The woman didn't have the money so she had to go with the sick child to the house. Her child is sick because she can't afford it … it's not right. (F, 22, IDI)

While participants found the pharmaceutical problem to be quite frequent, there was a deeper discomfort with the health insurance coverage of blood transplants. The idea of paying for bodily fluids, something more personal and connected to a holistic idea of health, was seen to be especially problematic:

> I have noticed that sometimes when you go the hospital there is the issue of blood. If you are a patient and in need of blood, normally they ask you to buy it. But that's just not right. We will look for somebody who is a close relative who will be ready to donate. (Male, FGD)

In sum, those participating in the FGDs and IDIs expressed disillusionment with the NHIS' continuation of the commodification of health. Participants had expressed hope that enrolment would alleviate them from having to think of health in this way, and yet found that the mindset of 'buying health' continued from pay-per-service into the new SHI model.

## Discussion

While it is recognised that there are indeed many great benefits that health insurance schemes have brought to developing countries, we must be careful in how these benefits are presented. SHI models are an obvious improvement from the pay-per-service health care that swept developing countries in the 1980s and 1990s. Pay-per-service models exclude those who are most vulnerable and most in need of health care, and put others at risk of falling into debt to cover their health care costs. In contrast, SHI models can enable access to health care for those who previously did not have access and help prevent catastrophic spending should someone become ill.

Ghana's NHIS in particular has been demonstrated to rectify many of the hardships under the pay-per-service era. Witter and Garshong (2009), for instance, have found that the introduction of the NHIS increased access to healthcare by taking away the cost of curative care. Additionally, there has been some preliminary evidence to suggest that members of the scheme are more likely to utilise healthcare (Blanchet et al. 2012; Sekyi and Domanban 2012), though these studies are quite limited by both geographic scope and sample size. Compared to a 2009 national average outpatient visit of 0.81 per person, the average outpatient visit per NHIS member was found to be between 1.4 and 1.5 per person (Apoya and Marriott 2011). Other studies suggest that when enrolled NHIS members become ill, they are more likely to seek care in a timely manner and within the formal health care system when compared to their non-enrolled counterparts (Health Systems 20/20 2009; Sulzbach et al. 2005), and Mensah, Oppong and Schmidt (2010) found that NHIS improved access to maternal care as well as increased the number of deliveries at hospital facilities. Simply put, the NHIS does indeed hold much promise for Ghanaians.

However, the rhetoric surrounding health insurance models seem to falsely equate SHI with a socially inclusive health insurance. In addition the commodification of health, as evident in the design of the SHI models, means that such enterprises do not lend themselves to effectively dealing with illness and wellbeing and also mask underlying societal causes of ill-health that should otherwise form the primary target of policy. From this perspective, it can be seen that health care makes up only a single contribution to the factors that impact an individual's health, and it is false to believe SHI alone can solve the health problems developing countries face. Just as the WHO's Commission on Social Determinants of Health (CSDH, 2008) recommends universal health care as one piece of a larger effort to improve daily living conditions, we too emphasise health insurance is only one tool that can be used towards the broader goal of creating health.

We have also argued here that the SHI model makes assumptions about health that are problematic. The SHI model conjures an image of publicly funded and equitable health finance arrangement. However, while avoiding the designation of a private scheme, it still remains mired in the very assumptions of the insurance market economy. We have punctuated this argument with the voices of real people experiencing the SHI model in Ghana's UWR. Ghana's NHIS has been a success in many ways, and this point should not be brushed over. However, we also must not lose sight of what 'health' is, and whether it can truly be secured by a narrow range of commodified practices that place emphasis on individuality rather collective wellbeing and social causes. Human beings are social creatures, embedded in economic, political, cultural, and community contexts and meaningful health approaches must correspond to the totality of human experience and existence.

Just as Bezner Kerr and Mkandawire (2012) have questioned the usefulness of the neoliberal underpinnings in Malawi's fight against the HIV/AIDS epidemic, we would like to question the continuation of neoliberal individualistic notions in the 'shiny' new health insurance based approaches to financing healthcare in Ghana, or more broadly sub-Saharan Africa and developing countries. Why is it that we are still relying on market based solutions for health when we *know* that health is a collective, intangible social good?

This approach is perhaps even more problematic in a cultural landscape of highly integrated extended families and communal living. The results from this study have highlighted a few of the ways that this individualism clashes with cultural collectivism:

how do mothers choose between their own children? How do husbands choose between their wives? How does a village come to terms with saving some and not others? What does it mean to 'pay' for health? Why does healthcare not actually 'fix' what makes us ill? These are some of the many questions that were especially poignant to the participants in our study context, but presumably will become more common questions as SHI schemes expand in developing countries.

To conclude, we return to our original question: *can these institutions which are rooted in the ideology of free markets and private property rights genuinely support health reforms that are founded on the ethic of collective wellbeing and social inclusion?* The evidence we have presented in this chapter suggests the answer to this question is at best uncertain. However, we do not think that this means we should be 'giving up' on Ghana's NHIS, or SHI schemes in developing countries. Again we would like to emphasise that the progress Ghana and others have made in opening access to health care is to be admired. Instead, at such an early point on the journey to healthcare reform we argue that this provides excellent opportunity to remain vigilant and try to incorporate our knowledge of the SDH into health polies, and social policies more broadly, as they unfold.

Perhaps this means Ghana needs to consider more inclusive ways in how its citizens can participate in the NHIS – by household unit or village unit? Perhaps too there should be much more leniency given for the core poor, as others have suggested (Dixon, Tenkorang and Luginaah 2011)? Or, if universal health coverage really is the 'third global health transition' as recently described by Rodin and de Ferranti (2012) in the Lancet, than maybe the NHIS should be considered the first step along Ghana's path to truly universal access to healthcare? Beyond just questions of access, our chapter aims to reiterate and highlight that true health is much more than a visit to the doctor. The NHIS is a piece of the puzzle, but only becomes successful along with other social policy measures that take aim at the reasons people become ill in the first place. So without interrogating, for instance, the underlying economic, cultural, political circumstances influencing a woman to be out dawn to dusk gathering wood to take to market and try to sell for a small amount of money, wearing on her body and not receiving proper nutrition – well then we are not going to make much of a difference to that woman's health by just enrolling her in the health insurance and prescribing her painkillers. Understanding *that* is the challenge going forward.

## References

Agyepong, I. and Adjei, S. 2008. Public social policy development and implementation: a case study of the Ghana National Health Insurance scheme. *Health Policy and Planning*, 23, 150–60.

Agyepong I. and Nagai, R. 2011. 'We charge them; otherwise we cannot run the hospital': Front line workers, clients and health financing policy implementation gaps in Ghana. *Health Policy*, 99, 226–33.

Aikins, M. and Dzikunu, H. 2006. *Utilization by and Cost of Health Care of the Insured Poor in Saboba-Chereponi District Northern Region.* Accra, Ghana: Danida Health Sector Support Office.

Anyinam, C. 1989. The social cost of the IMF's adjustment programs for poverty: the case of health care in Ghana. *International Journal of Health Services*, 19, 531–47.

Apoya, P. and Marriott, A. 2011. *Achieving a Shared Goal: Free Universal Health Care in Ghana.* London: Oxfam International.

Asante, F. and Aikins, M. 2007. *Does the NHIS Cover the Poor?* Accra, Ghana: Danida.

Avotri, J.Y., and Walters, V. 1999. 'You just look at our work and see if you have any freedom on earth': Ghanaian women's accounts of their work and their health. *Social Science & Medicine*, 48(9), 1123–33.

Bezner Kerr, R. and Mkandawire, P. 2010. Imaginative geographies of gender and HIV/ AIDS: moving beyond neoliberalism, *Geojournal*, 77, 459–73

Blanchet, N.J., Fink, G. and Osei-Akoto, I. 2012. The Effect of Ghana's National Health Insurance Scheme on Health Care Utilisation. *Ghana Medical Journal*, 46, 76–84.

Coovadia, H., Jewkes, R., Barron, P., Sanders, D., and McIntyre, D. 2009. The health and health system of South Africa: historical roots of current public health challenges. *The Lancet*, 374(9692), 817–34.

CSDH. 2008. Closing the gap in a generation: health equity through action on the social determinants of health. Final Report of the Commission on Social Determinants of Health. Geneva: World Health Organisation.

Dixon, J. 2000. Social Determinants of Health. *Health Promotion International*, 15(1), 87–9.

Dixon, J., Tenkorang, E.Y. and Luginaah, I. 2011. Ghana's National Health Insurance Scheme: helping the poor or leaving them behind? *Environment and Planning C: Government and Policy*, 29, 1102–15.

Earickson, R. and Meade, M. 2010. *Medical Geography*. New York: Guilford Press.

Gilson, L., Russell, S. and Buse, K. 1995. The political economy of user fees with targeting: developing equitable health financing policy. *International Development*, 7, 369–401.

Gottret, P. and Schiebar, G. 2006. *Health Financing Revisited: A Practioner's Guide.* Washington, DC: World Bank.

Health Systems 20/20 Project and Research and Development Division of the Ghana Health Service. 2009. *An Evaluation of the Effects of the National Health Insurance Scheme in Ghana.* Berthesda, MD: Abt Associates Inc.

Health Systems 20/20 Project and Research and Development Division of the Ghana Health Service. 2009. *An Evaluation of the Effects of the National Health Insurance Scheme in Ghana.* Bethesda, MD: Health Systems 20/20 project, Abt Associates Inc.

Hsaio, W. and Shaw R.P. 2007. *Social Health Insurance for Developing Nations.* Washington, DC: World Bank.

Hutchful, E. 2002. *Ghana's Adjustment Experience: The Paradox of Reform.* Geneva: United Nations Research Institute for Social Development.

Jehu-Appiah, C., Aryeetey, G., Spaan, E. et al. 2011. Equity aspects of the National Health Insurance Scheme in Ghana: who is enrolling, who is not and why? *Social Science and Medicine*, 72, 157–65.

Kalipeni, E., Craddock, S., Oppong, J. and Ghoshi, J. 2004. *HIV and AIDS in Africa: Beyond Epidemiology.* Oxford: Blackwell.

Konadu-Agyemang, K. 2000. The best of times and the worst of times: structural adjustment programs and uneven development in Africa: the case of Ghana. *The Professional Geographer*, 52(3), 469–83.

Marmot, M. and Shipley, M. 1996. Do socioeconomic differences in mortality persist after retirement? 25 year follow up of civil servants for the first Whitehall study. *BMJ*, 313, 1177–80.

Marmot, M. and Wilkinson, R.G. (eds) 1999. *Social Determinants of Health.* New York: Oxford University Press.

Marmot, M., Shipley, M. and Rose, G. 1984. Inequalities in death – specific explanations of a general pattern. *Lancet*, i, 1003–6.

Mensah, J., Oppong, J. and Schmidt, C. 2010. Ghana's National Health Insurance Scheme in the context of the health MDGs: an empirical evaluation using propensity score matching. *Health Economics*, 19, 95–106.

MOH. 2009. *Pulling Together Achieving More. Independent Review: Health Sector Programme of Work 2008.* Accra: Ministry of Health, Government of Ghana.

Oppong, J. 2001. Structural adjustment and the health care system, in *IMF and World Bank Sponsored Structural Adjustment Programs in Africa: Ghana's Experience 1983–1999*, edited by K Konadu-Agyemang. Aldershot: Ashgate, 357–70.

Peters, D.H., Garg, A., Bloom, G. et al. 2008. Poverty and Access to Health Care in Developing Countries. *Annals of the New York Academy of Sciences*, 1136, 161–71.

Rodin, J., and de Ferranti, D. 2012. Universal health coverage: the third global health transition? *Lancet*, 380, 861–2.

Saltman, R.B. and Dubois, H. 2004. The Historical and Social Base of Social Health Insurance Systems, in *Social Health Insurance Systems in Western Europe*, edited by R.B. Saltman, R. Busse, and J. Figueras. Maidenhead: Open University Press, 21–32.

Sekyi, S. and Domanban, P.B. 2012. The Effects of Health Insurance on Outpatient Utilization and Healthcare expenditure in Ghana. *International Journal of Humanities and Social Science*, 2, 40–49.

Sen, A. and Williams, B. (eds) 1982. *Utilitarianism and Beyond.* Cambridge: Cambridge University Press.

Strauss, A and Corbin, J. 1998. *Basics of Qualitative Research Techniques and Procedures for Developing Grounded Theory* (2nd edition). London: Sage Publications.

Sulzbach, S., Garshong, B. and Owusu-Banahene, G. 2005. *Evaluating the Effects of the National Health Insurance Act in Ghana: Baseline Report.* Bethesda, MD: The Partners for Health Reformplus Project, Abt Associates Inc.

Turshen, M. 1999. *Privatizing Health Services in Africa.* New Brunswick, NY: Guilford Press.

Waddington, C. and Enyimayew, K. 1989. A price to pay: The impact of user charges in Ashanti-Akim district, Ghana. *International Journal of Health Planning and Management*, 4, 17–47.

WHO (World Health Organisation). 2005. *Sustainable Health Financing, Universal Coverage, and Social Health Insurance.* Agenda Item 13.16, 58th World Health Assembly, Geneva: World Health Organization.

Witter, S. and Garshong, B. 2009. Something old or something new? Social health insurance in Ghana. *International Health and Human Rights*, 9.

World Bank. 1993. *World Development Report 1993.* New York: Oxford University Press.

Xu, K., Evans, D., Kawabata, K. et al. 2003. Household catastrophic health expenditure: a multicountry analysis. *Lancet*, 362, 111–17.

## Chapter 7

# From Effective Cure to Affective Care: Access Barriers and Entitlements to Health Care Among Urban Poor in Chennai, India

Christina Ergler, Patrick Sakdapolrak,
Hans-George Bohle[1] and Robin Kearns

In 2011 the world's seven billionth person may have well been a girl, born in India, a country in which most people continue to live in poverty. Poor people in cities are the ones who suffer most from the numerous environmental, economic and social risks that shape health status in a rapidly urbanising environment (Harpham and Molyneux 2001; Krafft et al. 2003). In this respect, this girl is very likely to grow up in poverty and fall ill in one of the major slums in an Indian megacity. She may encounter various infectious diseases associated with poverty (e.g. tuberculosis, cholera or typhoid), but she will also be prone to 'lifestyle' diseases such as diabetes (Patel et al. 2011). India, like many other developing countries, is at the brink of a health transition as the result of complex societal and economic changes. Their health care systems deals, or will have to deal, with this health transition in diverse ways. By way of example, they increasingly need to cater for the needs of people suffering from not only communicable but also non-communicable diseases, while the (financial) resources have not be adjusted to deal with this double burden (Patel 2007). So what are the girl's entitlements to health care?

Along with many others from the growing Indian population, the girl and her parents may seek help for her illnesses – as they are entitled to – in the easily accessible public health care system, but it is also very likely that the family will decide on treatment from a private practitioner. In India, private sector health care resources, which tend to be concentrated in urban areas, are commonly accessed by impoverished users (Peters et al. 2002; Akhtar 2004). For example, a study from Delhi reveals that impoverished residents mainly attend private sector facilities involving out-of-pocket payments despite the provision of care at subsidised government facilities, which are meant for those with fewer resources (Gupta and Dasgupta 2003). Thus, even geographical availability and physical proximity of public facilities do not necessarily imply better access for poorer urban residents as other factors also play a role (Penchansky and Thomas 1981; Andersen 1995). In the case of the girl introduced earlier, it will be important for her present and future health-seeking behaviour where facilities are located and how she and her parents feel about, experience and remember these visits; it will also be important to consider how the health service, as a place for cure and care, is represented (Ergler et al. 2011). If the family follows the example made by numerous other Indians of a similar location and social class, their preference will lie in the private sector.

---

1   Prof. Dr Hans-Georg Bohle, who taught and supervised the first and second authors, sadly and unexpectedly died in September 2014.

In this chapter, we address the apparent paradox of poorer residents using fee-for-service health care by drawing on a case study from the megacity city of Chennai in the South of India. We offer a geographical perspective on the health care landscape of Chennai and how providers and impoverished users present and negotiate the complex nature of entitlements to health care. The chapter offers a snapshot of the local connections between poverty, health and health care, which we embed in the health care accessibility literature (Pechansky and Thomas 1981) in combination with insights from Amartya Sen's (1981) entitlement approach. This theoretical framework allows us to take into account the space-centred approach to health care provision of medical geography and the more place-sensitive approach of contemporary health geography (Gesler and Kearns 2002). The result is an opportunity to consider inequalities within the health care system and their impact on the provision of both affective and effective care through the lens of 'private preference' in health services.

## Entitlements to Health Care: A Research Framework

In *Poverty and Famines* (Sen 1981) and elsewhere Sen and colleagues (Drèze and Sen 1997) emphasise the connection between the availability of food and entitlements to this resource. They argue that availability does not guarantee the prevention of famines. Rather, inequalities in distribution and accessibility may generate famines even if overall food supplies are sufficient. Consequently, they shift their focus to access and entitlements instead of supply. This approach has been successfully used to explain access issues in different contexts. For example, Leach et al. (1999) introduced environmental entitlements to discuss sustainable resource management, whereas Fünfgeld (2007) considered access to resources in the context of violent conflicts in Sri Lanka. By analogy, just as the mere availability of food cannot prevent famine, we argue that the presence of (public) health care services cannot guarantee good health status for slum inhabitants. Rather, it is residents' entitlements to health care that shape their access to facilities and affect their wellbeing. According to Sen (1984), entitlements are 'the set of alternative commodity bundles that a person can command in a society using the totality of rights and opportunities that he or she faces' (479).

Sen's approach is legalistic, economic and descriptive, but not normative. Therefore, entitlements refer not to what people *should* have, but to the range of possibilities they *can* have depending on various structural factors, such as individual capabilities, the state health care system, societal organisation (see below for more detail) (Leach et al. 1999). Entitlements originate in the transformation of endowments (e.g. land or labour) into a set of opportunities. Accessing these entitlement relations is based, for example, on production, trade or inheritance (Sen 1981). Consequently, Sen is interested in the extent to which people in different contexts are able to transform their endowments into entitlements in order to improve their capabilities and wellbeing. People are more vulnerable to disease if their entitlement set does not include a commodity bundle with adequate access to health care facilities, or if their endowment or exchange entitlements decline such that they become unable to acquire a commodity bundle with the necessary access to health care or to be able to cope with diseases (Watts and Bohle 1993). It is important to note that impoverished citizens in India are, in principle, entitled to free access to public facilities and pharmaceuticals. However, these entitlements are declining due to structural adjustment programmes which have resulted in a decline of funding for the public sector (see next section). But, command over health-related goods and services depends upon more than just legal or formal rights.

Leach et al. (1999) refine and extend Sen's approach to include 'the whole range of socially sanctioned, as well as formal institutional mechanisms for resource access and control' (233). Hence, they account for the often-levelled critique that Sen's approach focuses solely on property and legal rights (Fünfgeld 2007) by including an institutional dimension in their framework. Institutions are not stable entities; rather they are (re)negotiated on a regular basis and may entail formal and informal relationships (Etzold et al. 2012). Consequently, we see cultural and historical settings as well as social interactions (e.g. patterns of obligation and duty within and among communities, households and state systems) as central to the context of entitlements to health care (see also Agarwal et al. 2006). Following Watts and Bohle (2003) we regard entitlements to health care as being socially constructed and unstable. As Watts (2002, 12) explains, both 'social networks and positionality determine whether and what sorts of entitlements are available'. Our approach, therefore, considers not only the political, economic and structural factors that are central to Watts and Bohle's (1993) vulnerability framework, but we also include gender, social and cultural dimensions and the subjective, emotional and psychological perspectives of the urban poor and stakeholders in the health care system as determinants shaping access to health care (Nussbaum 2000; Agarwal et al. 2006). In brief, entitlements to health care refer to all alternative sets of utilities derived from goods and services over which social actors have legitimate effective command and which are instrumental in achieving wellbeing. In other words, the entitlement approach we use is a potential tool for improved understanding of the opportunities and constraints poor people face in transforming their endowments into entitlements to health care. In order to address accessibility, we integrate ideas from Pechansky and Thomas (1981) into our framework (see Figure 7.1). These authors identified five factors that influence the realisation of health care: *availability* refers to the adequate supply of health care infrastructure, whereas *accessibility* depends on the spatial and geographical location of health care providers and their users, whereby travel cost and time are taken in account. The term *accommodation* describes the organisational structures of health care services (e.g. waiting time or opening hours, and the patient's ability to cope with these structures). The need for patients to have the financial means to use the available health care is termed *affordability*. Lastly, the relationship between users' attitudes towards the providers and vice versa is summarised under the umbrella of *acceptability*.

We consider the ways the five factors influence access to health care as potential entitlement barriers. But given our focus on their endowments (Sen 1981) we are interested in how poor people can surmount these access barriers in order to gain health care entitlements. Thus, a more disaggregated entitlement approach considers how a range of institutions and structural factors mediate the relationship between different actors and components of the health care system. Therefore, as Andersen (1995) notes, it is important not only to know the characteristics of the population utilising the health care system, but also the characteristics of the system itself. Applying the entitlement approach in this way stretches it further than Sen's original concept and its adaptations (e.g. Watts and Bohle 2003; Agarawal et al. 2006), by seeking insights into not only formal entitlements and the use of services, but also the experiences and feelings of patients themselves (i.e. the affective dimensions of health care use). Emotions appear not to have been taken into consideration in the entitlement approach before Nussbaum (2000) first introduced this domain into her list of capabilities. In addition to the entitlement concept, we therefore draw on the literature associated with emotional geographies (Davidson et al. 2005), which

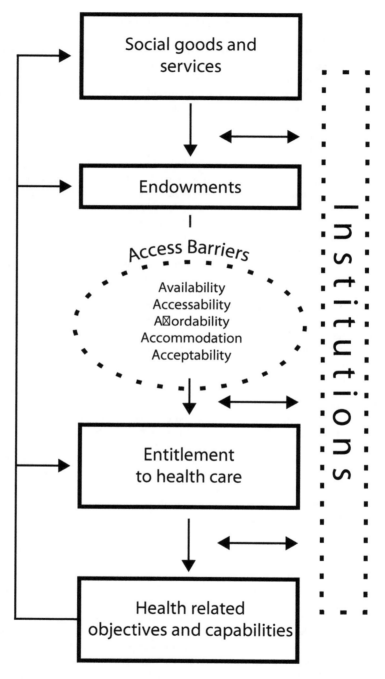

**Figure 7.1**     Conceptual framework adapted from Leach et al. (1999, p. 234)

further complements Pechansky's and Thomas' (1981) idea of acceptability. This move allows us to explore how space, place and time interact in producing and reproducing the practices which are related to meanings and experiences of the health care system. In this way, we can begin to identify new insights into the health care system and its dynamics.

*Including Sen's Ideas into a Research Design*

Our approach for investigating entitlements to health care is twofold: firstly, mapping the distribution of facilities around two slum settlements to understand the local availability of facilities; and secondly, giving voice to stakeholders and impoverished users regarding the latter group's entitlements to health care for gaining an improved understanding of the access to these entitlements.

In an initial phase of fieldwork, the first author mapped health care facilities available within a 400 metre radius of the two study sites (Anju Kudesai and Kalyanam Puram), which are located in the heart of the colonial part of Chennai. This buffer size was chosen in consultation with local advisors who recommended that this distance would be manageable for most sick or injured people using active transport. We included the location of pharmacies, private, public and not-for-profit sector health care services, and shops selling surgical supplies. This step provided a general understanding of the local landscape of provision in the old colonial part of Chennai and reflects the spatial determinants of health. In Sen's words, we tried to understand the connection between the availability of health care facilities and entitlements to this resource by first determining whether a lack of facilities can be attributed to an influence.

In a second step, to complement the maps and reveal the latent meanings embedded in the health care infrastructure and entitlement perspectives on this resource, semi-structured interviews were conducted after oral consent was obtained. Interviewees included members of the slum settlements as well as public, private and third sector stakeholders such as researchers, policy advisors, practitioners, pharmacists (see Ergler et al. 2011 for more details). Stakeholders were asked about the function of their organisation in the health care system, their main focus and aims as well as their personal role and experiences. Practitioners were invited to reveal their experiences in treating poor people, whereas interviews with residents themselves covered their access and health-seeking experiences within the health system.

*Chennai, its Inhabitants and the Health Care System*

Chennai (formerly Madras), the capital of Tamil Nadu, is located at the Bay of Bengal in South India. Of its approximately 7.5 million (official) inhabitants, more than one third live in marginal slum conditions (Gupta et al. 2009). The true slum population is assumed to be considerably higher due to in-migration from rural areas. With increasing globalisation and its associated negative implications, it is not surprising that both communicable and non-communicable diseases coexist (Bharucha and Krafft 2008). Impoverished residents are doubly affected by this health transition: they suffer not only from lifestyle-induced diseases, but also from environmentally related infectious health threats that are exacerbated, for example, by over-crowding, difficult working conditions, and severe pollution; and these conditions are worsening annually (Gupta et al. 2009). In turn, these living and working circumstances aggravate already existing inequalities within the city. In terms of health outcomes Chennai mirrors a national trend with intra-urban health inequality worsening. This was revealed in the National Family Health Survey (2005–2006) and was foreshadowed in earlier such surveys (Singh et al. 2004).

To cater for those needing treatment in Chennai, a highly complex health care system has evolved over the years consisting of dominant allopathic and minority traditional Indian components (Liebeskind 2002). The city and its various administrations since colonial times have attempted to establish a three-tier health care system analogous to the British model (Berman 1998). Until the 1990s the main emphasis was on free and publicly funded health care that has been complemented by a small private for-profit and not-for-profit sector. Various health care structures exist in parallel and the state, the city, private and third sectors operate largely independently of each other (Rao et al. 2011). By way of example, some of the corporate hospitals are of international standard and mostly used by elites and a growing number of 'health tourists' (Mudur 2004).

Given the city's role and status as a military and trade base in colonial times, as well as being capital of Tamil Nadu state, Chennai is still better equipped with health infrastructure than most other parts of India (Pati and Harrison 2006) despite the decline of public funding in the health sector since India began its structural adjustment programme. Aligning to a global trend of neoliberal reforms from the 1980s onwards that called for a 'rolling back of the state' and a greater reliance upon market mechanisms for service delivery, the budget for the public health sector declined in real terms (MoHFW 2002; Ergler 2007). A large and unregulated private health sector evolved which is now the major source of treatment (Misra, Chatterjee and Rao 2003; Balarajan et al. 2011). As a consequence of budget cuts and the loss of staff to the private sector and to wealthier overseas countries, the highly bureaucratic and overburdened public system seems increasingly unable to care for the steadily growing impoverished population (e.g. MoHFW 2002; Patel et al. 2011). Although this group relies on public health care for chronic or severe illnesses, patients increasingly seek out private facilities for minor *as well as* major health issues. According to a national survey, up to 80 per cent of outpatient treatments occur in the private sector (National Sample Survey Organisation 2006), whereas the not-for profit sector plays only a minor role. Direct and indirect costs of illness both in the public and private sector impact negatively on household welfare and many are reduced to poverty (Sakdapolral et al. 2013). With a greater reliance upon market mechanisms the situation of the poor has become problematic despite their legal entitlement to access 'free' public health care.

## Views on Entitlements in the Changing Landscape of Service Delivery: A Stakeholder Perspective

In this section we reveal how stakeholders involved in providing health care present and negotiate the complex nature of entitlements in Chennai. We also consider self-perceptions, and the perceptions of others, in the context of service delivery and accessibility, and the way these in turn impact upon entitlements to health care for poorer householders (e.g. structural violence in terms of reputation and stigma).

All interviewees agreed that public and private not-for profit sectors targeted poor people. One health administrator in a corporate hospital maintained that poverty and profit are not compatible. In his view, the facility he worked for was a 'power-profit hospital' and had to be seen as a business that maximises its profits for stockholders. The fees poorer patients are able to afford are below those expected by investors who are neither interested in the cure nor care of urban poor residents themselves. He associated expensive fees with high-quality treatment and this is reflected in his comment that their patients get 'some of the best care and therefore it is not cheap'. The *best care*, as defined by representatives of for-profit private health care providers, is invariably unattainable for poorer residents. They may be entitled to free care in the public sector, but they may not necessarily be entitled to the best care when they are unable to pay the required fees, which further cements existing inequalities. (Although occasionally the private sector raises funds for charity reasons, a prerequisite for treatment is invariably ability to pay.)

With the adaptation of a free market for health care provision under the banner of neoliberalism, and a shift towards individual choice, providers seem to distinguish between people's financial ability and the provision of care they offer. An officer from a public child welfare organisation highlighted that 'not all can afford to pay money and go to a private practitioner [to receive the best care]. ... It is expensive'. Equity in being entitled to access such care does not exists when a person does not have the necessary funds (Balajaran et al. 2011). Andrews and Crooks (2010, 9) discuss this issue in terms of making accessibility morally 'fair'. In turn, these perceptions imply that the quality of treatment in the public sector is less well regarded than similar treatment in the private sector and therefore discussed by many stakeholders as simply 'good enough' for slum dwellers. It is not surprising that, according to a zonal health officer, the 'patients coming to the dispensaries [local public primary health facilities] [for free treatment] are mostly from slum areas'. The delivery of care is influenced by this reputation of the public sector and further affected by declining public funds, as well as a growing number of patients and a perceived decline in the quality of treatment since structural adjustment programmes began to play out (Peck 2011, Rao et al. 2011).

Nonetheless, some public sector employees challenged the poorly regarded quality of treatment in the public sector, pointing towards the reinforcing and stigmatising discourse in their care provision, which in turn impacts on the entitlements to health care. A health officer highlighted that 'the public health system had improved a lot' in the past 20 years with the adaptation of structural adjustment programmes and a redistribution of allocated funds (e.g. equipment). Likewise, a public servant in a children's hospital stated that the 'public sector offers the same treatment [as the private sector], but at a lower cost. However, people do not realise that'. Underscoring this view, Misra et al. (2003) point to inconsistencies of quality within the public sector. One reason for the variability in perceived care provision may be attributed to the fact that income, career opportunities and working conditions appear more attractive in the private sector, thereby leaving the public and non-profit sectors with less qualified health care personnel and, in turn, merely adequate service provision. '[O]ur hospital used to be a very good hospital. Now because the outside opportunities for doctors are so much better ... we are having not very good doctors now' (Director of a Trust). However, despite the variability in the perception of health care delivery and possible explanations by stakeholders, they also highlight that neither the public nor the private sector delivers the best care; rather, there seems to be variability within at least the public sector. It was considered that changes in the public sector and the upgrading of facilities could not reverse the perception of its users and other sector providers. The public sector attempts to meet the needs for treatment as far as possible within its financial limits and its stakeholders might be able to notice the positive changes, but this sector still does not meet the expectations of its users.

Although a director of a private teaching hospital stated that the 'public sector has too much bureaucracy to perform well', there are few effective structures which monitor the quality of treatment and whether (or even if) poorer people can effectively access their entitlements to health care. Regulations are lacking and interviewees expressed an urgent need for policy on costs and quality assurance for all health providers. A director of an insurance company disclosed 'At the moment there is no health regulator [...] Even similar conditions in two patients, okay? Should cost only this much. There is no benchmark or guideline'. This gap had been previously identified by the Ministry of Health and Family Welfare in 2002 but, according to our respondents, no remedial actions were undertaken (see also Patel et al. 2011), which in turn undermines entitlements to health care.

While the private and public sector seem to be primarily occupied with the treatment of patients and regulations, the third sector often sees its role as addressing holistic welfare issues by focusing on prevention. They seem to fill a gap in service provision, as a community health worker revealed: 'NGOs are very necessary because they are working for the community development. [...] You know for prevention activity [instead of only cure ...] the government doesn't directly work with the people, they have institutions, structures, but they don't go along with the people understanding their needs.' The private non-profit sector clearly promoted their role for stepping in and taking a more people-centred and holistic approach for improving the health situation of the impoverished. Entitlements in this respect are not limited to access to care; rather they view poor people as entitled to a dignified and productive life.

In this section we have offered a snapshot of the socially sanctioned processes and formal institutional mechanisms that, at times violently determine the entitlements to health care for poorer people in Chennai. Providers and patients seem to be disconnected. Their problems and issues with the health care system do not seem to intersect, which may in turn contribute to the poor state of access to the best care for many. According to our findings, health care providers are more interested in effective cures rather than care *per se*. Most health care practitioners we spoke to were concerned about highlighting the standard of their treatment and differentiating their type of cure from other sectors (e.g. the availability of the latest medical equipment). Thus, health care providers appeared to be caught up in market dynamics and were concerned with maximising their profit and reputation. The result was that they seemed to be neither particularly interested in the needs and desires of their patients nor in making entitlements morally fair.

## Geographies of Entitlements to Health Care in Chennai: The Dimensions of Private Preference

In this section we address the preference for private health care through presenting and interpreting empirical findings on entitlements, organised according to the dimensions of access discussed earlier and addressing the space and place centred inquiry into health care services.

### Availability and Accessibility of Health Care Facilities

To obtain an understanding of the availability of health care facilities within walking distance, we follow the tradition of space-centred inquiry into health care provision (Phillips 1990). Our mapping activities suggested that there are sufficient health care facilities located within walking distance of the two case study sites, the slum settlements Anju Kudesai and Kalyanam Puram (see Figure 7.2).

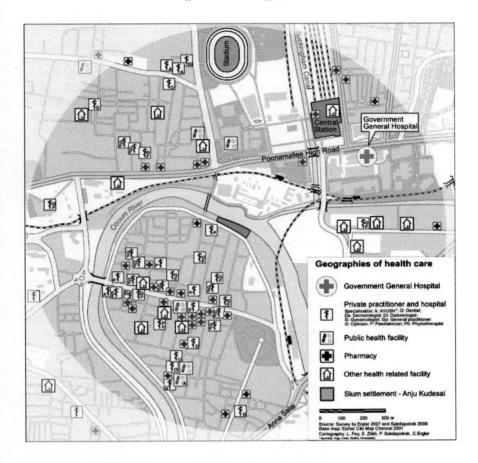

**Figure 7.2     Geographies of health care – Anju Kudesai**

Facilities ranged from primary health care services to more specialised services such as oncologists and also entailed secondary and tertiary care services. Perhaps unsurprisingly slum dwellers were satisfied with the availability of facilities around their settlement, as a 22-year-old mother and housewife stated:

> Yes, I am highly satisfied with the health facilities. There are many private doctors and
> medical shops. There is also the corporation clinic and the General Hospital nearby. There
> is also the 24 hour clinic where doctors are always available.

Thus, in principle at least, poor people are able to access a nearby health care provider and they can even exercise a choice between the for-profit private, non-profit private and public sectors. Drawing on the entitlement framework we outlined earlier, the availability of health care facilities is necessary, but may not be a precondition for satisfactory access. Only a handful of public facilities provide free health care for poorer citizens. They resemble the physical manifestation of the structural adjustment programme and reduced public funding within a city that attracts hundreds of new inhabitants each year. One of the opportunities for care in the public sector is the General Hospital, incorporating Chennai's and Tamil Nadu's largest public outpatient department. This facility is within a 400 metre radius of Anju Kudesai and is frequently used by residents of Kalyanam Puram. Patients walk, bus or use other options such as ox-carts to travel to the hospital. Transportation and its associated costs were not deemed by interviewees to be as much of a concern as we had anticipated, since it took patients an average of only 20 minutes to travel to their facility of choice (Sakdapolrak et al. 2013).

*Preference for Private Facilities: Two Examples of Health Seeking Behaviour*

Since our interviewees were all able to access nearby facilities, or those within convenient distance to their residence or workplace, proximity was not the key determinant underlying their utilisation decision, but rather their entitlements to health care were influential. Two examples can assist by way of illustration:

---

Example 1:
A widow in her fifties, living alone in Anju Kudesai in a small squatter shed in which all her countable belongings and cooking utensils are neatly organised on the floor next to her sleeping mat suffers from a chronic disease. She regularly consulted a private doctor until she ran out of money. She then sought treatment in the outpatient department of the General Hospital. She lost all connection with her two sons and extended family as her medical bills, along with her husband's alcoholism, brought the family to the brink of ruin. As she earned only 90 rupees a day as a street food vendor, she considered money to be the main obstacle to her treatment of choice:

*Suppose we have much money, we will go the doctor for putting injection. In the case of less money we go to a medical shop and tell ... I have headache, fever ... I will tell I only have 20 rupees. According to the 20 rupees give me the tablet ... Suppose if I don't have money, from the house I will get pepper. We will boil with water. Then we drink that water and get cured.*

Interestingly, although the public sector offered free health care, it did not figure among the options she used when she was ill and had little or no money available. Later in the interview she disclosed that the public sector is invariably her last resort. Not being satisfied with the way treatment is provided and communicated were her main reasons to disregard the public sector as a genuine option if her endowments allowed. We discuss these barriers to entitlements outlined in our framework in more detail under the umbrella of acceptability below.

---

Example 2:
A family in Kalyanam Puram comprising of a newly married and pregnant daughter, her husband, a teenaged brother attending secondary school and her parents, collectively earns approximately 300 rupees a day. Both husbands are the main breadwinner and support the extended family with their coolie jobs. During the interview they all observed that they see disease itself as the main driver of utilisation. As one householder remarked:

*First I will use only house remedies, when I cannot get cured I am going to a doctor. ... [S]uppose I get stomach pain, I will ask the medical shop to give me tablet. Medical shop owner will not giving, because you have to meet the doctor. ... [After begging] he will give. ... [For welfare issues, such as family planning or pregnancy, we consult a public facility, the health post] For malaria we can't go anywhere else as to malaria [clinic, a public facility]. It is very near. Then you get tablets from there itself. But if they tell the result you didn't have malaria, we go to a private doctor. ... Because we get immediate cure!*

The decision on where, and to what extent, professional help is sought appeared to depend on what symptoms are presented and the family's entitlements and endowments. For this household, treatment for protracted illnesses occurred in public facilities such as the health post or malaria clinic, suggesting that chronic diseases are too expensive for treatment in the private sector (Russel 1996; Peters et al. 2002; Patel et al. 2011). For any minor symptom which cannot be cured with in-house remedies there is a tendency to consult a pharmacist. Indian law prohibits selling some medications without prescription, but the reality is different. Some convince a pharmacist to provide remedies given their entitlements (e.g. social connections). Consulting a private doctor is generally only possible when income permits, but is preferred for major symptoms due to a widespread perception that recovery will occur more quickly.

The participants in both examples highlight a preference for private facilities, but explain their reasoning differently. In the first narrative the availability of money is ostensibly the most decisive factor. For this woman, using private care is a luxury to be sought only when circumstances allow. However, when money is in short supply, other and lower status remedies are sought. Thus, at least among poorer residents there appears to be no cohort of consistent users of private care. Rather, such care is sought by way of preference when it is affordable. This situation is seen in the second example, but here it is symptoms that trigger the treatment options. For acute and severe symptoms we found that interviewees sought cure in the private sector due to the perception of a shorter convalescence, which in turn means they can return earlier to work or school (as explained in more detail below). This engagement with the private sector may entail borrowing or pawning assets. Protracted, chronic or non-communicable diseases and pregnancy-related care involving frequent visits is unaffordable in the private sector as households lack the necessary financial endowments (see also Balajaran et al. 2011).

Financial constraints are seen as the major factors underlying not seeking treatment which, on face value, may seem odd as residents are entitled to free health care and public facilities should be within easy reach. According to McIntyre et al. (2006) an expenditure of more than 10 per cent of the household income on health costs is a severe burden since they then have to cut back on nutritious food in order to afford the medical treatment. Expensive treatments can drive people deeper into poverty, which in turn can negatively impact on their health status (Sakdapolrak 2010). Taking this risk into consideration, it seems unreasonable for householders to consult private practitioners when treatment in the public system is available for free. However, they clearly do seek care in the private system, which leads us back to the question: *why is there a preference for private health care?*

*Affordability: Costs of Seeking Care*

In Chennai, the difference between public and private facilities is simply the fees. As shown above slum residents have – no matter what ailments – the choice of practitioners at different price ranges. This availability satisfies their demand for private health care, which is seen as a synonym for quality care. According to the local doctors we interviewed, consultation fees are typically between 50 and 100 rupees but can range between 5 and 1,200 rupees depending on the treatment and education of the doctors.[2] In turn, Sakdapolrak et al. (2013) show that consultation costs can rise to 13,000 rupees in a private health care facility for treating severe diseases. On average our participants spent 173 rupees for treatment in the private sector. These varying costs are also an outcome of an unregulated health system (see also Singh 2009; Vaishnavi and Dash 2009).

People's preference for the private sector contrasts with the perception offered by a corporate hospital manager: 'People who can't afford any money, they prefer going to the public.' Poor residents seek private health care as they perceive there to be shorter convalescent times and hence they can maximise their most important endowment, their ability to work and earn money. As a mother of two adolescents states: 'suppose if I go to dispensary it takes ten days to get cured. But if we go to private doctor within three days we are getting cured.' Given that all doctors receive the same education in public medical colleges,[3] this perception is surprising and seems highly subjective, especially as private practitioners can also vary in quality (Thaver et al. 1998). While excellent care is provided by some, the general picture contrasts with the private sector's self-perception in Chennai. One lecturer teaching western medicine whom we interviewed, however, suspected ulterior motives for these views: 'Probably they want to say they have better care obviously because they pay more.'

Nevertheless their perception has consequences for poor people's health-seeking behaviour. According to their reasoning, it is cheaper to invest in private care, be cured in a shorter time and therefore also be able to return to work and earning potential again. On average, income earners lost two days of productive working time when they fell ill (Sakdapolrak et al. 2013). They can often only spend as much on treatment as they earn per day:

> Six o'clock [in the evening] he [father] will come [home from work], get the money from him. What ever he earns. Then we used to go to medical shop. Mostly in the evening time.
> (Adolescent male, secondary school student)

This response represents a quest for effective care and an attempt to convert their endowment into what is perceived to be their best entitlement option. The strong feeling that effective care can only be found in the private sector forces poorer residents to develop coping strategies such as borrowing money from friends or family members to consult a private practitioner as even small treatment fees cannot always be covered by their daily income. When their own endowment does not allow overcoming barriers, householders draw on their networks, in an attempt to increase their entitlements:

> I borrow mostly from my brother, relatives or neighbours. I have no savings. Otherwise I pledge some tiny jewels in the pawn shop and get money. We try to collect money from two or three sources. (Woman, 30, divorced, 2 children, housewife)

For acute ailments (e.g. fever, diarrhoea) residents seek treatment in private facilities as there are also indirect costs involved for seeking cure in the public sector (see discussion

---

2   In May 2007, US$1 was equal to 40 rupees and GBP£1 was equal to 80 rupees. The median income per worker is 1,500 rupees per month in the case study sites (see also Sakdapolrak et al. 2013).

3   Private medical colleges are only a recent phenomenon as Rao et al. (2011) document.

below). Furthermore, although the public system is meant to be free, bribing to see a doctor or get a hospital bed is common in the Indian health care system:

> In the government hospitals the staff is already paid by the government. In addition they demand poor patients for pushing stretchers or for other services. Don't they have the guilty feeling to demand money from the poor? (Woman, 38, abandoned, 2 children, maidservant)

According to Transparency International one quarter of patients paid informal payments in the public sector (Thampi 2002). Although they are entitled to receive free public health care, people can end up paying to get treated. They seek treatment for protracted illnesses in the public sector, but for acute ailments they prefer the private sector as other barriers seem more important than affordability, especially as activating their social capital can often overcome these barriers.

*Accommodation: Opening Hours, Waiting Time and Pharmaceuticals*

Inconvenient opening hours prevent those willing to seek treatment in the public sector from doing so. Many public facilities open for consultations later than poor people typically start their working day and then close earlier than they can easily access them (in general, 8am–12pm and 2pm–5pm). This situation forces poorer people to consult a private practitioner as they may not be able to bear discomfort until the next day when the facility opens again. It is common practice that public sector employees run their own private practice before and after their duties offering alternative treatment to the public sector for a small fee.

If residents are not familiar with symptoms, they might also interpret even minor ailments as life-threatening diseases, which require immediate attention. Such feelings regarding illness and the relative urgency of seeking care cannot be ignored. As Davidson and Bondi (2004, 373) put it 'emotion has the power to transform the shape of our life-worlds'.

> Suppose if I go to General Hospital and only morning time I can see. Evening time only accident cases they will see in the evening. Suppose I go in the evening, they will tell tomorrow morning we can see. How can you sleep with a disease? Tomorrow morning we can see you. They won't see. That is why lending money from our neighbour house to see a private doctor to save our lives. (Woman, 50, widowed, street vendor)

Further, this interviewee explained that even if she waited till the next morning, there would not be a possibility to see the doctor immediately, as the queues in a public facility can be so long that it might take two days before they are able to consult a doctor as they always get told to 'wait, wait, wait'. Entitlement barriers, as we discussed earlier, have to be seen within a broader picture. As a result of structural adjustment programs and chronic underfunding the public system cannot keep up with the demands of its users. On average seeking help in a public facility took 2–4 hours, while they often spent less than 55 minutes in a private facility (Sakdapolrak et al. 2013). Therefore it is understandable that patients spend a considerable portion of their income in the private sector – often with the support of their social networks, and prompted by the public system delaying access to treatment.

> They'll go to private sector where they spend a huge amount of money. Emergency.
> For emergency, government sector is not good … [D]elay causes so much of damage.
> (Employee, Communicable Disease Hospital)

Such conditions are unacceptable for people who are labourers and rely on their daily income. Time spent waiting in a public facility is lost income. Although they are entitled to free public care, many cannot access this care. However, some find it convenient to go to a public facility close to work and collect their medicine at a quieter time during the day, if their employer allows them to leave. In this example, their entitlement depends on both the goodwill of an employer and the health staff knowing the patient and their medication requirements.

> I don't have any problem coming here every two days. In the morning I can come and
> get the tablets. Then go to work no problem. It makes me feel better. (Male, 55, married,
> children unknown, coolie)

Such social endowments are very helpful as they reduce the costs associated with waiting in a facility or sometimes even the need to visit a facility at all. This situation can be illustrated with another example provided by a widow in which an orderly in the General Hospital collected the pills for his neighbours with illnesses. These social networks significantly reduced the 'costs' of visiting a public facility by removing travel and waiting time. Usually a patient suffering from a chronic disease has to see a doctor on a weekly or daily basis as a full course of drugs is not dispensed at one time. But if they know the nurses or orderlies they have two advantages: getting medication for a longer time period and seeing a doctor immediately.

> I was waiting one or two hours. Because of influence of that man, I can see doctor now
> immediately. … That man telling the doctor. Take care of her, she is from our area. … She
> is very poor. … So she can not come [every day]. You have to give tablets for 15 days.
> (Woman, 50, widowed, 2 children, street vendor)

Accommodation as an entitlement barrier involves not only with the immediate effect this has on health seeking behaviour, but also how it relates to the way unhealthy environments are experienced and especially remembered as we discuss in more detail below.

*Acceptability: Effective Cure and Affective Care*

Contrary to expectations however, seeking a cure in the private sector does not always pay off. On the one hand, patients feel that their ability to pay for treatment affects the way the doctor is treating and curing them. As a 50-year-old widow stated: 'If I will give more money to the private doctor, then he will take more care of us. […] So according to money he is treating me.' We observed that some doctors differentiate between patients, a practice admitted to by a director of a private teaching hospital. He saw this action as positive, since poorer people pay less or nothing compared to those with sufficient funds, and he believed the attention granted to patients and the outcome of the consultation was not affected. Others, however, clearly saw a difference in care and thereby affirmed the experience many patients had of a decline in their entitlements to health care, which amounts to a breach of the Indian Medical Council Act of 1956. As one hospital employee observed:

> [E]ven the surgeon who operates in the operation theatre, there is an ear-phone attached. So any problem in his practice, he discusses it. He spends time for that [while treating a patient in the public sector]. (Employee, Communicable Disease Hospital)

Notwithstanding the reputation of the quality of the private health care sector, the expected recovery is often slow or never occurs. As a woman in her fifties explained 'the disease increased not decreased. Only increased, that is not a proper treatment'. The widespread perception of a quicker cure in the private sector did not live up to this patient's expectations nor did it amount to the best available treatment. Unfortunately, by the time patients realise their precarious situation, they may have spent much of their own savings as well as that of their supporters (Peters et al. 2002). In turn, this situation can mean friends or family members will reduce or remove financial support from them and their entitlements will further decline leaving an ill person without an important coping system: their support network. Their choice of last resort is then the public system in which they have little trust. A consequence can be that they try to cure themselves as the same interviewee disclosed:

> I got money from my sons ... so, I went to a [private] doctor. ... [As my sons] left me ... I went to government hospital. In government hospital I got more tablets. But not good. I did not feel good. They are not taking care of us. In General Hospital also. Now I do myself. I put the kerosene to treat the pain or when I have more money I buy tylom [ayurvedic medicine]. It costs only 1 rupee. (Woman, 50, widowed, 2 children, street vendor)

This choice reflects an underlying distrust in the diagnosis of doctors, which might be associated with the fact that public sector practitioners are unable to give much attention to their patients due to the high numbers they have to treat daily. As one doctor, reflecting on his time as a public sector employee, disclosed:

> We [40 doctors] used to handle around an average of 500–600 patients a day. ... So not much of qualitative care used to go into it. It's only the quantitative care that used to go into it. (Director, private teaching hospital).

As discussed elsewhere (Rao et al. 2011), understaffing of the public sector has clearly impacted upon doctors' ability to provide adequate free health care. This is an important point, as the decline of public funding can lead to existing staff being unable to provide adequate health care both in terms of results (e.g. cure) and responsiveness towards the needs of their patients. Poorer patients are not only looking for *effective cure*, but also *affective care*, that is the feeling that a doctor or the government at large is concerned about their health and cares about them (Lee et al. 2010). Therefore the absence of attention from authorities was a central theme:

> Most of the doctors in the General Hospital are careless and don't even touch us and diagnose. (Woman, 26, married, 3 children, housemaid)

Due to the high patient load for public doctors, their time with each patient is very limited, and in the eyes of the poorer residents, doctors are 'not interested' (Woman, 40, married, 2 children, housewife) in their patients or the private practitioners are 'concentrating only on money' as her husband a coolie explained (Atkinson et al. 1999). Patients clearly noticed and highlighted the differences in the delivery of care they experienced since the introduction of structural adjustment programmes in the public sector:

> Twenty years back, doctors were really good, taking care of the patients. ... doctor used to ask what kind of problem do you have, eye problem, paining, systematically they asked. Nowadays we have to tell. (Woman, 50, widowed, 2 children, street vendor)

Despite these well-known problems in the public sector, little has changed so far (see Peters et al. 2002; Rao et al. 2011).

> The only thing is ... the attitude of the nurses, the doctors to the patient has to be improved. That's all. The nursing care and the doctor's medical care, the time they spend with the patient always comes first. (Employee, Communicable Disease Hospital)

In this respect, doctors observe that impoverished patients are increasingly aware of diseases and its implications. Consequently, they often consult a doctor in the early stages of a disease, which then affects their entitlements to health care positively. This 'awareness entitlement' is bestowed on the patients through state education or media campaigns and advertisements.

> Because of the TV and media, they will ask us questions also. They're quite aware now. ... Before they'll come when they're very bad, sick. Now they come even when one sneezing, one cold they come running [laughs]. (Doctor, Indian Red Cross Society)

However, some private and public practitioners remain scornful poor people with one telling us 'you can't explain to them and make them understand because education is very less. You can only cure them'.

The doctor–patient relationship is important for impoverished city-dwellers to feel taken seriously. Doctors usually take notes and keep these for future consultations. If, however, 'they are not writing in the papers' (Woman, 40, married, 2 children, housewife), poor people feel that doctors are not fully involved in their case and whatever care they receive is not 'good' or the 'digital things' used 'feel unhealthy' (Woman, 19, married, pregnant, housewife). Attending to the needs of patients seems equally important to explaining the procedures in a appropriate way. Quality of care therefore not only involves achieving cure, but also includes *how* the care on the journey to cure is delivered to the patient or how treatment is explained. People were found to be accustomed to being questioned about their health, which was then documented. However among interviewees, there was a strong feeling that it is *their* responsibility to explain ailments to doctors. Thus, in their perspective the doctor-patient role has been inverted, with the patient having to take the assertive role, a position which may contribute to the decision for seeking self-treatment among some. Over time it seems poor city-dwellers adjusted to elements of the neoliberal health model. They have 'learned' to take individual responsibility for their health as the state continues to shift focus towards the private sector, changing the landscape of health care delivery (Peck 2011).

Although poor residents of Chennai access both paid and free health care, few were satisfied with *how* the care is delivered once they consulted a practitioner. The importance of showing respect to your patients and getting involved not only in addressing a current ailment, but also in being available to discuss other issues and problems, is demonstrated by a female doctor working for the Indian Red Cross Society:

> If I show a cold shoulder to the parent ... they won't send their children here. Some ways it's a rapport. ..., like we get involved in their families. ... So it's a family doctor concept. So any problem they'll come to us. Any, not only [maternal issues].

Entitlement barriers to health care facilities in Chennai do not stop once a patient enters a facility. Rather the style of delivery influences how comfortable they feel seeking treatment in a facility. To this extent the link between emotion, place and style of care is potent. For instance, one interviewee started to cry while explaining that:

> ... in General Hospital entrance a lot of bloods. Ambulance will come, bring new patients. Sitting just next to you. So I get frighten. Inside the patients' room, a lot of blood. ... Even when I come home at night time, I have to think about the hospital. (Woman, 40, married, 2 children, housewife)

Hence, a focus on a more affective style of care would enhance the attitudes of poorer residents such that they would be more likely to engage in health-seeking within the public sector. One interviewee stated that the public sector is 'miles away' from being a therapeutic setting for cure as it 'will not be so clean and hygienic and you know very attractive. So many will not like it' (Staff member, NGO working on communicable disease).

## Moving Towards Affective Care

Our approach has provided an analytical framework for examining entitlements to health care for poorer residents. We have combined the insights of users and providers to explain why poor people still prefer being treated in the private sector despite this preference potentially exacerbating their poverty when, in fact, they are entitled to free public health services. Thus, we shifted the focus from merely identifying barriers to considering the various ways poor people can transform their endowments into entitlements and overcome at least some of the well known barriers. For example, income and social networks influence both the choice of health care sector and the experience of the medical care received. Length of waiting time, inconvenient opening hours and a perceived longer recovery time in public facilities underlie the use of private facilities, but these barriers are experienced differently when poor residents transform their endowments into entitlements to health care (e.g. 'queue-jumping', bribery, borrowing money to attend private sector). Moreover, illuminating access barriers with an entitlement approach has allowed us to discuss not only how slum residents experience inequalities of access, but also how inequalities are reproduced through stakeholders' actions. Entitlements to health care are not only determined by the structure of the health care system and the way doctors treat patients and pay attention to their specific needs but also by how stakeholders regard the socially-sanctioned and institutionalised rights of impoverished users. Slum dwellers might be entitled to receive treatment, but they may not in fact receive the best cure in many stakeholders' eyes, a view which questions equity in access to the perceived *best* cure both in the eyes of patients and providers.

While the stakeholders seemed more interested in the cure of patients, we revealed not only that outcome or 'cure' is important to patients, but also illustrated that *how* the prospect of 'cure' is experienced is of importance. We showed that not only effective, but also affective dimensions of health care utilisation are important for impoverished users and determined by stakeholders' actions and dominant beliefs. Feelings can influence how care is both received and delivered, as well as which discourses on the part of both service providers and users are reinforced (e.g. the tarnished reputation of the public sector). Consequently, feelings about health care influence the health-seeking behaviour of poorer people. In this respect, trust and being taken seriously are just as valid health-care issues as the treatment itself. We moved beyond the meanings and experiences of the health care system to reveal its human dynamics within our case study areas. Emotional experiences influence health care utilisation and, in turn, lead to a preference for using private medicine. In conclusion, we note a need to complement conventional analyses of affordability and physical access to health care facilities (the dimensions of cure) in developing countries with attempts to better understand the emotional dimension of health care utilisation.

### Acknowledgements

An earlier version of this chapter was published as Ergler, C. et al. 2011. 'Entitlements to health care: Why is there a preference for private facilities among poorer residents of Chennai, India?' *Social Science and Medicine*, 72(3), 327–37. http://www.sciencedirect. com/science/article/pii/S0277953610007203. The authors are grateful for permission of the publisher to draw on and extend the original article.

### References

Agarwal, B. et al. 2006. *Capabilities, Freedom, and Equality: Amartya Sen's Work from a Gender Perspective.* New Delhi: Oxford University Press.

Akhtar, R. (ed.) 2004. *India: Health Care Pattern and Planning.* New Delhi: APH Publishing Cooperation.

Andersen, R.M. 1995. Revisiting the behavioural model and access to medical care: Does it matter? *Journal of Health and Social Behavior*, 36, 1–10.

Andrews, G.J. and Crooks, V.A. 2010. Geographies of primary health care. *Aporia: The Nursing Journal* 2(2), 7–16.

Atkinson, S., Ngwengwe, A., Macwng'gi, M. et al. 1999. The referral process and urban health care in sub-Saharan Africa: the case of Lusaka, Zambia. *Social Science and Medicine*, 49, 27–38.

Babu, B., Swain, B., Mishra, S. and Kar, S. 2010. Primary healthcare services among a migrant indigenous population living in an eastern Indian city. *Journal of Immigrant Minority Health*, 12, 53–9.

Balarajan, Y., Selvaraj, S. and Subramanian, S.V. 2011. Health care and equity in India. *The Lancet*, 377, 505–15.

Berman, P.A. 1998. Rethinking health care systems: Private health care provision in India. *World Development*, 26(8), 1463–79.

Bharucha, E. and Krafft, T. 2008. Urbanization and urban health inequalities in India. *Source*, 11, 70–76.

Chandrasekhar, S. and Gebreselassie, T. 2008. Exploring the intra-urban differences in economic well-being in India, in *India Development Report 2008*, edited by R. Radhakrishna Delhi. Oxford: Oxford University Press, 87–95.

Davidson, J. and Bondi, L. 2004. Spatialising affect; affecting space: an introduction. Gender, Place and Culture, 11(3), 373–4.

Davidson, J., Bondi, L. and Smith, M. 2005. *Emotional Geographies*. Aldershot: Ashgate.

Drèze, J. and Sen, A. 1997. *The Political Economy of Hunger: Selected Essays*. Oxford: Claderon Press.

Ergler, C. 2007. *The Health Care System in Chennai/South India – Structure and Development Tendencies Focusing on the Urban Poor*. Unpublished Masters thesis. Rheinische-Friedrich Wilhelms University, Bonn Germany.

Ergler. C., Sakdapolrak, P., Bohle, H.-G., Kearns, R. 2011. Entitlements to health care: Why is there a preference for private facilities among poorer residents of Chennai, India? *Social Science and Medicine*, 72(3), 327–37

Etzold, B., Jülich, S., Keck, M. et al. 2012. Doing institutions. New trends in institutional theory and their relevance for development geography. *Erdkunde*, 66(3), 185–95.

Fünfgeld, H. 2007. *Fishing in Muddy Waters: Socio-Environment Relations under the Impact of Violence in Eastern Sri Lanka*. Saarbrücken: Verlag für Entwicklungspolitik.

Gesler, W.M. and Kearns, R.A. 2002. *Culture/Place/Health*. New York: Routledge.

Gupta, I. and Dasgupta, P. 2003. Health-seeking behaviour in urban Delhi. An exploratory study. *World Health and Population*. [Online]. Available at: http://www.longwoods. com/product.php?productid=17580andcat=388andpa ge=1 [accessed: 4 April 2010].

Gupta, T., Arnold, F. and Lhugdim, H. 2009. *Health and Living Conditions in Eight Indian Cities. National Family Health Survey (NHFS-3)*. Mumbai: International Institute for Population Science.

Harpham, T. and Molyneux, C. 2001. Urban health in developing countries: A review. *Progress in Human Geography*, 1(2), 113–37.

Krafft, T., Worf T. and Aggarwal, S. 2003: A new urban penalty? *Environmental and Health Risks in Delhi*, 147(4), 20–27.

Leach, M., Mearns, R. and Scoones, I. 1999. Environmental entitlements: Dynamics and institutions in community-based natural resource management. *World Development*, 27(2), 225–47.

Lee, J.Y., Kearns, R.A. and Friesen, W. 2010. Seeking affective health care: Korean immigrants' use of homeland medical services. *Health and Place*, 16(1), 108–15.

Liebeskind, C. 2002. Arguing science: Unani tibb, hakims and biomedicine in India, 1900–50, in *Plural Medicine, Tradition and Modernity 1800–2000*, edited by W. Ernst. London: Routledge, 58–75.

Longhurst, R. 2003. Semi-structured interviews and focus groups, in *Key Methods in Geography*, edited by N. Clifford and G. Valentine. London: Sage Publications, 117–38.

McGranahan, G., Songsore, J. and Kjellén, M. 1999. Sustainability, poverty and urban environmental transitions, in *The Earthscan Reader in Sustainable Cities*, edited by D. Satterthwaite. London: Earthscan, 107–30.

McIntyre, D., Thiede, M., Dahlgren, G. and Whitehead, M. 2006. What are the economic consequences for households of illness and of paying for health care in low- and middle-income country contexts? *Social Science and Medicine*, 62(4), 858–65.

Misra, R., Chatterjee, R. and Rao, S. 2003. *India Health Report*. New Delhi: Oxford University Press

MoHFW 2002. *National Health Policy*. Delhi: Ministry of Health and Family Welfare.

Montgomery, M.R., Stern, R., Cohen, B. and Reed, H. 2004. *City Transformed: Demographic Change and its Implication in the Developing World*. Washington: National Academy Press.

Mudur, G. 2004. Hospitals in India woo foreign patients. *British Medical Journal*, 328, 1338–9.

National Sample Survey Organisation. 2006. *Morbidity, health care and conditions of the aged – sixtieth round (January–June 2004)*, Report No. 507(60/25.0/1). New Delhi: Ministry of Statistics and Programme Implementation, Government of India.

Nussbaum, M.C. 2000. *Women and Human Development: The Capabilities Approach*. Cambridge: Cambridge University Press.

Patel, R. 2007. *Stuffed and Starved: The Hidden Battle for the World Food System*. New York: Melville House Publishing.

Patel, V., Chatterji, S., Chisholm, D. et al. 2011. Chronic diseases and injuries in India. *The Lancet*, 377, 413–28.

Pati, B. and Harrison, M. (eds) 2006. *Health, Medicine and Empire: Perspectives on Colonial India*. Delhi: Orient Longman.

Peck, J. 2011. Global Policy Models, Globalizing Poverty Management: International Convergence or Fast-Policy Integration? *Geography Compass* 5(4): 165–81.

Penchansky, R. and Thomas, J.W. 1981. The concept of access: definition and relationship to consumer satisfaction. *Medical Care*, 14(2), 127–40.

Peters, D.H., Yazbeck, A.S., Sharma, R.R. et al. 2002. *Better Health Systems for India's Poor: Findings, Analysis, and Options*. Washington: World Bank.

Phillips, D. 1990. *Health and Health Care in the Third World*. Harlow: Longman.

Planning Commission 2008. *Percentage of population below poverty line by states and UTs for 61st (2004–05) rounds*. New Delhi: Planning Commission, Government of India.

Rao, M., Rao, K.D., Kumar, A.K. et al. 2011. Human resources for health in India. *The Lancet*, 377, 587–98.

Russel, S. 1996. Ability to pay for health care: Concepts and evidence. *Health Policy and Planning*, 11(3), 219–37.

Sakdapolrak, P. 2010: *Orte und Räume der Health Vulnerability. Bourdieus Theorie der Praxis für die Analyse von Krankheit und Gesundheit in Megaurbanen Slums von Chennai, Südindien*. Saarbrücken: Verlag für Entwicklungspolitik.

Sakdapolrak, P., Ergler, C. and Seyler, T. 2013. Burdens of direct and indirect costs of illness: Empirical findings from slum settlements in Chennai, South India. *Progress in Development Studies*, 13(2), 135–51.

Sen, A. 1981. *Poverty and Famines: An Essay on Entitlement and Deprivation*. New York: Oxford University Press.

Sen, A. 1984. Rights and capabilities, in *Resources, Values and Development*, edited by A. Sen. Oxford: Blackwell, 307–24.

Singh, C.H. 2009. The public-private differentials in health care and health-care costs in India: The case of inpatients. *Journal of Public Health*, 17, 401–7.

Singh, S., Barua, N., Mukundan, K. et al. 2004: *The Health of the Urban Poor: Directions for Strategy*. H.D.U.S. Asia. Delhi: World Bank.

Thampi, G.K. 2002. *Corruption in South Asia: Insights and Benchmarks from Citizen Feedback Surveys in Five Countries.* Transparency International. Available at: http://unpan1.un.org/intradoc/groups/public/documents/APCITY/UNPAN019883.pdf [accessed 7 December 2009].

Thaver, I., Harpham, T., McPake, B. and Garner, P. 1998. Private practitioners in the slums of Karachi: what quality of care do they deliver? *Social Science and Medicine*, 46(11), 1441–9.

Vaishnavi, S. and Dash, U. 2009. Catastrophic payments for health care among households in urban Tamil Nadu, India. *Journal of International Development*, 21, 169–84.

Watts, M. 2002. Hour of darkness: vulnerability, security and globalization. *Geographica Helvetica*, 57, 5–18.

Watts, M. and Bohle, H.-G. 1993. The space of vulnerability: The causal structure of hunger and famine. *Progress in Human Geography*, 17(1), 43–67.

Watts, M. and Bohle, H.-G. 2003. Verwundbarkeit, Sicherheit und Globalisierung, in *Kulturgeographie – Aktuelle Ansätze und Entwicklungen*, edited by H. Gebhardt, P. Reuber and G. Wolkersdorfer (eds). Heidelberg: Spektrum Akademischer Verlag, 67–82.

# Chapter 8

# Human Resources for Health: Challenges Facing Sub-Saharan Africa

Gavin George, Candice Reardon and Tim Quinlan

## Introduction

The World Health Organisation's (WHO) 'Framework for Action' provides a guide for resolving the human resource challenge (WHO, 2007). It describes six building blocks: health service delivery, health workforce (that is human resources), health financing, medical products, vaccines and other technologies, health information, and leadership and governance. The guideline was compiled in reference to contemporary global health challenges but it does not represent a departure from the underlying and long-standing premises of public health care. We refer here to the model of decentralised health care (Tabibzadeh 1990; Bossert 1998; Mills, Vaughan, Smith and WHO 2003), key principles of which are the co-ordination and integration of health care services. These principles guide efforts to marshal resources within and between service programmes (Hoffmarcher et al. 2007; Walt et al. 2008; Shiffman 2009), for example, incorporation of 'prevention of mother to child (HIV) transmission' (PMTCT) in maternal and child health services and 'task shifting', the delegation of tasks and responsibilities (Zachariah 2008).[1]

The WHO's advocacy of a 'people-centred' approach (WHO 2008) represents a refinement and, significantly, infers need for more investment in human resources. In the past, the decentralised model of health care and its key principles were justified primarily as means to enable effective and efficient use of resources for the delivery of services (WHO 2003; 2008; UNAIDS 2004; 2005). In contrast, the 'people-centred' approach endorses health policies that go beyond focusing on individual patient care, to incorporate families' and society's needs and expectations of health services. Indeed, the people-centred approach encourages the development of health systems that confront the underlying social, economic and political causes of poor health. In other words, it elaborates the existing approach, emphasising the need for a comprehensive perspective on public health and outcomes of services as a criterion for assessment of service efficiency and effectiveness. This approach has been evolving in Africa, particularly in the field of HIV/AIDS care. For example, the recruitment of patients and ensuring adherence through the development of social support mechanisms has bracketed clinicians' focus on the biophysical demands of treatment. More generally, the concepts of 'comprehensive care' and 'continuity of care' articulate the social as well as the clinical demands of HIV/AIDS treatment. There is therefore, some experience with

---

1   Task shifting: '… a process of delegation whereby tasks are moved, where appropriate to less specialised health workers. By reorganising the work force in this way, task-shifting can make use of the human resources currently available. For example, when doctors are in short supply, a qualified nurse could often prescribe and dispense therapy. Further, community workers can potentially deliver a wide range of services, thus freeing the time of qualified nurses' (WHO 2006b).

the human resource ramifications of this approach (Chen et al. 2004; Honogor and McPake 2004; Schneider et al. 2006; Bärngihausen, Bloom and Humair 2007; Huicho et al. 2008; Van Damme, Kober and Kegels 2008; George et al. 2010). Firstly, it potentially exacerbates the problem of staff shortage because the onus is on health services to address social as well as clinical prescriptions of health care. Secondly, it requires additional and appropriate training of staff. Thirdly, it requires deployment of staff with multiple or different skills or the re-organisation of duties and responsibilities of facility staff.

Whilst the shortage of staff in Africa is a significant problem, the context does not suggest that the problem can be resolved simply by increasing the number of staff. The human resource needs in Africa are changing as the burden of disease changes and as health strategies evolve. Therefore, any assessment of the staff shortage problem needs to take these factors into account.

One consistent focus was, and still is, to build up and sustain the human resources necessary to provide health care. This challenge is the focus of this chapter. It seeks to qualify what is commonly perceived to be a problem of staff shortages, that is a lack of the required number of service delivery staff, such as doctors and nurses, to serve the health care demands of a national population. Specifically the chapter explores anomalies in a large yet fragmented body of information on the human resource challenges to illustrate the actual nature of the staff shortage problem.

Compared to many African countries South Africa is relatively wealthy, has a sophisticated health service infrastructure and it has received considerable international assistance to combat HIV/AIDS. However, the human resource challenges have not been resolved despite a range of interventions to date.

**Human Resources for Health (HRH) Situation in Sub-Saharan Africa**

In 2006, the WHO reiterated concerns about the shortage of health service staff (WHO 2006a, 2006b, 2006c). It estimated that there were 59.8 million staff globally but a shortage of 4.2 million overall and critical shortages in 57 countries (WHO 2006a). Furthermore, the WHO highlighted a global shortage of professional health service delivery staff, that is 2.4 million doctors, nurses, and midwives in total. Putting these estimates in context, the WHO (2006a, 2006b) estimated that sub-Saharan Africa had 11 per cent of the global population yet only 3 per cent of the global health workforce but bore 24 per cent of the global disease burden; and that the health expenditure by African countries was less than 1 per cent of the global amount. Table 8.1 summarises the WHO's assessment. Reasons for the shortage of HRH vary between regions, with common factors being retirement, migration, death, low production rates, and poor working conditions.

The regions with the largest health workforces are identified in Table 8.1, namely the Americas and Europe. Africa, in comparison, has a HRH density of 230 per 100,000 of the population, with roughly three-quarters (78.2 per cent) of African countries experiencing a critical shortage of HRH. A HRH-to-population ratio of 230:100,000 has been proposed by the WHO as the level under which a critical shortage of HRH can be determined. According to the World Health Report (WHO 2006b), countries with a HRH to population ratio of less than 230:100,000 will be unlikely to achieve adequate coverage rates to attain the health-related Millennium Development Goals (MDGs) as well as an 80 per cent coverage of skilled birth attendants. In order for Africa to overcome its shortage of HRH (817,992), the WHO predicted that the total health workforce will have to expand by 139 per cent.

**Table 8.1    Shortage of HRH by region**

| WHO region | Total health workforce | | Number of countries with critical shortages | | Counties with shortages | | % govt. health expenditure paid to HRH* |
|---|---|---|---|---|---|---|---|
| | Number | Density per 100,000 | Total | With shortages | Estimated shortage | % increase required | |
| Africa | 1,640,000 | 230 | 46 | 36 | 817,992 | 139% | 29.5% |
| Eastern Mediterranean | 2,100,000 | 400 | 21 | 7 | 306,031 | 98% | 50.8% |
| South-East Asia | 7,040,000 | 430 | 11 | 6 | 1,164,001 | 50% | 35.5% |
| Western Pacific | 10,070,000 | 580 | 27 | 3 | 32,560 | 98% | 45% |
| Europe | 16,630,000 | 1,890 | 52 | 0 | NA | NA | 42.3% |
| Americas | 21,740,000 | 2,480 | 35 | 5 | 37,886 | 40% | 49.8% |
| World | 59,220,000 | 930 | 192 | 57 | 2,358,470 | 70% | 42.2% |

*Sources:* WHO, 2006a; 2006b; 2006c.

*Note:* This figure consists of the wages, salaries, and allowances of HRH as a percentage of government health expenditure. Not all countries in region had data available on the proportion of government expenditure that was allocated to HRH.

However, the health workforce within Africa receives the lowest proportion of government expenditure (29.5 per cent) in comparison to other regions, which suggests that government expenditure on HRH will be forced to increase dramatically in order to overcome the HRH crisis in Africa. According to the WHO (2006b), a typical country will allocate roughly 42 per cent of its health expenditure to paying for the salaries, wages, and allowances of its health workforce (WHO 2006b). As is shown in Table 8.1, African countries generally spend considerably less on its HRH than the average amount of health expenditure paid by other countries.

Regional shortages of HRH are particularly significant when examined in relation to the burden of disease afflicting these areas. The World Bank has estimated that a country with 15 per cent adult HIV prevalence rate can expect to lose up to 3.3 per cent of its health care providers from AIDS annually (WHO 2006b). In particular countries with the lowest disease burden possess the largest health workforce, whilst countries that carry the greatest burden of disease have the smallest numbers of HRH (WHO 2006b). For example, sub-Saharan Africa currently faces a devastating shortage of HRH, while it is home to 11 per cent of the global population, it carries 24 per cent of the global disease burden and has 3 per cent of the global health workforce. Furthermore, it receives less than 1 per cent of global health expenditure (WHO 2006a).

Whilst Africa, as a whole, has the minimum ratio set by WHO, there remains considerable variation across the continent. It reported critical shortages in 36 African countries (78 per cent), representing also the majority (63 per cent) of all countries in the world where this is the case.

South Africa, Namibia, Botswana do not have staff shortages in terms of the WHO's global assessment. For example, WHO's calculations presented in Table 8.2 show that these three countries exceed the minimum required ratios, of 20 medical practitioners and 120 nurses respectively per 1,000,000 people (WHO 2006b). Updated estimates for 2010 have put the number of doctors (GPs and specialists) currently working in South Africa at 17,801 and 9,630 respectively, which implies a doctor to patient ratio of 55 medical doctors per 100,000 population. However, South Africa and Botswana fall well below the doctor to population ratio for middle income countries set by the World Bank (180 per 100,000), nearing the ratio level expected for low-income countries of 50 doctors per 100,000 population. Moreover, South Africa and Botswana's doctor to population ratio falls way below countries with a similar level of economic development such as Mexico (198 per 100,000) and Brazil (185 per 100,000) (Econex 2010a).

Staff shortages have been identified as a critical problem in sub-Saharan Africa; primarily in terms of a skewed distribution of human resources between the public and private health sectors, between rural and urban areas, low recruitment and retention rates and the changing demands imposed on the public health services by the introduction and expansion of large scale HIV/AIDS prevention and treatment programmes (McIntyre and Klugman 2003; Shishana et al. 2004; Couper, de Villiers and Sondzaba 2005; Lehmann Schneider et al. 2006; Bateman 2007; Van Rensburg et al. 2008; Breier 2008; 2009; Sanders and Lloyd 2009).

## Migration

Whilst South Africa possesses the largest proportion of medical doctors, we find that it experiences a significant migration of its doctors and health workers more generally. In

**Table 8.2     Cross-country comparison of physician and nurse rations per 100,000 population**

| Country | Medical practitioner | Nurse |
|---|---|---|
| | ratio per 100,000 people | |
| Mozambique | 3 | 21 |
| Zambia | 12 | 174 |
| Namibia | 30 | 306 |
| Botswana | 40 | 265 |
| South Africa | 77 | 408 |
| United States of America | 256 | 937 |
| United Kingdom | 230 | 1212 |

*Source:* WHO (2006b).

terms of actual migration flows, there has been significant growth in the inflow of doctors to the UK as shown by work permit data, and supported by the registration data for 2001 and 2002. In 2002, nearly half of new full registrants on the UK General Medical Council (GMC) register were foreign (Buchan 2007), out of which 3,509 were South African doctors. In the same year 1,950 South African doctors were reported to be living in the United States (Pagett and Padarath 2007). In 2002, 2,884 South African nurses were documented to have emigrated from South Africa to the UK (Breier, Wildshut and Mgqolozana 2009), which decreased to 1,418 South African nurses in 2003 (Buchan 2004). By 2004, 7 per cent of the total nursing workforce in South Africa had left South Africa to work in seven Organisation for Economic Co-operation and Development (OECD) countries, while slightly over a third of South African doctors, (37 per cent, n=12,136) trained in South Africa, were living in eight OECD countries (Breier et al. 2009). Moreover, by 2006 the proportion of South African doctors who had left the country rose to a staggering 40 per cent (Pagett and Padarath 2007). Other statistics reported that almost 9000 (n =8,921) South African doctors and 6,844 nurses and midwives were practicing abroad in 2006 (Wadee and Kahn 2007).

South African doctors are highly concentrated in English speaking, first world countries (Breier et al. 2009). For instance, a follow-up investigation into the whereabouts of University of Witwatersrand medical school graduates in 1998 revealed that approximately 45 per cent of graduate doctors since 1975 were located abroad, mostly in North America, the UK, Canada, Australia and New Zealand (Breier et al. 2009). In the town of Saskatchewan in Canada, alone, between 17 and 20 per cent of physicians were found to be from South African medical schools (Grant 2006). 2006 figures reflect that 9.7 per cent and 7 per cent of the foreign trained doctor workforces in Australia and the UK, respectively, are made up of South African doctors (Long 2007). In 2006, popular destination countries such as the United States, Canada, New Zealand, and Australia held a combined total of 6,993 South African doctors who were registered in their workforces, comprising 18.5 per cent of the 30,740 registered physicians in South Africa (Long 2007). More recent estimates suggest that in 2010 about 29.4 per cent (12,108) of physicians trained in South Africa emigrated (Tjadens et al. 2012).

In addition to those health professionals who have left the country, many more are considering emigration, influenced by the prospects of a better life in their destination country (Crush, Pendleton and Tevera 2005). Crush et al. (2005) found that a substantial proportion of South African health professionals had already taken active steps to emigrate, such as applying for work permits and professional registration. Similar findings have been found in other studies. At the time of data collection for their study, Pendleton, Crush and Lefko-Everett (2007) found that 7.1 per cent of South African nurses and doctors in the sample had applied for work permits, 7.8 per cent were in the process of applying, roughly 3 per cent had applied for and were applying for a permanent residence permit in their destination country, and roughly 4 per cent had already applied for or were applying for citizenship in their country of destination. In their study, South African health professionals showed a preference for destination countries such as Australia, New Zealand, the UK, Europe, North America and Canada (Pendleton et al. 2007).

A large proportion of health sector students in South Africa, as well as students further afield in Africa, contemplate leaving Africa. Research has found (Pendleton et al. 2007) a high degree of emigration potential among health sector students in southern Africa, with 65 per cent indicating that they would like to emigrate within five years after graduating. Health sector students in the study were noted to have given more thought to moving to another country and were inclined to want to stay in their destination country for a longer period of time than non-health sector students. Although lower than the proportion found by Pendleton et al. (2007), a study amongst 194 medical students in the province of KwaZulu-Natal, showed that roughly one in five students (n = 27, 18.5 per cent) intended to emigrate to practice medicine abroad after graduation, while fewer wished to pursue postgraduate training abroad (n= 10, 7.6 per cent) (Van Wyk, Naidoo and Esterhuizen 2010). Emigration considerations were also prevalent amongst a sample of 9,743 students from sub-Saharan Africa, 4,532 of which were South African students. Approximately four in five students (79 per cent) had thought about moving to another country, and for 35 per cent there was the possibility this could happen in the next six months. The proportion of final-year students in the study, however, who had actually taken active steps to leave the country was much smaller; 19 per cent had applied or were in the process of applying for work permits abroad, while 11 per cent were applying for permanent residence elsewhere or for citizenship (Crush et al. 2005). The UK was a favoured destination country for this sample of students. More recently, George and Reardon (2012) found that 37 per cent of medical and nursing student respondents in their sample planned to seek for employment abroad after their studies, the majority of whom (67 per cent) were planning to emigrate within five years of graduation.

## Factors that Play a Role in Health Professionals' Decisions to Emigrate Abroad

Factors influencing individuals' decisions to migrate to other countries are commonly grouped into push and pull factors depending on whether the factor is located in the source or destination country. Prominent push factors that can encourage health professionals in sub-Saharan Africa to leave their home country include resource-limited health care systems, deteriorating work environments, human resource shortages, low salaries, political tensions and upheaval, gender discrimination, lack of personal security, HIV/AIDS, and deteriorating quality of life and social systems such as education and welfare. Salient pull factors attracting health professionals to developed countries abroad often relate to the availability of jobs in the destination country, more manageable workloads, high remuneration, better working conditions, safer living environments, better quality of life and a more economically and politically stable country (Oberoi and Lin 2006; Labonte Packer and Claasen 2006; Hamilton and Yau 2010). Although few studies have explicitly set out to determine the variation of push and pull factors across age groups, it is interesting to note that Maslin (2003) found that young health professionals in South Africa between the ages of 20 and 29 were more likely to cite deteriorating working conditions as a reason for wanting to leave, while older respondents (<60 years old) were less likely to identify heavy workloads as a reason for wanting to emigrate.

Further research amongst South African heath workers revealed that financial factors, better job opportunities for themselves and schooling opportunities for children abroad as well as the high crime rate in South Africa were significant factors encouraging these health workers to emigrate abroad (Bezuidenhout Joubert, Hiemstra and Struwig 2009). The opportunity to gain international experience is an important pull factor that has been found to attract South African health professionals, and in particular doctors, to overseas countries (Maslin 2003). According to Oberoi and Lin (2006), however, push factors motivating health professionals to leave South Africa can exert a more powerful influence on their emigration decisions than the factors attracting them to their destination country. The major push factors that emerged most frequently in their interviews with South African doctors that had emigrated to Australia were poor remuneration, lack of job satisfaction, lack of future prospects for further education and career development, poor working conditions, HIV/AIDS and poor quality of life (Oberoi and Lin 2006).

## International Codes of Practice Governing Health Worker Migration and Employment

Several codes of practice on the international recruitment of health workers have been developed over the past few years with the aim of better protecting migrant health workers, and minimising the negative impact of out-migration of health personnel for the source countries.

In the early twenty-first century developed countries became increasingly engaged in large-scale targeted international recruitment of health workers from developing countries to address domestic shortages. Although experience working within developed nations can provide health care professionals with an enriching experience, enhanced skills and expertise, and a chance to increase their quality of life, there has been great concern about the impact this may have upon the health care systems of developing countries. In view of this several codes of practice for the international recruitment of health workers have been developed over the past few years with the aim of better protecting migrant health workers, and minimising the negative impact of out-migration of health personnel on source countries. These codes are not legally binding, but they set out agreed voluntary principles and responsibilities. These are so far limited in their geographical scope (for example the Commonwealth Code of Practice from 2003, the Pacific Code of Practice from 2007, the UK Code of Practice from 2001/2004 and the Scotland Code of Practice from 2006), or focused on specific health services (for example EPSU/HOSPEEM Code of Conduct for health personnel working in hospitals within the EU). The WHO code of practice is the first code with a worldwide scope applicable for both source and destination countries (Luckanachai and Rieger 2010). This international code has a worldwide impact and was agreed upon in 2010 (Hamilton and Yau 2010).

The Code of Practice for the International Recruitment of Healthcare Professionals was the first country level policy instrument that was designed to moderate international recruitment activity. The UK Department of Health first established guidelines in 1999 (Department of Health 1999), which required National Health Service (NHS) employers not to target South Africa and the West Indies. It then introduced a Code of Practice for the International Recruitment of Healthcare Professionals for NHS Employers in 2001 (Department of Health 2001). This code of practice was extended in 2004 to cover recruitment agencies, temporary staff working in the NHS, and private sector Organisations providing services to the NHS (Department of Health, 2004). In its current form the Code of Practice for the International Recruitment of Healthcare Professionals still prohibits its NHS Organisations from actively recruiting health workers from Africa, thus promoting high standards of practice in the ethical international recruitment of health care professionals (Department of Health, 2004). The key points contained within the 2004 revision of Code of Practice for the International Recruitment of Healthcare Professionals include the following:

1. Developing countries should not be targeted for active recruitment by the NHS unless the government of that country formally agrees;
2. NHS employers should only use recruitment agencies that have agreed to comply with the Code of Practice;
3. NHS employers should consider regional collaboration in international recruitment activities;
4. Staff recruited from abroad have the same legal protection as other employees;
5. Staff recruited from abroad should have same access to further training as other employees (Buchan, Baldwin and Munro 2008).

The overall impact of the UK Code of Practice is difficult to assess, given data limitations, and the fact that the Code does not 'ban' inflow, but attempts to moderate active recruitment. It has provided local NHS employers with 'good practice' guidelines and information on which countries are acceptable targets for international recruitment (Buchan 2007). The Code does not prevent health professionals taking the initiative to apply for employment in the UK or to come to the UK for training purposes (Buchan et al. 2008). Thus, it has not ended the inflow of African nurses to the UK (Buchan et al. 2008) but, as we indicate later, it has reduced the numbers finding work there.

*Changes to UK Immigration and Employment Policies for Health Professionals*

In recent years a number of policy changes in relation to the recruitment, immigration and employment of foreign health professionals in the UK have taken place. These policy changes have made it increasingly difficult for South African health professionals to secure work opportunities in the UK, although the actual impact of these policy changes on immigration flows does not seem to have been researched in much detail to date. The various policies serve to discourage or decrease the numbers of health workers emigrating to the UK by making the process of application for visas and work permits more difficult and stringent. In May 2010, the UK government announced their intention to review the immigration system to ensure that net migration reduces between 2010 and 2015 to the levels previously seen in the 1990s (National Health Service 2011).

The UK government's new five tiered visa system for assessing immigrants recently instituted has made it increasingly difficult for African nurses and doctors to enter the UK for work purposes (Buchan et al. 2008). Tier 2, the relevant visa for which South African health professionals are eligible, is an employer-led category, which means employers must sponsor any skilled workers from outside the European Economic Area (EEA) they wish to recruit in order to fill vacancies that cannot be filled by a British or EEA worker. Hence, UK employers cannot employ a foreign person outside of the UK or EEA when a suitable UK or EEA candidate exists (National Health Service 2011), which limits the employment opportunities of South African health professionals' in the UK. In addition, the Tier 5 visa allows UK employers to recruit individuals from outside the EEA for up to 24 months under the temporary worker or youth mobility categories. This was a popular visa for young Africans in the past to gain entry into the UK to work and travel for a two year period. However, in mid-2008 changes were made to this visa, which now prohibits Africans from qualifying for it (National Health Service 2011).

Other policy changes include the introduction of two Professional and Linguistics Assessments Board (PLAB) tests for South African doctors, which the doctors have to pass in order to gain employment in the UK. The high cost of writing the second PLAB test in the UK presents a definite obstacle to African doctors wanting to emigrate to the UK, especially given the fact that doctors have no guarantee of securing a job in the UK even after passing the PLAB exams.

## Curbing the Loss of HRH: Lessons from South Africa

*Bilateral Agreements and Economic Incentives*

Various initiatives have been put in place abroad to reduce the emigration of health professionals from South Africa and to alleviate the negative effects of the emigration of South African health professionals. The Memorandum of Understanding (MOU) between the UK and South Africa and The Commonwealth Code of Practice for the International Recruitment for Health Workers have played an important role in reducing the significant inflows of South African health professionals to the UK in earlier years, while the Bilateral Agreements between the South African government with Tunisia and Cuba have also played a role in strengthening rural health care systems in South Africa weakened by the internal migration of health professionals from public to private sectors and away from South Africa. The South African government has introduced financial incentives to encourage health professionals to remain in rural areas and within the public service, including the Occupational Specific Dispensation (OSD) and two types of allowances: (1) the scarce skills allowance which benefits medical doctors and certain categories of professional nurses (operating theatre nurses, critical care/intensive care nurses and oncology nurses), regardless of rural or urban place of employment, and (2) the rural allowance which benefits those health workers in specific rural areas.

South Africa has a great imbalance of health workers between rural areas and urban areas. In 2008 it was reported that 34 per cent of rural medical practitioner posts and 40.3 per cent of rural nursing posts were vacant (Health Systems Trust 2009). The problem was recognised a decade earlier when, in 1999, the government instituted a rural allowance in an effort to attract more health professionals to rural areas. It is applicable to all areas or 'nodes' as defined by the Integrated Sustainable Rural Development Strategy (ISRDS), as well as rural areas as designated by the Public Service Bargaining Chamber (PSBC). In ISRDS, rural medical doctors receive a rural allowance which amounts to an additional 22 per cent of their salary, while professional nurses receive an allowance of 12 per cent of their monthly salaries. For those in PSBC nodes, an 18 per cent allowance is given to medical doctors and an 8 per cent allowance is given to professional nurses (Reid, 2004).

The development and implementation of the OSD in the mid-2000s for health professionals in South Africa was based on the recognition that the improvement in the conditions of service and remuneration for health professionals constituted the most urgent priority. The objectives of the OSD are to improve the public services ability to attract and retain employees, to provide differentiated remuneration dispensations for the vast number of occupations in the public service, to cater for the unique needs of the different occupations, to provide a unique salary structure per occupation, to prescribe grading structures and job profiles to eliminate inter-provincial variations and to provide adequate and clear salary progression and career pathing opportunities based on competencies, experience, and performance. Dispensations for specific occupational categories include unique salary structures for each identified occupation in the public service, centrally determined grades and job profiles, career progression opportunities, and other employment practices (Mahlathi 2009, in George et al. 2009).

Announced in 2007, the OSD has resulted in some categories in the public service being re-graded according to their qualifications and years of experience and remunerated accordingly. The fact that not all categories of nurses are benefiting from the OSD has raised much contention amongst nurses and other health professionals. It was agreed that nursing would be the first profession to benefit from the OSD in 2007, followed by remuneration increases for medical, dental, specialists, pharmacists, and emergency medical service staff in 2008. However, due to inadequate funding, the proposals were fully implemented only by 2010, but there were still discrepancies due to inconsistent implementation by provincial governments (Bateman, 2010).

The introduction of community service for all categories of health professionals aimed to alleviate staff shortages in rural and under-served areas. Community service for professional nurses was instituted in 2008, with an initial cohort of approximately 200 nurses. The extent to which community service will encourage health professionals to remain in such areas, and even in the public sector after completion, is questionable. It is arguable that the introduction of community service has not stopped doctors from leaving after their year to spend time overseas. Reid (2004) found that an increasing proportion of community service students between 1999 (34 per cent) and 2001 (43 per cent) intended to work overseas after their community service year. Of Reid's sample, 20 per cent said they would consider working in rural or under-served areas in the future, which he argues is adequate reason for the government to implement an appropriate and systemic set of incentives that could encourage these health professionals to practice in rural areas and thus obviate the need for young health professionals to have to endure their year of obligatory service. He cautioned that community service may actually defeat its own end because young doctors assume that after their community service, they have fulfilled their duty and compensated society for the costs of their study (Reid 2004).

*The Bilateral Agreement between the UK and South Africa*

South Africa has entered into a number of bilateral agreements with foreign governments that have been aimed at moderating the outflow of South African health professionals and alleviating health worker shortages that have worsened due to internal migration within South Africa and emigration itself. The Bilateral Agreements that will be discussed in the following paragraphs include the MOU between the UK and South Africa as well as the Bilateral Agreements between the South African government and the governments of Cuba and Tunisia.

In the 1990s, the South African government began placing pressure on the UK to refrain from recruiting South African doctors. In 1999, the former president of South Africa, Nelson Mandela, publicly accused the UK of poaching South Africa's health professionals (Rogerson 2007). This culminated in the endorsement of a MOU between the UK and South Africa in 2002 as a policy response to the recruitment of health workers from developing countries. This was announced by South Africa's Minister of Health at a meeting with Commonwealth Ministers of Health in May 2002. The MOU takes a dynamic flexible approach to encouraging ongoing dialogue between the UK and South Africa around human resources for health, health care capacity and development with regular assessment and adjustment by both countries (Robinson and Clark 2008). Bilateral agreements are widely regarded as effective mechanisms for promoting health worker flows that can be beneficial to both source countries and receiving countries (Hamilton and Yau 2010). The MOU established between the government of South Africa and the government of the UK has, thus, focused on the reciprocal educational exchange of healthcare concepts and personnel. The MOU covers a wide range of areas with a view to sharing and disseminating best practice between the two countries. It also offers the opportunity for nationals from both the UK and South Africa to benefit from time limited placements in either country, thereby creating trans-cultural opportunities for clinical personnel and healthcare managers (Maslin 2003; Rogerson 2007). However, it has been criticised by some health professionals who argue that it has limited employment opportunities for South Africans in the UK due to the prohibition of active recruitment of South African health professionals. Notably, statistics documenting the inflow of South African nurses to the UK show a marked decrease in the number of nurses entering the UK between 2000 and 2006 (Mills et al. 2008; Robinson and Clark 2008)

*Bilateral Agreements between South Africa and Other Developing Countries: Cuba*

The problem of the maldistribution of health personnel in South Africa is well known and documented. Researchers have argued that the shortage is historical, attributing it to the apartheid regime which failed to invest in the provision of health care personnel for the rural, largely Black population (Awases, Gbary, Nyoni, and Chatora 2004). Many countries in Africa, including South Africa, have had agreements with Cuba and have received groups of Cuban doctors for deployment in rural and under-resourced areas (Dovlo 2004). The arrival of Cuban doctors within rural areas in South Africa has not been without controversy, as some researchers argue that the reliance on Cuban doctors to fill the vacant posts in rural areas has resulted in non-advertisement of these posts to local South African doctors (Lee 1996, cited in Awases et al. 2004).

In 2004, there were close to 500 Cuban doctors practicing in rural areas and townships around South Africa (Southern African Migration Programme 2004). According to Fidel Radebe, director of communications for South Africa's Department of Health, there were 134 Cuban doctors in the country in 2008 (Nieuwoudt 2008). The Bilateral Agreement between South Africa and Cuba also provides for the medical training of South Africans at training facilities in Cuba. A total of 470 South African medical students were enrolled in the medical training programme in Cuba between 1996 and 2007, as part of an agreement signed between the two nations in 1995 (Nieuwoudt, 2008). After being selected for the training programme, the South African students study for five years in Cuba. The South African students then return to South Africa in their sixth year to do their final clinical year and internship in various South African health facilities, particularly those in under-resourced areas. The students then sit for a South African examination with the rest of the country's medical students to qualify as doctors (BizCommunity New, 2007).

*Tunisia*

The Tunisian Agency for Technical Cooperation has a pool of more than 2,000 health professionals that are available to work in countries that have cooperation agreements with Tunisia. South Africa's cooperative agreement with Tunisia was signed in 1999 and reaffirmed in 2004 during a visit by the former Minister of Health, Dr Manto Tshabalala-Msimang to Tunisia. Recruitment of Tunisian doctors was one of the short-term measures taken by the Department of Health to address the challenge of an inadequate supply of doctors locally (BizCommunity New, 2007). Representatives of the Tunisian Agency for Technical Cooperation have been in South Africa to inspect public health facilities, as part of a drive to help recruit Tunisian doctors to work in South Africa's under-served areas.

Between 2000 and 2002, Tunisian ophthalmologists visited South Africa to perform eye operations. A total of 234 operations were performed in 2000, 260 in 2001 and 176 in 2002. In January 2007, 171 eye operations were performed by Tunisian ophthalmologists at Butterworth Hospital in eGcuwa, in the Eastern Cape. South Africa and Tunisia continued the ophthalmologist programme between 2008 and 2011. These initiatives affirm the commitment of both countries to the South development agenda and to further strengthen cooperation in other areas of health. South African remuneration packages were found to be competitive with the amount Tunisian doctors would be paid in their home country; a little more than a thousand dinars per month (Tunisia.com, 2006).

*The Role of Africa Health Placements in Recruiting Doctors to Rural and Under-resourced Areas*

Africa Health Placements (AHP) is a recruitment Organisation that recruits South African health professionals from private into public health facilities, as well as foreign health professionals into public rural and under-resourced health facilities around the country. In addition, AHP currently offers a consulting service where they assist health facilities with improving the level of human resource management in their facilities.

In recent years, the AHP has played an important role in strengthening rural health care services in South Africa. After taking into account the number of newly qualified doctors who will emigrate or work in the private sector, South Africa is left with approximately 150 graduate doctors who will enter the public service each year, 35 of which will work in rural areas of South Africa. However, in 2009, AHP placed 7 times this amount of foreign doctors in rural hospitals around South Africa. Since the AHP's inception in 2006, they have filled 548 permanent government health workers posts in rural and under-resourced areas. AHP have consultants based in the UK and USA that enable it to recruit foreign health professionals from further afield. The recruitment consultants based in the UK and North America enable AHP to recruit foreign health professionals from Belgium, the Netherlands and Scandinavia, as well as Canada, Australia and New Zealand (AHP 2010).

AHP have also been instrumental in assisting South African health professionals abroad to return to the country. AHP's expertise in this regard is being utilised by the Homecoming Revolution, an NGO that has been established to encourage and facilitate the return of South Africans in foreign countries back to their home country. AHP's ability to streamline and fast track the administrative process involved in bringing foreign health professionals or South African health professionals back to the country is made possible by having individuals contracted to them within the Department of Health and Health Professions Council of South Africa (HPCSA).

**Recommendations**

This chapter reviewed sub-Saharan Africa's HRH capacities as well as lessons learnt from the South African context. It is evident that the absolute shortage of HRH as well as the maldistribution of HRH constrain efforts to achieve targeted health outcomes. In the absence of effective and immediate actions, the shortages which exist within certain HRH categories will jeopardise the attainment of health targets through their negative impact on the delivery of these services. Current production levels of medical practitioners and nurses will be unable to fulfil the HRH requirements for the achievement of country health targets. The impact of HIV and AIDS on HRH, increasing rates of migration, and an ageing nurse population are factors which exacerbate the shortages of HRH within sub-Saharan Africa.

Several policies and strategic actions have been undertaken to address the HRH crisis and strengthen efforts to achieve HIV prevention targets in South Africa. The implementation of task-shifting practices as well as increased production of mid-level cadres and highly skilled HRH have been identified as priority interventions of the South African government. Measures to retain HRH through improving work conditions and remuneration packages have also been undertaken through the OSD and rural and scarce skills allowances. The institution of community service for all categories of health professionals is expected to alleviate some of the HRH shortages within rural areas of the public health sector. Shortages in the public health sector and within rural areas, in particular, could be further addressed with the recruitment of foreign health professionals through government-to-government agreements with other countries, although the South African government's restriction on the proportion of HRH employed in the public health sector will dramatically diminish the number of foreign HRH currently employed in the public health sector. These are lessons that can be adopted by other African countries.

Researchers proposing recommendations to overcome the HRH crisis within Africa have underscored the importance of developing comprehensive strategies to alleviate shortages that can be implemented within short, medium, and long-term time horizons (Lehmann 2008; Sanders and Llyod 2009; Wildschut and Mgqolozana 2009). Initiatives to overcome the HRH crisis in South Africa, according to Wildschut and Mgqolozana (2009), should be aligned with correctly identified shortages. For instance, in recognition of the absolute shortage and the maldistribution of HRH that exists within South Africa, they assert that initiatives spanning the entire spectrum of responses should be put in place to provide a comprehensive response to the different types of nursing shortages experienced. They argue that the most pressing need is to rectify the maldistribution of nurses between public and private sectors and rural and urban areas. Thus, strategies aimed at ameliorating the impact of nursing shortages should concentrate on:

1.  The retention of nurses being produced;
2.  Recruiting nurses now practicing in other fields back into the profession;
3.  Identifying specific areas and provinces where shortages exist, as well as where shortages are in the public and private sectors (Wildschut and Mgqolozana 2009). To alleviate identified shortages in rural areas, Sanders and Lloyd (2009) have advocated for the selection of trainees and mid-level workers from rural areas because of the strong possibility that they will return to work in rural areas after their training. Further, they underscore the importance of improved management and support for rural health professionals operating in under-resourced areas, which can include better accommodation, infrastructure, and amenities and rotating visits from specialists.

Secondly, Wildschut and Mgqolozana (2009) assert that congruence should exist between different strategies to ameliorate nursing shortages. Currently, there is a contradiction inherent to the Department of Labour's Master List of scarce and critical skills, which implies the importance of training more professional nurses, whereas the National HRH plan strongly proposes the increased production of lower levels of nurses, more specifically enrolled nurses and nursing assistants.

A range of initiatives to address the shortage of HRH have been proposed by Wildschut and Mgqolozana (2009) as well as other researchers. These include the following;

*Short-term Initiatives:*

1.  These can entail importing health professionals from other countries and using retired nurses (Wildschut and Mgqolozana 2009);
2.  The regulation, integration and better utilisations of Community Health Workers (CHWs) within health services (Lehmann, 2008; Sanders and Lloyd 2009);
3.  Task shifting of selected activities from health professionals to CHWs and mid-level workers, which will require redefining the scope and practice of health professionals. In the Short-term the skills gap in PHC implementation in rural areas should be primarily filled by appropriately trained CHWs and mid-level workers (Sanders and Lloyd 2009).

*Medium-term Initiatives:*

1.  The implementation of recruitment, and retention initiatives: e.g. the WHOs' 'Treat, Train, and Retain' initiative to increase the number of HRH and give them better resources to fight HIV and AIDS. This can include the offering of retention bonuses and efforts by the South African Government to limit recruitment of South African HRH by developed countries (Sanders and Lloyd 2009; Wildschut and Mgqolozana 2008);
2.  The implementation of scarce skills and rural allowances;
3.  Improved remuneration structures such as the OSD.

*Long-term Initiatives:*

1.  The accelerated production of health professionals and mid-level cadres (Lehmann 2008). Sanders and Lloyd (2009) emphasise that the rapid production of nurses is an urgent necessity and, further, that they should be trained and oriented to practice in low-resourced environments;

2.  Comprehensive curriculum audits that result in a revision of training curricula of health professionals where necessary (Lehmann 2008; Sanders and Lloyd 2009);
3.  Increasing the number of public-private partnerships (for example, like that which formed between the Gauteng Department of Health and Life Health Care for the introduction of a new neo-natal ICU nursing training programme in 2003);
4.  Increasing the amount of bursaries given to students;
5.  Increasing South Africa's training capacity by reopening previously closed nursing colleges and increasing the capacity of educational institutions to train more nurses (Wildschut and Mgqolozana 2009). Honogor and McPake (2004) suggest that South Africa should make increasing use of the existing capacity in the developed world to train and produce health professionals. Twinning medical schools in developing countries with those in developed countries, which can provide training support in the form of training staff in neglected areas, is one potential option. The promotion of distance learning, particularly in non-clinical areas by public health schools in the developed world is another option.

## Conclusion

The number of nurses and doctors that have left sub-Saharan Africa and who consider emigration is worryingly high, given the imbalance of health workers between urban and under-resourced health facilities in the country. We have learned that despite several responses and initiatives by the South African government to reduce the number of health professionals wanting to leave the country or to alleviate its negative effects, emigration still persists. Health professionals leave South Africa driven by a desire to escape negative and unfulfilling working and living conditions in South Africa and attracted by the prospects of a better life abroad. In spite of the difficulty of gaining access into developed nations such as the UK in terms of stringent policies around immigration, recruitment and employment of foreign health professionals, South African health workers still emigrate to the UK. Despite advances, South Africa along with other African countries have to do more to improve working conditions, salaries and job satisfaction of health workers to encourage African doctors and nurses to remain in the country, as well as to bring back those health workers that have emigrated abroad.

## References

Africa Health Placements. 2010. *The doctor is not yet in: Africa Calling the Challenge.* [Online]. Available at: http://www.afdb.org.

African Health Placements. 2010. *African Statistical Yearbook 2010.* [Online]. Available at: http://www.afdb.org/fileadmin/uploads/afdb/Documents/Publications/ADB_Yearbook_2010_web.pdf.

Awases, M., Gbary, A., Nyoni, J. and Chatora, R. 2004. Migration of health professionals in six countries: A synthesis report. *World Health Organisation Document.*

Bärngihausen, T., Bloom, D.E. and Humair, S. 2007. Human resources for treating HIV/AIDS: needs, capacities, and gaps. *AIDS Patient Care and STDs,* 21(11), 799–812.

Bateman, C. 2007. Slim pickings as 2008 health staff crisis looms. *South African Medical Journal,* 97(11), 1020–34.

Bateman, C. 2010. Occupational Specific Dispensation – A Hapless Tale. *South African Medical Journal*. 100(5), 268–72.

Bezuidenhout, M.M., Joubert, G, Hiemstra, L.A and Struwig, M.C. 2009. Reasons for doctor migration from South Africa. *South African Journal of Family Pratice*, 51(3), 211–15.

Bizcommunit.com. 2007. Medical – SA & Tunisia Agreement, 17(12). [Online]. Available at: www. bizcommunit.com.

Bossert, T. 1998. Analysing the decentralisation of health systems in developing countries: Decision space, innovation and performance. *Social Science Medicine*, 47, 1513–27.

Breier, M., Wildshut, A. and Mgqolozana, T. 2009. *Nursing in a New Era: The Profession and Education of Nurses in South Africa*. Cape Town: HSRC Press.

Buchan, J. 2007. International recruitment of nurses: policy and practice in the United Kingdom. *Health Research and Education Trust*, 10(1111), 1475–6773.

Buchan, J. and Dovlo, D., 2004. *International recruitment of health workers to the UK: A report for DFID*. DFID Health Systems Resource Centre, 1–44.

Buchan, J., Baldwin, S. and Munro, M. 2008. Directorate for Employment, Labour and Social Affairs. *Organisation for Economic Co-operation and Development Health Working Paper*, 38. Migration of Health Workers the UK Perspective.

Chen, L., Evans, T., Anand, S. et al. 2004. Human resources for health: overcoming the crisis. *Lancet*, 364(9449), 1984–90.

Couper, I., de Villiers, M. and Sondzaba, N. 2005. Human resources: district hospitals, in *South African health review 2005*, edited by P. Ijumba and P. Barron. Durban: Health Systems Trust. [Online]. Available at: http://www.hst.org.za/sahr.

Crush, J., Pendleton, W. and Tevera, D.S. 2005. *Degrees of uncertainty: Students and the brain drain in southern Africa*. Southern African Migration Project, 1–24.

Department of Health. 1999. Guidance on International Recruitment. Department of Health, London

Department of Health. 2001. Code of Practice for NHS Employers involved in international recruitment of healthcare professionals. Department of Health, London.

Department of Health. 2004. Code of practice for the international recruitment of healthcare professionals. Department of Health, London.

Development Bank of South Africa. 2008. DBSA roadmap process. [Online]. Available at: http://www.dbsa.org/Research/Documents/Health percent20Roadmap.pdf.

Dovlo, D. 2004. The brain drain in Africa: An emerging challenge to health professionals' education. *JHEA/RESA*, 2(3), 1–18.

George, G., Quinlan, T. and Reardon, C. 2009. *Human resources for health: A needs and gaps analysis of HRH in South Africa*. Health Economics and HIV & AIDS Research Division (HEARD), 2–70.

George, G. Atujuna, M., Gentile, J. et al. 2010. The impact of ART scale up on health workers: Evidence from two South African districts. *AIDS Care*, 22, 77–84.

George, G. and Reardon, C., 2013, 'Preparing for export?: Medical and nursing student migration intentions post-qualification in South Africa', *African Journal of Primary Health Care Fam Med*. 5(1), 9pp.

Grant, H.M. 2006. From the Transvaal to the Prairies: the migration of South African physicians to Canada. *Journal of Ethnic and Migration Studies*, 32(4), 681–95.

Hamilton, K. and Yau, J. 2010. *The Global Tug-of-War for Health Care Workers*. Migration Policy Institute.

Hoffmarcher, M., Oxley, H. and Rusticelli, E. 2007. Improved Health System performance through better care Coordination. OECD Working Paper No. 30.

Honogor, C. and McPake, B. 2004. How to bridge the gap in human resources for health. *The Lancet*, 364 [Online]. Available at: http://www.thelancet.com.

Huicho, L., Scherpbier, R.W., Nkowane, A.M. and Victoria, C.G. 2008. How much does quality of child care vary between health workers with differing durations of training? An observational multicountry study. *The Lancet*, 372, 910–16.

Junior Doctors Association of South Africa (Judasa). 2010. Internship and Community Service Report August 2010. [Online]. Available at: http://www.judasa.org.

Lehmann, U. 2008. Strengthening human resources for primary health care, in *South African Health Review 2008*, edited by P. Barron and J. Roma-Reardon. Durban: Health Systems Trust. Available at: http://www.hst.org.za/sahr.

Luckanachai, N. and Rieger, M. 2010. Research project making migration a development factor, the case of North and West Africa: A review of international migration policies. *International Institute for Labour Studies*, 4–45.

Maslin, A. 2003. *Databank of Bilateral Agreements*. The Aspen Institute – Global Health and Development.

McIntyre, D. and Klugman, B. 2003. The human face of decentralisation and integration of health services: Experience from South Africa. *Reproductive Health Matters*, 11(21), 108–19.

Memorandum of Understanding. 2008. *Memorandum of Understanding between the Government of the United Kingdom of Great Britain and Northern Ireland and the Government of the Republic of South Africa on the Reciprocal Exchange of Healthcare Concepts and Personnel.*

Mills, A., Vaughan, J.P., Smith, D.L. and Tabibzadeh, I. 1990. *Health System Decentralization: Concepts, Issues and Country Experience*. Geneva: World Health Organization.

Mills, E.J, Schabas, W.A, Volmink, J. et al. 2008. Should active recruitment of health workers from sub-Saharan Africa be viewed as a crime?. *The Lancet*, 371, 685–8.

National Health Service. 2011. [Online]. Available at: http://www.nhsemployers.org.

Nieuwoudt, S. 2008. *South Africa Welcomes Cuban doctors*. IPS – Inter Press Service Africa.

Oberoi, S.S. and Lin, V. 2006. Brain drain of doctors from southern Africa: Brain gain for Australia. *Australian Health Review*, 30(1), 25–33.

Pagett, C. and Padarath, A. 2007. *A review of codes and protocols for the migration of health workers*. Health Systems Trust.

Pendleton, W., Crush, J. and Lefko-Everett, K. 2007. *The hemorrhage of health professionals from South Africa: Medical opinions*. Southern African Migration Project, 47, 1–38.

Reid, S. 2004. *Monitoring the effect of the new rural allowance for health professionals*. Health Systems Trust, 2–7.

Robinson, M. and Clark, P. 2008. Forging solutions to health worker migration. *The Lancet*, 371, 691–3.

Rogerson, C.M. 2007. Medical Recruits: The Temptation of South African Health Care Professionals. *Southern African Migration Report*, 45, 1–39.

Sanders, D. and Lloyd, B. 2009. *Major and focused investment in health personnel is needed to solve the Health Care Crisis*. [Online]. Available at: http://www.amandlapublishers.co.za/special-features/the-nhi-debate?start=15.

Schneider, H., Blaauw, D., Gilson, L. et al. 2006. 'Health Systems and Access to Antiretroviral Drugs for HIV in Southern Africa: Service Delivery and Human Resources Challenges'. *Reproductive Health Matters*, 14(27), 12–23.

Shiffman, J. 2009. A Social Explanation for the Rise and Fall of Global Health Issues. *Bulletin of the World Health Organisation*, 23(5), 308–17.

Shishana, O., Hall, E.J., Maluleke, R., Chauveau, J. and Schwabe, C. 2004. HIV/AIDS prevalence among South African health workers. *South African Medical Journal*, 94(10), 846–50.

South African Department of Health. 2004. Minutes of SA-UK Bilateral Forum Ministerial Meeting, 25 August 2004. [Online]. Available at: www.doh.gov.za/docs/pr/2004/pr0825.html.

Southern African Migration Programme. 2004. *Migration Resources: Brain drain resources.*

Tunisia.com. 2006. [Online]. Available at: http://www.Tunisia.com.

Tjadens, F., Weilandt, C. and Eckert, J., 2012. Mobility of Health Professionals: Health systems, work conditions, patterns of health workers' mobility and implications for policy makers, MOHProf summary report, viewed 12 September 2013, from http://www.mohprof.eu/LIVE/DATA/National_reports/national_report_Summary.pdf.

UNAIDS. 2004. *Three Ones Principles: Coordination of national Responses to HIV AIDS Guiding Principles for National Authorities and their Partners.* Geneva: UNAIDS.

UNAIDS. 2005. *The Three Ones in Action: Where We are and Where we go from Here.* Geneva: UNAIDS.

Van Damme, W., Kober, K. and Kegels, G. 2008. Scaling-up antiretroviral treatment in Southern African countries with human resource shortage: How will health systems adapt? *Social Science & Medicine*, 66, 2108–21.

Van Rensburg, D.H.C.J., Steyn, F., Schneider, H. and Loffstadt, L. 2008. Human resource development and antiretroviral treatment in Free State province, South Africa. *Human Resources for Health*, 6(15).

Wadee, H. and Khan, F. 2007. Human resources for health, in *South African Health Review 2007*, edited by S. Harrison, R. Bhana and A. Ntuli. Durban: Health Systems Trust. [Online]. Available at: http://www.hst.org.za/sahr.

Walt, G., Shiffman, J., Schneider, H. et al. 2008. Doing Health Policy Analysis: Methodological and Conceptual Reflections and Challenges. *Health Policy and Planning*, 2(6), 58–67.

Wildschut, A. and Mgqolozana, T. 2009. Nurses, in *Skills Shortage in South Africa: Case Studies of Key Professions*, edited J. Erasmus and M. Breier. Cape Town: HSRC Press.

WHO. 2003. The World Health Report 2003: Shaping the Future. Geneva: World Health Organization.

WHO. 2006a. The global shortage of health workers and its impact. [Online]. Available at: http://www.who.int/mediacentre/factsheets/fs302/en/index.html.

WHO. 2006b. The World Health Report 2006: Working together for health. Geneva: World Health Organisation, 2006. [Online]. Available at: http://www.who.int/whr/2006/en/.

WHO. 2006c. Taking stock: health worker shortages and the response to AIDS. [Online]. Available at: http://www.who.int/hiv/pub/advocacy/ttr/en/index.html.

WHO. 2007. Everybody business: strengthening health systems to improve health outcomes: WHO's framework for action. [Online]. Available at: http://www.who.int/healthsystems/strategy/everybodys_business.pdf.

WHO. 2008. Universal access report. [Online]. Available at: http://www.who/int.

Zachariah, R., Ford, N., Philips, M. et al. 2008. Task-shifting in HIV/AIDS: opportunities, challenges and proposed actions for sub-Saharan Africa. *Royal Society of Tropical, Medicine and Hygiene*. Available at: doi:10.1016/j.trstmh.2008.09.019.

# Chapter 9
# Wanting to Care:
# A Comparison of the Ethics of Health Worker
# Education in Cuba and the Philippines

Robert Huish

## Introduction

Global health inequity has never been worse. As a global community we live in a perverse geography lacking 4.3 million health workers while 2 billion people have no access to quality health care. Fifty thousand people die each day due to completely preventable causes (WHO 2006). Against such perilous health inequity the ability for a nation to train and retain health workers is imperative. Yet, many countries are unable to provide accessible and affordable health services for their populations, let alone keep hold of health professionals. In Cape Verde 54 per cent of physicians leave for service in other countries (World Bank 2011). One in every two physicians leave Fiji, and in Ethiopia, a country of 77 million people with a paucity of human resources for health and one of the highest incidences of maternal deaths in the world (19,347 mothers died in 2007), 25.6 per cent of physicians migrate (World Bank 2011; Gapminder 2012). It is widely assumed that difficult working conditions in resource poor countries, coupled with lucrative remuneration opportunities in countries like the US, Canada, the UK, Australia and New Zealand explain why so many physicians are involved in global migration. This narrative suggests that the migration of health professionals is the consequence of a spontaneous pipeline of health professionals who independently make rational choices to seek better work elsewhere (Ceniza Choy 2003). But the global movement of health workers is more dynamic. In some cases skilled professionals move between countries in the global South, and occasionally graduates from wealthy countries take positions in lower and middle-income countries.[1] While factors such as working conditions, lifestyle and remuneration are important, institutional cultures of medical education have been largely overlooked as important enablers of health worker migration. Medical education has a transformative effect on geographies of health and health care on a global scale.

While many countries in the global South struggle to maintain human resources for health, some nations have taken to specialising in training health workers for overseas service. Over 97 per cent of graduates from medical schools in Grenada and Dominica leave (World Bank 2011). Wealthier nations like Ireland and Israel are now taking to

---

1 Admittedly, this is a small number in comparison to the massive outpouring of physicians from countries like India. However there is an increasing trend for health workers to practice in the Gulf States, like Qatar or the UAE, or to work in the private 'medical tourism' sector in India or Thailand. In some cases these health workers are nationals returning home after having received medical education in the global North.

recruiting high-paying medical students from the United States so that they may return to practice in North America under International Medical Graduate programmes (Sullivan 2000). In other cases, medical schools like Dalhousie University in Halifax, Nova Scotia, Canada have sold out their own medical school seats, usually reserved for nationals, to Saudi Arabia even though those spaces could help to ease the tension of 50,000 Nova Scotians who are without family doctors (Moultan 2002; Birchard 2011). While these schools have put a particular focus on building health worker capacity from affluent medical students who would then work in affluent settings, two countries in the global South have positioned their health worker training programmes to address broader geographies of health and health care.

Since the 1960s, both Cuba and the Philippines have worked to develop human resources for health for service abroad. While the geographies served by both countries vary significantly, there is an analogous tendency for these governments to encourage the training of human resources for health for service abroad with the understanding that it produces domestic benefits. In the Philippines this is meant to come in the form of remittance, while in Cuba compensation comes through a more complicated socio-political process best titled 'medical internationalism' (Huish and Kirk 2007). In both countries the institutional ethics of medical education is important in designing the patterns of outmigration of health workers, and also in influencing, if not determining, domestic geographies of health equity. This chapter looks at the impacts Cuba and the Philippines are having on the global health landscape. Both countries are harnessing their domestic capacity for outreach, but they are doing so under two unique economic and political rubrics. As a result, both Cuba and the Philippines are playing a role in negotiating uneven geographical development both abroad and at home.

Cuba and the Philippines have situated the training of health care workers as an opportunistic response to a massive global need for health care professionals. The strategies of both countries are seemingly a means of furthering their own national interests while trying to respond to a pressing global demand. The ability to generate remittance, remuneration, building capacity, and global solidarity are sought after goals in both cases. Yet there are noticeable differences. Namely Cuba's state-organised medical internationalism address health care inequities in marginalised areas of the global South through bilateral cooperation in a way that affords benefits to its own domestic health service. On the other hand the 'Overseas Filipino Worker' (OFW) programmes in the Philippines employ free-market principles to bring in enormous remittance contributions. The Philippines ranks number four in countries that receive the most remittance dollars. China and India receive about $21 billion each in remittance. Mexico brings in $18.1 billion, and the Philippines garnered in $11.6 billion in 2004 (Castles and Miller 2009, 60). These payments and the catered training of health workers, most notably nurses, may benefit the national economy through increased purchasing power of individuals and families, but cash does little to address growing social inequities within the country's own domestic health sector. As this chapter will show, the Filipino model of exporting health services is widely recognised as generating much-needed income for the country, but Cuba's managed medical internationalism may be a better situated approach to alleviating global health inequity while furthering its own national health needs. The value of this comparison is that at a time when many nations, rich or poor, are struggling to fulfil their human resources for health needs, the Philippines model may be more greatly recognised as an income earner, but the Cuban case presents an important example of cross-border health cooperation that goes beyond income generation to address dire socio-economic inequities that result from neoliberal globalisation.

## A Global Conundrum

The World Health Organisation estimates that 4.3 million health workers are needed in order to ensure global health care equity (WHO 2006). Wealthy countries have a far better chance of coping with uneven development, as they are often better positioned to retain their own health workers and to receive internationally trained workers. In 2000 India, a country with one physician for every 1,886 people lost 20,000 physicians to emigration. The Philippines, with a similar ratio of one physician to 1,724 people, lost 9,000 physicians that same year. South Africa has lost half of its medical graduates (Pang 2002) and some estimates suggest that 30 per cent of the South African physician workforce has left for Europe, North America and Australia (Ncayiyana 1999). Chen et al. found that of 146 medical schools in 40 sub-Saharan African countries, 26 per cent of physicians emigrated from their home country within five years of their graduation (Chen et al. 2012). Over 20 per cent of the Haitian physician workforce left in 2000, and in Somalia one in every four doctors leaves. In a country where there is one physician for every 25,000, the exodus of one doctor makes a dire health care landscape all the more hopeless (World Bank 2011).

The migration of health workers from the global South to the global North has increased dramatically in the last decade. A broad range of issues explains this. Austerity measures in many health systems in the global South have resulted in poor paying, exhausting and demoralising work environments for skilled health workers. A Ghanaian physician claimed that he was expected to see 200 patients a day in his clinic over a 12-hour period (personal communication 2012). The disparity in earnings between low-paying salaries in the global South compared to lucrative fee-for-service health care systems in Europe and North America is enormous. While a general practitioner working for the public system in Ecuador may receive $300 a month in salary, a family doctor in Ontario, Canada can easily bill a provincial health system $16,000 a month (CMAJ 2004). The economic benefits of outmigration to individuals and their families are significant when such an increase in earnings is involved. The World Bank figures that emigrants contributed $75 billion annually to remittance (World Bank 2011). While there is no way to break down the figure to show how much is contributed by health workers alone, it is clear that there is an ever-increasing number of international health workers who participate in remittance trends.

Despite economic distribution of wealth to the South through remittance, the social consequences of outmigration of health workers have been devastating to many countries in the global South. The United Nations Commission for Trade and Development estimates that each health worker to leave Africa brings an economic loss of $184,000, when considering the amount of public resources that goes into training the health professional (Oyowe 1996). The hopeless doctor to patient ratios of one physician for every 50,000 in countries like Malawi or Mozambique are inconceivable against ratios of one physician for every 227 people in Italy, or one physician for every 256 people in Israel – a system that provides universal health care access for its citizens. This division is only furthered in many countries in the global South, as private fee-for-service care becomes a prohibitive measure against ensuring universal access for the poor. As well, the retention of practicing physicians is one challenge, an even greater dilemma is how to retain medical instructors (Mufunda et al. 2007). The Gambia was completely without capacity to train medical professionals until 2000, thanks to Cuban cooperation.

The working conditions of many health centres in the global South can be demoralising. Wards with three patients per bed, poorly stocked pharmacies, lacking diagnostic equipment, poor cleaning standards for internal medicine equipment and in some cases the conscientious placement of the morgue next to the maternity wing.[2] All of these factors combine to create a working culture of martyrdom, for which the health care worker must bear onerous strain in order to provide the most basic level of service. The organisation of space within many poorly funded health care systems in the global South directly challenges the capabilities of health care professionals to properly care for patients. In many poorly-funded systems, the organisation of medical space is more conducive to providing limited care, furthering suffering and ultimately demoralising health workers.

### Cosmopolitan Ethics of Migration

While the consequences of the migration pipeline of health workers out of resource poor countries are devastating to the capacity of health systems in the global South, the brain drain is still largely tolerated, if not encouraged. Many health systems justify the recruitment of physicians out of resource-poor areas as a noble move, one that will provide salvation and empowerment to the fortunate migrating health worker (Ineseon and Seeling 2005). The underlying assumption is that because health systems in the global South are so dire it must be a natural desire for workers to want to leave. Ineson and Seeling have even suggested the idea of a 'medical passport' that expedites the migration process of workers from the South into northern health systems. Because many health care systems in the South are underfunded and inadequate to satisfy the quality of life desired by physicians, accepting health workers from resource-poor nations is meant to facilitate one's fundamental right to work and to enjoy an adequate standard of living (Labonte et al. 2006).

This justification of brain drain employs Rawls' Equality of Opportunity principle (Rawls 1999). If a qualified physician working in sub-Saharan Africa is just as capable as a Swiss physician, then why should he or she be denied the appropriate remuneration and quality of life as his or her European colleague? The cosmopolitan notion of equality of merit, regardless of location, provides the ethical justification for brain drain. Some medical schools, according to Astor et al. go as far as intentionally prepping and streaming their students for migration out of their country (Astor et al. 2005). For cosmopolitans it would be unethical to restrict the movement of a skilled individual to pursue their craft in the best-situated location of their free choosing. Indeed, the restriction of movement for an individual can present numerous ethical challenges. Some countries like Cuba or Jamaica have stringent exit requirements for skilled personnel that may involve the denial of a passport or expensive exit visas. In other cases some health worker licensing boards require mandatory service contracts for graduates in order for them to receive their qualifications. Nurses in the Philippines are now required to spend two years in domestic service before migrating abroad (ANSAP 2008). In Ecuador, physicians must contribute one year to a rural service post in order to be fully licensed within the country (Huish 2008). While these policies are intended to maintain national capacity, there are limitations to the long-term effectiveness of forced retention. First, state-level restrictions on the movement of skilled individuals do not necessarily guarantee that health workers will practice in their field or

---

2    When visiting a medical centre in Western Uganda I was informed that having the morgue next to the maternity wing made sense from the point of view of hospital administration, as that is where the highest rate of mortality occurred.

in areas where they are needed. Second, forced retention for qualification of a license or a degree has serious limitations on building long-term sustainable health care in marginalised communities. Often forced retention involves recently graduated, and at times, under confidant, health workers placed in extremely challenging rural or poverty-stricken areas. Many persons in forced-retention programmes are there because of necessity rather than desire. When reluctant health workers face demanding expectations in the field the result is resentment of the placement rather than eagerness to seek out long-term sustainable practice. For marginalised communities, the primary line of health care services is limited to novice health workers who would have their sights set on work elsewhere.

Under the cosmopolitan framework there are clearly normative dilemmas in suggesting that a health worker's movement should be restricted. If an individual yearns to seek out their personal ambitions and desires, state or bureaucratic mandates to prevent them mobility access to their good life are clearly taken as an authoritarian limitation on individual liberties. Cosmopolitanism can also suggest that it would be appropriate to ensure that the good life of the European physician could be made available in Malawi. This might include the creation of rewarding work environments, access to resources, leisure and cultural engagement. Indeed, this argument could be employed to call for greater retention programmes and greater spending to create the sort of affluent conditions in the South that are often thought to be desirable in the North.

What if, however, a health worker wants to work in a marginalised area? What if it is the ambition and desire for a health worker to serve a vulnerable community? The dismissive response may be to say, 'what is stopping them?'. If a health worker wants to serve the marginalised there is certainly plenty of need for it, and in some cases little competition. But can a health worker practice in a marginalised area so that he or she can fulfil professional obligations and pursue a good life? The cosmopolitan approach suggests that if it is the desire of an individual to serve the poor, then it is morally justified to seek policies that transform geographies so he or she can do so without excessive burden or personal risk. But some caution is needed here. If the material conditions in Switzerland are to be reproduced in Malawi then it could involve the influx of costly resources, equipment and commodities in order to mirror the quality of Swiss life. For a country like Malawi it would be incredibly burdensome to reposition health spending to improve the comfort of life for its current 266 physicians on the lifestyle expectations of a physician in Geneva, all the while the majority of the 12.8 million Malawians remain isolated and removed from reliable access to health care (WHO 2006). The more fitting question then is whether it is possible to position policy so that the quality of life for a Malawian physician can be one that satisfies the moral grounds of happiness in the job, quality care, leisure time and self-fulfillment, rather than just looking at the material differences in lifestyle to that of the European colleague? Can the cosmopolitan approach go beyond advocating for better quality of life for the health worker to actually improving the conditions of care in marginalised settings?

Indeed it can, if there is an acceptance that the needs of care in marginalised communities do not require costly infrastructure inputs in order to meet patient's needs and in order for health care workers to achieve a good life. The constrains against health care delivery in marginalised areas often comes down to the lack of basic infrastructure, poor community-level education, social support for health workers, and integration of care into urban or centralised health systems. Often the health worker faces long hours, poor resources, meagre pay and an inability to fulfil patient's needs over simple dilemmas such as a lack of medicine, a lack of clean water, or a lack of decent housing. Such service embodies sacrifice and detracts from an individual's professional commitments and moral responsibilities to care for individuals. It inhibits the good life of health workers, but for reasons that require minimal inputs in infrastructure or community-level support. Because health care to the marginalised falls short of meeting patient's needs, or fulfilling health worker expectations, it is not often a choice that allows individuals to seek out the good life on the same moral level as health workers who practice in affluent centres. In the current global health landscape service to the marginalised is often closer to personal sacrifice albeit martyrdom.

Considering the cosmopolitan position that individuals should be able to fulfil the good life where and how they want, then it is possible to interpret the lacking social and infrastructural support in marginalised communities as a restriction of choice for health workers. Rawlsian thinkers would identify policies that restrict movement of health workers as incongruent to the values of the global equality of opportunity principle. Likewise, a lack of conditions to fulfil a doctor's good life would be seen as a failure to this principle. But the same case can be made to suggest that the lack of supportive policies to enable health workers to practice in vulnerable communities is an infringement on their choice, their potentials and their abilities to fulfil their vision of the good life. Because service to the marginalised entails numerous hardships to the health worker, it is hardly an even keeled moral choice. Governments and medical schools have responded for the call of health workers to leave resource-poor settings, but exceptionally little has been done to facilitate the choice for health workers to stay in those settings. How can measures be taken to allow health workers the choice to serve the vulnerable that allows individuals to fulfil the good life, but does not necessarily require the reproduction of elaborate lifestyle expectations of affluent health workers in the global North?

Looking at policies in Cuba and the Philippines can illuminate the question of quelling the global migration pipeline. These countries have sought to control and disperse human resources for health abroad. In both cases, efforts are made to facilitate the broader range of a health worker's desire to serve in a global context. The Philippines has structured its OFW programme in a manner that greatly affords 'free choice' of health workers to immigrate, but does very little to address geographies of health inequity at home. Cuba, on the other hand maintains steadfast attention to its domestic health needs while positioning a portion of its health workforce into global service. While market-based choice for individual health workers is limited in the Cuban case, compared to the Philippines, the benefits for career fulfilment, national priorities and strategic positioning appear to be far stronger.

## Chronicles of Care from the Philippines

Filipino nurses represent 50 per cent of all internationally educated nurses in the United States, 46 per cent in the United Kingdom and 30 per cent in Canada. An estimated total of more than 150,000 Filipino nurses work in over 80 countries (Lorenzo et al. 2007). The Philippines has been the number one source of international nurses in the last 50 years (Ceniza Choy 2003). Since the 1960s the Philippines has worked to develop the expansion of OFW nurses. Along with other countries like Turkey, the Philippines positioned its capacity to train professionals for export in the hope that remittance payments from OFWs would stimulate economic growth at home (Castles and Miller 2009, 51). A weak currency and a comparatively low cost of living help to facilitate the economic benefit of remittance income. There have been cases of bilateral recruitment from the British National Health Service, the Irish health system, and in recent years by Canada, South Korea, Saudi Arabia and other gulf states. Hospitals in the United States have participated in the direct recruitment of Filipino nurses (Lorezno et al. 2007). The annual salary of a nurse working in the public system in the Philippines can range between $2,000 and $2,400 annually. Comparatively a Filipino nurse working in San Diego can expect to receive between $48,000 and $62,000 a year in salary. By sending two days' pay home a month, OFW nurses can double the earnings he or she would have made working in country.

According to Ceniza Choy, the emphasis for the outmigration of Filipino nurses extends beyond economic development strategies in the 1960s to earlier processes of US imperialism. The establishment of nurse training programmes in the Philippines begins at the turn of the twentieth century with American women taking on education roles after the 'Spanish-American War'.[3] As Ceniza Choy suggests, establishing nursing schools 'provided White American women a sense of purpose in the new colony' (Ceniza Choy 2003, 23). For American women nurse training in the Philippines was taken as 'an international avenue for heroism', yet it reinforced dominant colonial mentalities of health and wellbeing (Ceniza Choy 2003, 23). The establishment of early nurse training programmes created the dominant narrative of Filipino nurses being competent, compassionate and caring. As Tan suggests, there is a stereotype of Filipino nurses being 'joyous, smiling, yet dedicated and committed' to their practice (personal communication with Tan 2009). These cultural attributes facilitated a targeted demand for nurses in Europe and North America by the 1960s. The need for skilled nurses was outstripping local capacities in countries like the United Kingdom and the United States, and as a result Filipinos provided a 'critical source of labour' for industrialised countries (Ceniza Choy 2003, 2).

A cultural acceptance in the global North of Filipino nurses as compassionate caregivers, coupled with modernist economic development strategies to bolster Gross Domestic Product (GDP) through remittance services positioned Filipino nursing schools as fulfilling a global market demand. Between 1995 and 2000, over 34,000 Filipino nurses were OFW. In 2003, 163,756 Filipino nurses were working in 80 countries. Meanwhile only 29,466 nurses remained in country to meet the needs of roughly 94 million people, which is one nurse for every 3,199 people (Lorenzo et al. 2007). By comparison Canada, a country close to one third of the population of the Philippines has 252,000 registered nurses, which is one nurse for every 142 people. There are currently over 460 nurse colleges that offer degrees in the Philippines. Over 20,000 nurses graduate in the country every year (Lorenzo et al. 2007). In 2008, 31,275 nurses passed the Philippines Nurse Licensure Examinations. Yet only 2,500 domestic positions were available to them (DOLE, 2012). The government contributes a paltry 1.4 per cent of the national budget to health care (Gapminder.org 2012). Even though there is enormous domestic need for Filipino nurses, along with health workers, the government does not position capacity building towards local needs. Parts of the country such as Malapasuca Island have no licensed physicians and the nearest hospital is several hours away. In 2010 seven out of every 10 Filipinos died without seeing a health professional (Harris Cheng 2009).

Because the push for remittance is so strong within the Philippines, accounting for 12 per cent of the GDP, the government has not acted to position health worker services for domestic needs (World Bank, 2011). The ethics of health worker education in the country,

---

3    The commonly adapted name to this conflict saw US forces battle Spanish troops in the Americas and South East Asia. In the Philippines the greatest loss of life was with Filipinos slaughtered by US troops. The number of Spanish casualties in this conflict was incredibly low by comparison.

notably for nurses, directly encourages graduates to seek employment abroad. Within the training process it is assumed that the top students will seek employment elsewhere, and that to stay within the country, serving poor regions for poor pay, is a failure of merit and expectations. In some cases entire communities will pool their monetary resources together in order to train a young girl as a nurse in one of the costly private nursing schools in Manila. The expectation is that she will migrate abroad, repay the debt, and contribute a steady stream of remittance to the local community. Furthermore, many nursing programmes are sensitive to building cross-cultural competency for nurses. This includes education in English, or caring for patients in Islamic centres. Ultimately when a nurse migrates and begins to send remittance home she or he is venerated as a national hero. Even in the Manila airport OFWs are given preferential treatment through security and customs.

The Philippines has the greatest nurse training capacity anywhere on the planet. Yet they also suffer from a dangerous lack of human resources for health to the point where most Filipinos can expect to die without the care of a skilled health worker. The choice to train thousands of nurses for export reflects a moral perception that it is in the national interest to garner a portion of the GDP from foreign remittances rather than direct health care capacity for the immediate needs of the population. This is a telling example of how governments choose to value economic progress to the direct consequence of their population's health needs. For 12 per cent of the GDP the consequence is that 70 per cent of Filipinos will have no medical assistance on their deathbeds. The 12 per cent GDP contribution does not meet the needs of the marginalised, nor will it trickle down to help those in need (Asis 2008). The Philippines have fulfilled the cosmopolitan value of enabling movement abroad, but it has not created the conditions to meet the needs of those who want to stay in the country. When a health worker leaves the Philippines, and he or she is venerated as a national hero to further the national economy the poor are expected to take on an enormous sacrifice from the lack of quality care that they can expect to receive.

The outpouring of Filipino nurses continues. The United States is still the largest receiver of Filipino workers, at about 3.5 million residing in the country. Saudi Arabia has over 1.1 million working in health, construction and domestic service although the Saudis instituted a hiring freeze on maids (The Economist 2011). Malaysia is the third largest émigré community with roughly 900,000, and countries including Canada, Japan, Australia, Qatar and Spain have over 250,000 OFWs within each country. Still, the demand of OFWs continues to grow. The new government in Libya has posted a request for 1,700 Filipino nurses (Jaymalin 2012).

The migration process for a nurse to enter a new country and obtain licensed accreditation is much more straightforward than it is for physicians. A physician who immigrates to the United States could have to spend as much as four years re-qualifying under local licensing and practice boards. A nurse, however, can be pre-accepted to a position in the United States provided that he or she has written and passed the qualifying exams. This has led to a curious phenomenon in the Philippines of physicians retraining as nurses in order to enter the migration pipeline. As of 2003, 3,000 physicians had qualified as nurses. As of 2006 another 4,000 physicians were in nursing programmes, many of them catered to the physician's schedule so they can attend classes on weekends. The Public Health Authority of the Philippines estimates that 80 per cent of public sector physicians have qualified as nurses (Lorenzo et al. 2007). Not only does this career-change exodus represent the dominant cultural push for health workers seeking options elsewhere, it also greatly endangers the sustainability of the health care system in the Philippines. With such an enormous flight out of the public health sector, the country stands against great odds in being able to maintain the basic structures of a functioning health care system, let alone meet the needs of the marginalised.

In a sense the push to invest in migration has brought the Filipino health care system near collapse. Not only has the intensive outmigration drained the country of much-needed human resources for health; it has also compromised the retention of highly-skilled physicians and administrators to manage the complex needs of a national service. The end result from this process is that the Philippines have effectively compromised domestic capacity through economic models that favour out migration for remittance as an inherently positive driver of national wealth. While the income per capita in the Philippines may have doubled from $1,500 per person in 1960 to $3,200 in 2009, the rate of economic growth has not transformed into effective policy decisions to improve, let alone maintain, basic social services. A half century after the big push for OFWs, the Philippines remains fixed into the migration pipeline with detrimental results for social capacity and inequitable geographies of health and health care.

## The Cuban Alternative

Since about roughly the same time that the Philippines has been exporting its human resources for health Cuba has developed an ambitious programme best labelled 'medical internationalism'. Since the onset of the Cuban revolution, this resource-poor country has been sending its own human resources for health overseas to some of the most vulnerable communities in the world. Unlike the Filipino model where the motivation comes through remittance, the Cuban programmes retain health workers as employees and expect them to return home when their brigade (mission) is over. The Cuban model is not open to market forces in the same way as the OFW. Rather, Cuban medical internationalism is a carefully organised bilateral project that builds cooperation with other countries struggling to overcome underdevelopment (Feinsilver, 1993; Kirk and Erisman 2009). Some of these outreach programmes have been enormously costly, and at times have put strains and tensions on the Cuban system. Still medical internationalism has managed to achieve notable goals. First, it has facilitated access to health care in vulnerable communities abroad that have traditionally been overlooked. Second, it has worked to garner political and monetary gains through bilateral relations.

Cuba's first international medical outreach offering went to Chile in 1960 following a devastating earthquake that crippled Santiago. In 1961 Cuba sent its first international medical team to Algeria to provide care to combatants in the civil war. In 1970 a medical team travelled to Peru following an earthquake there. The team constructed six rural hospitals in the country and brought in over 100,000 units of blood. In 1972, despite enormous political hostility with the Somoza government, Cuba sent in a medical team, food, and medicines to assist in the aftermath of an earthquake that rocked Lima (Huish and Kirk 2007).

Neighbourly response and outreach to natural disasters is quite common in any region of the world. But there are two notable issues with the early Cuban response. First, Cuba was deeply isolated from many countries and international organisations like the Organisation of American States in the 1960s and the 1970s. The governments that Cuba sent emergency relief to were tremendously hostile to the Castro regime. Nicaragua went as far to provide military support and assistance for attacks against the Cuban government in the 1960s. Yet, Cuba's outreach acted as a means of health diplomacy (Feinsivler 1993).

Second, Cuba went through enormously challenging circumstances. In 1962, after it was announced by the government that Cuban physicians could no longer bill patients directly for services, half of roughly 6,000 physicians left the country (Feinsivler 1993). The University of Havana's medical teaching staff were reduced in number from over 200 to 12. This incredible loss to a medical and training system that had a century's long reputation as being the most advanced in Latin America was devastating. With the revolution's goal to provide universal health care to every Cuban citizen, regardless of location, each and every health worker mattered enormously. Still, the Cuban government chose to offer opportunities for physicians to work abroad in medical missions. The government embarked on an ambitious training campaign for human resources for health, which included commitments to assist other resource-poor countries facing similar struggles of under development.

Since the 1990s, Cuban medical internationalism evolved from providing emergency relief and technical assistance to building health care capacity in under-resourced settings. Following the collapse of the Soviet Union in 1993, Cuba faced brutal economic conditions. The country's GDP dropped by 35 per cent in a year. Cuba lost 87 per cent of its exports, and was denied credit to import basic goods like food and medicine. Hard currency became scarce and resource shortages plagued the entire nation. The country endured rolling black outs, lacked medicine, failed transportation sector, and enormous social hardships. Whereas most economists figured that Cuba would collapse under such economic pressure, the government defied traditional logic of austerity and actually scaled up its facilities to train human resources for health (Cole 1998). The country expanded medical school enrolment and did not close a single hospital or training facility. Before the crisis, Cuba had one physician for every 277 people. By 1998, thanks to the expansion of enrolment in medical schools, the country boasted one physician for every 189 people – the best doctor to patient ratio anywhere in the world.

With such a tremendous scaling up of training capacity for human resources for health, Cuba opened its cooperation efforts to include students from countries in the Caribbean and Africa. Foreign students trained alongside Cuban students in the county's 23 medical schools. In some cases foreign students paid modest tuition and in other cases the Cuban government provided scholarships.

In 1999, in response to Hurricanes Mitch and George that ravaged Central America and Haiti, Cuba constructed *The Escuela Latinoamericana de Medicina* (ELAM) to exclusively receive foreign students from affected regions for a free six-year medical education. The Cuban government converted a former naval academy into a medical school in under a year. Students were, and still are, offered a full scholarship, accommodation, meals, a small living allowance, supplies and clothing. The Cuban government does not restrict the movement of these students after graduation and has no forced retention projects. Instead, the school operates under a moral commitment to return students to areas of their home country where they are needed the most. Students initially came from the regions affected by the hurricane, but the scholarship later opened up to students from around the globe by 2001. As of 2013 ELAM received over 19,000 students from 110 different countries, including affluent countries like Canada and the United States.

Based on findings from a 2008 study, many graduates had difficulty securing placement in rural and vulnerable areas of their home countries. In Ecuador, students who returned to the country in 2006–2007 faced enormous difficulties in securing long-term rural service contracts. Due to austerity measures taken by the Ecuadorian government, ELAM graduates were not offered long-term contracts for rural service. As a result many had to seek alternative placements. For the graduates who returned to Ecuador some went to secure residency placements with Ecuadorian medical schools, others went to serve alongside outreach brigades in rural areas, others returned to Cuba for additional education, but none went to the private sector or sought out migration to countries like Chile – where Ecuadorian physicians are widely received.

Not only is ELAM scaling up the training of physicians to levels the world has never seen before by a single medical programme, the institutional ethics of the institution are repositioning health workers to seek out service in marginalised, albeit trying conditions. This is a stridently different sort of internationalism than that of the Philippines case. The Cuban model effectively piggybacks international outreach on its own domestic capacities. While ELAM requires significant financial resources from the government in order to operate, it does so without compromising domestic training programmes or limiting access to care for its own population. The Cuban government considers ELAM a strategy in diplomacy, outreach, and solidarity with other countries. There are numerous challenges in ensuring that ELAM graduates can secure employment in resource poor settings in their home countries, but the Cuban government does not get directly involved with the placements of graduates in other countries. Still, this is the beginning of a process of replenishing human resources for health in areas that have often been punished through the migration pipeline. It is, in the cosmopolitan sense, offering that choice to serve the poor rather than being solely pushed into furthering the brain drain.

In addition to ELAM, Cuba offers medical internationalism in a wide range of areas. Cuban doctors working with mission Milagro have restored eyesight to over 1.6 million people in the Caribbean, South America and Africa for no charge. Cuba's Henry Reeve Brigade has provided emergency relief for Guatemala, Pakistan, China, Bolivia, Indonesia and Haiti following disasters in those countries. After providing one year of relief services for Pakistan, Cuba offered 1,000 scholarships for Pakistani students to enrol in the ELAM programme. The brigade continues to provide assistance in Haiti alongside 2,000 Cuban health workers who will remain in Haiti on a rotating basis for 8 years. As well, Cuba currently has comprehensive health brigades and medical education cooperation with 76 countries. In 2012, 36,000 Cuban health workers were operating abroad. Over 19,000 workers are posted in Venezuela as part of a bilateral agreement. With all of these countries there is an expectation of bilateral cooperation. Most nations that have partnered with Cuba agree to take on certain costs. In the case of comprehensive medical brigades the host country is expected to cover transportation, accommodation, a living allowance, and salary for the health workers. The Cuban government also contributes to the physician's salary. In certain cases the government will make direct financial contributions to the Cuban government, but for resource poor nations like The Gambia or Haiti, little remuneration is expected. This model of shared responsibility positions Cuba's outreach not as aid, but as mutually responsible capacity building to alleviate resource shortfalls with income generation, even in modest amounts.

This enormous global outreach wins Cuba political favour throughout the global South. Medical internationalism has warmed relations with traditionally hostile countries like Guatemala, Uruguay, and even South Africa – a country Cuba was at war with during the Apartheid conflict in Angola. Beyond medical internationalism, Cuba has also set up cooperation programmes in sport, art, education, technical assistance, and business in 141 countries. Against the pressures of the US embargo, Cuba has a dedicated interest in building strategic partnerships with other nations in the global South. In some cases the bilateral cooperation can mount to political support in forums like the Organisation of

American States or the United Nations for policies favourable to Cuba, such as lobbying for the termination of the US embargo.

Cuba's internationalism is often conjoined to bilateral financial cooperation between countries. Other than the disaster and emergency relief programmes, Cuba's cooperation programmes do not run as pure aid. For the long-term service of health workers working abroad, Cuba negotiates financial retribution packages from the host government. Venezuela has offered Cuba preferential trading rights on oil, for the receipt of thousands of health workers. Cuba is able to import oil from Venezuela on an extremely generous line of credit. South Africa, China, Saudi Arabia, and Qatar all offer direct cash payments to the Cuban government for the services of their health workers, in addition to covering their salaries and costs of living. Lower- and middle-income countries may or may not pay Cuba directly in hard cash, but all are expected to offer some form of solidarity contribution that would alleviate economic strain in Cuba. In some cases this can be preferential purchasing of raw material or finished goods. For example in 2008, Guatemala exported commodities to Cuba at preferred rates, which supplied government-run stores across the country. Resource-poor countries like Haiti, Bolivia and The Gambia have benefited enormously from the presence of Cuban health workers in their countries. But, the Cuban government does not expect the sort of remuneration from these economically hobbled nations as it would from an oil-rich nation like Qatar. For receipt of hundreds of Cuban health workers, Bolivia has allowed Cuba to purchase Bolivian goods and resources in Bolivianos rather than US dollars. The Gambia has benefited from the presence of Cuban physicians who helped to establish the country's first medical school and who led an ambitious programme against malaria. The economically hobbled nation included Cuba as a preferred trading partner for its peanut exports. Haiti, a country that still struggles to develop from the brutal 2010 earthquake and that is still saddled with foreign debt does not pay Cuba for its services. Rather, the costs are offset through contributions and assistance from other Caribbean nations.

In sum, Cuba's outreach is dynamic, controlled, and at the political level seeks both monetary and political benefits for itself through altruistic cooperation. The funds raised on medical missions abroad contribute to public services in Cuba, primarily health care and education services. Cuban health workers who go abroad receive modest, but still greater salary than they would have if they had remained in country. The financial opportunities for doctors to work abroad are numerous, and for those who remain in country this can create tensions against colleagues who are earning significantly more than the contemptible $30 a month in-country salary. Because Cuba has maintained tight control of its medical internationalism, it has been able to obtain remuneration from overseas partners and direct it at national priority areas like health and education. Through this model of sharing its human resources for health with other countries in the South, Cuba is able to use its domestic capacity for transformative international outreach.

**Two Visions of Mobile Health Workers**

Cuba and the Philippines both position their health care workforce as willing and able to meet global demands. No other countries have trained more health workers for international service. In both cases the governments argue that it is in the best interests of the nation to have health workers leave home for service abroad. The contrasts between these two models are enormous. The Philippines yearns for economic growth through remittance, while Cuba seeks managed remuneration through cooperation with other countries in the global South. The Filipino workforce aims for opportunities in centres of affluence, while Cuban health workers journey to remote and marginalised areas of the global South. The Philippines is training its own nationals for export, while Cuba trains foreigners alongside its own nationals.

The Cuban model not only generates much needed revenue for the country, but also strategic political and trade alliances with other countries in the global South. It is in many ways a careful strategy of soft-power (Nye 2008). By positioning its own national strength into foreign policy, Cuba effectively built strategic alliances around the world. Still, Cuba continues to struggle with resource shortfalls and the perils of lacking infrastructural development. Material resources can run into short supply in Cuba, and this can have a negative effect on the quality of health care, or more broadly speaking, the functionality of social services in the country. Despite the continuous challenge to acquire wealth and resources, Cuba has not abandoned its social commitments to its population. Services may be short on material resources, but they are never completely forfeited. In essence, the Cuban government realised it had limited material resources and took steps to invest in human resources. The results have resulted in a global medical outreach and a robust domestic health sector that sends health workers to vulnerable and marginalised places.

By contrast the Philippines continues to bleed itself dry of human resources for health. Notably, the remittances do contribute to the overall economy of the country, but this development strategy fails to compensate for the deep social impacts of lacking domestic human resources for health. Remittances tend to gravitate to the individual or family level, and in some cases to the community level. But with such deep impacts on the health system, remittance alone cannot muster the capacity to retain health workers, let alone work to expand coverage. The laissez-faire approach to outmigration in the Philippines has created new proposals of bilateral cooperation from some of the Philippines leading health authorities.

Jaime Galvez-Tan, President of Health Futures Inc., a group dedicated to improving health outcomes and equity in the Philippines, has proposed that the country move towards forming bilateral agreements with destination countries (personal communication, April 2009). The agreements would call for greater transparency of the recruiting process, and for the establishment of bilateral relations to insist that destination countries compensate the Philippines for the massive exodus of trained professionals. This could occur through the construction of specialised training facilities, or through the financing of retention programmes for domestic service. Galvez-Tan's approach is to ensure that the needs of migrant workers are met, all the while ensuring greater compensation for the Philippines in the form of partnerships to offset the damage of too few human resources for health needs in the country. The focus of bilateral agreements would be to ensure that the rights of migrant workers are met. The value of remittance is still at the heart of the proposal, and by no means is it a step towards a Cuban approach to bilateral relations. Rather, this is the first step in realising that some sort of policy and regulation is needed to mitigate the damage of the brain drain. The unbridled release of human resources for health has come at the expense of the needs of the poor and marginalised.

## Concluding Thoughts

The global need for human resources for health is enormous. Both Cuba and Philippines have positioned their health care workforce to respond to international needs. In the Philippines case, the focus is on acquiring cash by having nurses serve the affluent. Cuba's approach is to garner monetary and political support through bilateral trade relations. As this chapter has shown, the Filipino model has devastated the domestic health care system, while the Cuban approach is better positioned to meet the needs of vulnerable populations abroad while maintaining health care integrity at home. Even though Cuba suffers from material resource shortfalls, the state's ability to manage and regulate its medical internationalism is ultimately beneficial to Cuba's national needs, when compared to the Philipines' system that encourages massive outmigration in the hopes of remittance payments.

The message from this comparison is that regulation of some form is needed in both managing the training of human resources for health and for placing health workers into international geographies of care. If it is possible for poor countries like The Gambia to contribute peanuts back to Cuba for the receipt of health care services, in this case the contribution is literally peanuts, then it should be possible for resource-flush nations that drive the brain drain to contribute assistance to countries like the Philippines that have contributed enormously to the migration pipeline. Health care inequity exists not only between rich and poor nations, but also between the rich and poor of all nations. Both Cuba and the Philippines demonstrate that it is possible to muster the political will to train a global health workforce. The challenge that remains is finding a way to regulate the system so that it is capable of offering the ability for health workers to serve the marginalised as much as it is wanting the receipt of wealth from the export care givers.

## References

Asis, M. 2008. How international migration can support development: A challenge for the Philippines, in *Migration and Development: Perspectives from the South*, edited by S. Castles and R. Delgado Wise. Geneva: International Organisation for Migration, 175–201.

Association of Nursing Service Administrators of the Philippines, Inc. 2008. *Standards of nursing service*. Quezon City: ANSAP – Committee on Nursing Practice.

Astor, A., Akhtar T., Matallana M.A. et al. 2005. Physician migration: Views from professionals in Colombia, Nigeria, India, Pakistan and the Philippines. *Social Science & Medicine*, 61(12), 2492–500.

Birchard, K. 2011. Dalhousie university says it will sell medical school places to Saudi Arabia. *The Chronicle of Higher Education*.

Castles, S. and Miller, M. 2009. *The Age of Migration*. New York: The Guilford Press.

Ceniza Choy, C. 2003. *Empire of Care: Nursing and Migration in Filipino American History*. Quezon City: Ateneo de Manila University Press.

Chen, C., Buch, E., Wasserman, T. et al. 2012. A survey of sub-Saharan African medical schools. *Human Resources for Health*, 10(4).

CMAJ. 2004. Physician billing highest in Ontario, lowest in Quebec. *Canadian Medical Association Journal*, 170(5), 776.

Cole, K. 1998. *Cuba: From Revolution to Development.* London: Pinter.

Department of Labour and Employment (DOLE). 2012. [Online]. Available at: http://www. dole.gov.ph/.

Feinsilver, J.M. 1993. *Healing the Masses: Cuban Health Politics at Home and Abroad.* Berkeley: University of California Press.

Gapminder Foundation. 2012. *Gapminder world.* [Online]. Available at: www.gapminder. org.

Harris Cheng, M. 2009. The Philippines' health worker exodus. *The Lancet,* 373(9658), 111–12.

Huish, R. 2008. Going where no doctor has gone before: The role of Cuba's Latin American school of medicine in meeting the needs of some of the world's most vulnerable populations. *Public Health,* 122(6), 552–7. Available at: doi:10.1016/j. puhe.2008.03.001.

Huish, R. 2009. How Cuba's Latin American school of medicine challenges the ethics of physician migration. *Social Science & Medicine,* 69(3), 301–4. Available at: doi:10.1016/j.socscimed.2009.03.004.

Huish, R. and Kirk, J.M. 2007. Cuban medical internationalism and development of the Latin American school of medicine and human-resource-based healthcare provision. *Latin American Perspectives,* 34(6), 77–92.

Ineson, S. and Seeling, S. 2005. The medical passport. *Continuing Education in the Health Professions,* 25(1), 30–33.

Jaymalin, M. 2012. Thousands of jobs await Pinoy nurses in Libya. *The Philippine Star.*

Kirk, J.M. and Erisman, M. 2009. *Cuban Medical Internationalism: Origins, Evolution and Goals.* New York: Palgrave MacMillan.

Labonte, R. et al. 2005. Managing health professional migration from sub-Saharan Africa to Canada: A stakeholder inquiry into policy options. *Human Resources for Health,* 4(22).

Lorenzo, F.M., Galvez-Tan, J., Icamina, K. and Javier, L. 2007. Nurse migration from a source country perspective: Philippine country case study. *Health Services Research,* 42(3 Pt 2), 1406–1418. Available at: doi:10.1111/j.1475–6773.2007.00716.x.

Moultan, D. 2002. Sorry, no new patients. *Canadian Medical Association Journal,* 166(4), 490.

Mufunda, J. et al. 2007. Challenges in training the ideal doctor for Africa: Lessons learned from Zimbabwe. *Medical Teacher,* 29, 878–81.

Ncayiyana, D. 1999. Medical migration is a universal phenomenon. *South African Medical Journal,* 89(1), 107.

Nye, J.S. 2008. *The Powers to Lead.* Oxford, New York: Oxford University Press. [Online]. Available at: http://ezproxy.library.dal.ca/login?url=http://www.DAL.eblib.com/EBLWeb/ patron/?target=patron&extendedid=P_415954_0.

Oyowe, A. 1996. Brain drain: Colossal loss of investment for developing countries. *The Courier ACP-EU,* 159(October), 59–60.

Pang, T.E.A. 2002. Brain drain and health professionals: A global problem needs global solutions. *British Medical Journal,* 324(7336), 499–500.

Rawls, J. and Rawls, J. 1999. *The Law of Peoples; With, the Idea of Public Reason Revisited.* Cambridge, MA: Harvard University Press.

Sullivan, P. 2000. Shut out at home, Canadians flocking to Ireland's medical schools – and to an uncertain future. *Canadian Medical Association Journal,* 162(6), 868–71.

*The Economist*. 2011. Philippines and remittances: The house that Saud built. *The Economist*, 21 July.

The World Bank. 2011. *The Migration and Remittances Factbook 2011*. Washington, DC: The International Bank for Reconstruction and Development.

The World Health Organisation. 2006. *The World Health Report 2006 – Working Together for Health*. Geneva: The World Health Organisation.

# PART III
# Environmental Influences on Health and Development

# Chapter 10

# Living in the Same Place, Eating in a Different Space: Food Security and Dietary Diversity of Youth Living in Rural Northern Malawi

Lauren Classen, Rachel Bezner Kerr and Lizzie Shumba

## Introduction

Adolescent nutrition has been called to center stage in international health circles. There is increasing evidence that adequate nutrition during adolescence may help reverse the detrimental effects of undernourished early childhoods, decrease susceptibility to disease, including HIV/AIDS, and break vicious cycles of intergenerational malnutrition, poverty and poor health in sub-Saharan Africa (WHO 2005). Additionally, research indicates that food habits formed during adolescence tend to last a lifetime (Bull 1992; WHO 2005), and will impact food practice and nutritional health in future generations, making this a critical life stage at which to instill the values of good nutrition. Current research on adolescent nutrition, dominated by international organisations including the United Nations and the World Health Organisation, is largely population-based, focused on the relationship between nutrition and physiological changes during adolescence. This approach neglects the 'private dimension' (Baro and Deubel 2006) of vulnerability to food insecurity and malnutrition, namely the psychosocial changes also common during this life stage (Dehne and Riedner 2001; WHO 2005). Broader examinations of the geographies of 'youth' evidence the importance of shifting socio-political contexts in the restructuring of youth cultures (Massey 1998; Ruddik 2003; Van Blerk and Ansell 2006) which in turn influence the psychosocial changes associated with the transition from childhood to adulthood. For example, several practitioners have looked at the effects of rural youth migration on youth cultures (Ansell and van Blerk 2004; Punch 2007). The vulnerabilities and agencies of African youth who have moved away from villages to urban contexts, such as street youth, are increasingly well recognised. There is little research, however, examining the geographies of rural youth (Evans 2008) and less still examining shifting youth cultures and health in rural villages where youth food security and dietary diversity is often subsumed in household-level analyses. In this chapter we explore some of the political, psychosocial, cultural and spatial dimensions of food insecurity and dietary diversity for rural youth in northern Malawi.

This chapter thus not only addresses the gap in attention to the complex factors influencing rural youth in food and nutrition research, but also responds to calls for creative methods for engaging young people in social and health research (Kesby 2007; Van Blerk and Kesby 2008). We use mixed methods, combining survey data with youth photos and narratives to tease apart the interactions among food and nutrition insecurity, changing social relations and expectations in rural villages, and youth perceptions of their conditions. This study reveals the complex assembly of social and political processes from which gender and age-related food inequalities in rural households emerge. We show that understanding the particularities of shifting youth labour, mobility and social relations in the contemporary climate of market liberalisation and expanding socioeconomic divide is critical to developing appropriate food security and nutrition programming for rural youth. In so doing, we affirm calls in social geography for recognition that 'young people may use and experience space in different ways to children, and that by failing to recognise this, young people's needs may not be met by policies providing for children' (Evans 2008, 1661).

## Literature and Context

Youth health in African contexts has been an increasingly important topic of academic research for several reasons. One is due to rising concerns about the risk of HIV. Forty-five per cent of newly infected adults in sub-Saharan Africa in 2007 were estimated to be aged 15–24 (UNAIDS 2008). Recent studies of youth sexual behavior and reproductive health range from national epidemiological surveillance of condom use (Munthali et al. 2004; Hendriksen et al. 2007) to qualitative studies exploring youth sexual decision-making (Varga 1997), and violence in romantic relationships among school-going youth (Swart et al. 2002). HIV prevalence rates in Malawi are estimated at 11 per cent with over 50 per cent of new infections occurring among those aged 15–24 years (GOM 2012). The Malawi National Human Development Report 2004 presents evidence that the infection rate of females aged 15–24 is 4–6 times higher than that of males (MDHS 2004).[1]

The importance of food security and nutrition among young women is compounded by early marriage and pregnancy in Malawi. One report in 2011 found that 50 per cent of Malawian girls aged 20–24 were married before the age of 18 (PRB 2011). Pregnancy closely follows marriage in this context and there is some evidence that girls' age at first marriage is decreasing due to perceptions of declining longevity in light of HIV, perceptions that younger brides are less likely to be infected and parental pressure driven by poverty (Ueyema and Yamauchi 2009). Twenty-eight per cent of girls in the northern region have their first child when they are between 15 and 19 years of age (NSO 2012a, 50).

Dietary diversity, that is, the range of types of foods consumed, is widely viewed as an important component of a healthy diet, and has been shown to be positively associated with nutrient intake, household income, food security and child growth in the Global South (Ruel 2003). Ensuring a diverse diet is considered a crucial strategy for addressing health and nutrition of vulnerable groups, including children, women of child-bearing age and people with HIV. Although links between food security, nutrition and HIV risk are well-established (Gillespie and Kadiyala 2005), studies exploring rural youth food security and nutrition are rare, with a few recent studies in Rwanda, Ethiopia and Nigeria (Brown et al. 2008; Oladoja 2008; Tefera et al. 2012). While examining some aspects of food security, these studies do not undertake to understand the more complex relations which underpin the food security and nutrition status of rural youth. This two-fold gap in studies specifically targeting rural youth and those which use qualitative methods to understand the complexities of food consumption patterns in rural households is due in part to the ways in which the recent youth-focus emerged in the social sciences in combination with academic

---

1   Whereas there is a slight difference between rural and urban rates overall, among young people no difference in prevalence rate was found (MDHS 2004).

inclinations towards agency and independence – which means that those who are embedded in the social context of the family are often overlooked (Panelli, Punch and Robson 2007; Durham 2008).

Malawi is a relevant case study for understanding links between rural youth food insecurity and social relations, in part because the majority of people live in rural areas and depend on agriculture for food provisioning. Dietary diversity in Malawi tends to be low, with a high level of maize consumption per capita and limited consumption of fruits, vegetables and animal products (Gibson et al. 1998; GOM and World Bank 2006). With an annual per capita income estimated at $340 (World Bank 2011), high debt load, high levels of child malnutrition and high reliance on a few agricultural products (namely tobacco) for foreign exchange, in many ways Malawi is 'typical' of many countries in sub-Saharan Africa.

Malawi is a particularly important context for studying rural girls' access to and quality of food consumption. As noted above, women frequently marry very early in Malawi, during adolescence, when their nutritional requirements can be more consequential than at other life-stages. Married women experience very low levels of health decision-making power; nearly 70 per cent of Malawian men make the healthcare decisions on behalf of their wives (PRB 2011). Very low levels of education may contribute to rural girls feeling unable to assert power in relationships. Twenty-one per cent of women in rural Malawi have never attended school (MDHS 2010, 11). While education levels of both women and men are higher in the northern region of Malawi where this research was conducted, only 3 per cent of urban and rural women in the northern region have completed high school, many undoubtedly from urban areas (MDHS 2010, 13). While decisions about reproduction, use of contraceptives, financial issues, education of children and agricultural decisions are largely made by men (Alumira et al. 2005), nonetheless, women play an important role in agricultural labour (Bezner Kerr 2005). Unequal gender relations are thus a crucial dimension of understanding food insecurity and nutrition, and gender relations among young people are largely unexplored.

In recent years, the Government of Malawi has been hailed as a 'model' for improved *national* food security through provision of agricultural input subsidies, which increased availability to commercial fertiliser and hybrid seeds for the majority of smallholder farmers (Denning et al. 2009). There is, however, a persistent level of *household* food insecurity and child malnutrition (NSO 2012b), calling into question the success of this model for addressing food access and inequality (Bezner Kerr 2012). At the same time, Malawian youth (15–24 years of age), who make up over 50 per cent of the national population, also have the highest rates of unemployment (NSO 2012b). Some champions look to Malawi as a globalisation 'success story' which draws on the neoliberal industrial agricultural model of increased reliance on intensive inputs of fertiliser, hybrid seeds and pesticides (Juma 2010). We, rather, use Malawi as a case study to highlight the 'friction' as Tsing (2005) has called the interplay between different actors and processes in the context of contemporary globalisation, to generate unexpected outcomes of state policy in specific populations. In the context of globalisation, Nayak (2003, 5) reminds us that 'Rather than witnessing the 'death of geography', through the annihilation of space and time, we find instead that place and geography matter more than ever (Massey and Allen, 1984). Global cultures, then, do not operate independently but connect and interact differently at national, regional or local scales' (McEwan, 2001). In the context of this research 'rural' implies a young population with limited access to public services including transport, hospitals and schools. It is also a context in which young people participate actively in the social and economic lives of their families, characterised by patrilineal (sons inherit land) and patrilocal (wives move to and raise their children in their husband's natal compound) kinship patterns.

Youth programming is extensive in Malawi, focusing on sexual and reproductive health, sports and recreation, and asset-building (Government of Malawi 2004). In the region of this research it is organised and funded by a combination of private NGOs, the local hospital, the Synod of Livingstonia, Church of Central Africa, Presbyterian (CCAP), Christian Aid, PLAN International, the National Aids Commission, and private philanthropists. Programmes are frequently established and worked through youth clubs in rural villages through which certain health-behaviours could be disseminated by key youth leaders to peers and elders in their home villages. While food security was not addressed directly by these programs, volunteer participation correlated with higher levels of food insecurity for reasons discussed below.

## Methods

This chapter draws on mixed-method survey data combined with ethnographic data, gathered from January 2008 to August 2009. A food security and dietary diversity survey was implemented by five young people trained in survey techniques, to 213 youth (11–29 years old) randomly selected from 10 villages in the Ekwendeni Catchment Area. The survey was conducted in February 2009, coinciding with the annual period of food insecurity in the region (Maleta et al. 2003). To assess food security status, the Household Food Insecurity Access Scale (HFIAS), developed by the Food and Nutrition Technical Assistance Project (FANTA) guided the development of questions to ask rural youth about individual experiences of anxiety around, access to, and consumption of food (Swindale and Bilinksy 2006).[2] The questions were analysed individually and as part of two composite scores, the Food Insecurity Access Score (0–21) and the Insufficient Food Intake Scale (0–15).

To assess nutrition, an adapted version of the Individual Dietary Diversity Survey developed by the Food and Agriculture Organisation (FAO 2007) was employed to elicit individual food recalls for food consumed over the previous 24 hours. Foods were categorised into 14 food categories (FAO 2007). Administered at the individual level, this tool measures nutrient adequacy across different groups and is able to account for the frequent consumption of foods outside of the house by young people relative to other family members in rural households.

---

2   The Food Insecurity Assessment Scale uses a Likert scale (never, rarely sometimes often) for questions related to three domains of food insecurity: anxiety and uncertainty about food supply, food quality and adequacy of food intake or consumption. To measure food anxiety respondents in this study were asked, 'Did you worry that you would not have enough food in the past 30 days?'. The question 'Did you ever eat food that you preferred not to eat/did not like because of lack of resources to obtain other types of food?' measured food quality. Five questions were used to measure adequacy of food intake: 'Did you ever go a whole day without eating anything except fruits, cassava and/or green maize because there was not enough food?'; 'Did you ever eat a small amount of food and not get satisfied because the food was insufficient?'; 'Did you ever go a whole day without eating anything but supper/ ate fewer meals because there was not enough food?'; 'Was there ever no food at all in your household because there were no resources to get more?'; 'Did you ever go a whole day and night without eating anything because there was not enough food?'

Data was entered into and analysed using SPSS software. Key grouping variables tested against food security and dietary diversity variables were: i) gender; ii) shared residence with someone who drinks alcohol excessively; iii) respondent education level; iv) caregiver participation with Soils Food and Healthy Communities (SFHC) project; v) kin relations (i.e.: home village – mother's, father's, other); vi) marriage; vii) relation to primary caregiver; viii) caregiver education; and ix) respondent participation with youth organisations/clubs. The latter five showed significant differences. Pearson's Chi Square and Fisher's Exact Test were used to test significant differences between groups for categorical variables. Student's t-test was used to compare mean food security and dietary diversity scores. Significance at 90 and 95 per cent confidence levels are reported in this chapter.

Our understanding of the complex relationships among youth obligations in rural households, mobility, gender inequalities, access to resources and food and nutrition security among young people emerged in ethnographic data gathered over the 18 months in two rural villages. A brief survey of the infrastructure and basic services available in the villages across the catchment area enabled purposive selection of these villages to represent 'typical' villages in the catchment area. They were located near one another, 15 km proximity to the nearest hospital, secondary school, and market and 10 km from the nearest public transport. Various Christian religious institutions were present in both villages and the two villages shared a health dispensary that held unpredictable hours. The rural youth involved in the research identified themselves with six tribal groups, Tumbuka, Ngoni, Nkhonde, Tonga, Chewa, and Yao, the first two being the most predominant in the research area. All the young people practiced patrilocality and patrilineality, with important implications for agricultural resource allocations and thus how they define their goals and prioritise their challenges.

The research was done in collaboration with the Soils, Food and Healthy Communities (SFHC) project, which carries out participatory research with smallholder farmers on sustainable agriculture options to improve food security and nutrition (Msachi et al. 2009). The SFHC project had previously noted a low level of youth participation in their sustainable agricultural programs, as well as high levels of gender inequality, and sought to understand youth perceptions, experiences and challenges related to food security and nutrition.

In addition to participant observation, focus groups, interviews, and community-mapping, a critical part of the ethnographic research was the use of a participatory tool, Photo-LENS (Life-Experience Narratives of Significant concepts), developed and piloted with 118 young people to engage shy, rural youth in the process of examining and discussing their perceptions of the health challenges they face. Relevant to this research were photography assignments asking them to capture and discuss 'what most makes them suffer'. These photographs provided opportunity to discuss and understand the nature and specificities of rural youth hunger and poor nutrition in relation to social and spatial dynamics in northern Malawi.

## Food Security and Dietary Diversity Results

In general those in the 10 communities surveyed experienced significant food insecurity and very low dietary diversity during the pre-harvest season in 2009. Sixty-six per cent of respondents experienced one or more behaviours indicating insufficient food intake and scored exceptionally low on the Food Insecurity Access Score[3] and Insufficient Food Intake Scale,[4] scoring 6.5 and 3.6 on the two scales respectively. Breaking this down, we find that over 50 per cent of the respondents indicated that in the past 30 days they ate a *small amount of food and did not get satisfied* due to insufficient food and 44.1 per cent and 48.4 per cent indicated that they *ate fewer meals due to food shortages* and *found no food in the house for an entire day* respectively, at least once in the past 30 days. Further, 62 per cent of those surveyed were forced to consume 'survival foods', or foods they preferred not to eat as a result of not having the resources to obtain preferred foods, a strong indicator of poor dietary quality.

Whereas food intake and quality were very low, comparatively fewer, 37.4 per cent, indicated that they worried about not finding food to eat. This is still a high number, but the difference in experience of 'food insufficiency' and 'anxiety/worry' about food access may reflect a lower feeling of responsibility to ensure there is food for the family among young people (relative to adults).

The young people surveyed consumed an average of 4.28[5] out of 14 food groups (30.6 per cent) on the Individual Dietary Diversity Scale (FAO 2007) during the 24 hour period prior to the survey. The bulk of foods consumed at home and outside of the house, apart from the family, fall into the categories, 'cereals', 'white tubers', 'dark, leafy-green vegetables' and 'fruits'. The latter 2 categories are often consumed in very small quantities, fruits mostly being wild fruits gathered and eaten while collecting firewood or herding animals. Thirty-four per cent of those surveyed ate nuts or legumes.

Key grouping variables tested against food security and dietary diversity variables were: i) gender; ii) shared residence with someone who drinks alcohol excessively; iii) respondent education level; iv) caregiver participation with the SFHC project; v) kin relations (i.e.: home village – mother's, father's, other); vi) marriage; vii) relation to primary caregiver; viii) caregiver education; and ix) respondent participation with youth organisations/clubs. Each of these factors will be discussed in turn.

No significant differences were found in food security or dietary diversity of respondent education level, nor household participation with the SFHC project within participating villages. This latter finding is particularly interesting. While a survey conducted simultaneously and in the same villages as the youth survey showed significant positive impacts on the household level of food security, dietary diversity and child growth of children under the age of two (Bonatsos et al. 2009; Bezner Kerr et al. 2010), this project had no apparent impact on food access or consumption by young people. In SFHC project villages, no significant differences were found in food security or individual dietary diversity of young people between SFHC participating and non-participating households.[6]

---

3  Possible score of 21 points calculated based on the sum of the frequency of occurrence for each of the 7 food security questions (Often = 3 points, sometimes = 2 points, sometimes = 1 point).

4  Possible score of 15 calculated based on the sum of the frequency of occurrence for each of the 5 questions in Domain 3 (Often = 3 points, sometimes = 2 points, sometimes = 1 point).

5  This result showed very little deviation around the mean; the standard deviation was 1.33.

6  There is a small but significant difference in youth food security between SFHC project communities and control communities with young people in control communities more frequently indicating they went at least one whole day without eating any food at all in the past 30 days (32.4 per cent) compared with non-participating households (16.1 per cent) and participating households (12.3 per cent) in intervention communities. Additionally, although differences between the control and intervention community mean Food Insecurity Access Score (0–21) and Insufficient Food Intake Score (0–15) were minimal, high standard deviations for control communities indicate significant variation

Project efforts to influence child care and related feeding practices of under two children, while significant for child growth and dietary diversity (Bezner Kerr et al. 2010) did not, it seems, have positive effects on youth food security.

This finding led us to take interest in which factors, if not agroecological improvements and participatory nutrition education, influence youth consumption and health in rural households. Key variables correlated with food insecurity among young people were living with grandparents and caregivers with low levels of education, living with paternal kin, marriage and youth club participation.

## Food Security

The data indicated that young people living with grandparents experienced greater food insecurity than those living with their parents and they showed significant food anxiety, worrying about where to find enough food relative to those living in any other circumstances. Food anxiety was not significantly affected by other factors. Access to adequate quantities of food was significantly influenced by caregiver education. As long as one caregiver had achieved some secondary level schooling, young people under their care experienced less food insecurity. Marriage and residence with matrilineal kin were also important factors in food quality and intake. Young people who were married were significantly more likely to eat smaller meals (63.6 per cent) than the unmarried living with biological parents (44.4 per cent). Unmarried girls living in their father's home village, as would be most common in this region where families practice patrilocal kinship, were slightly less food secure and significantly less likely to eat preferred foods. Young people participating in youth clubs were significantly more food insecure for five of the seven food security questions (Table 10.1).

## Dietary Diversity

The data showed no significant differences in dietary diversity between boys and girls in general, with both scoring about 4/14. Married young women, however, experienced significantly lower dietary diversity than unmarried girls of their same age. In fact, more than 40 per cent of married young women, compared to 16.7 per cent of unmarried girls, reported very low dietary diversity, consuming primarily maize, white tubers and very small amounts of green vegetables (Table 10.2). Interestingly, in the first years of marriage, although the dietary diversity of both boys and girls appeared to decline, the decline is significant only for girls. Whereas 16.7 per cent of single girls experience very low (0–3) dietary diversity scores, 41.7 per cent of married girls experience the same. This finding is consistent with girls who said their primary caregiver is their husband also experiencing significantly lower dietary diversity than girls who lived with one or both biological parents.

In the following section we examine the processes and relations that in turn influence which factors are most associated with youth food security and dietary diversity in rural Malawi.

---

around the mean score relative to intervention communities. This indicates higher variation in food security among the young in control communities relative to intervention communities, perhaps due to greater availability of legumes on the market in participating villages.

**Table 10.1    Key factors influencing experiences of food insecurity by rural youth**

| Group | | Domain 1: Food anxiety 'yes' | Domain 2: Insufficient quality 'yes' | Domain 3: Insufficient intake 'yes' | | | | | | Food Security Scores | |
|---|---|---|---|---|---|---|---|---|---|---|---|
| | | Q1 | Q2 | Q3 | Q4 | Q5 | Q6 | Q7 | | Food Insecurity Access Score (0–21) mean | Food insecurity Intake Score (0–15) mean |
| | | (Worried) % | (Eat food not preferred) % | (Only wild fruits) % | (Small amt food) % | (Fewer meals) % | (No food in house) % | (Whole day without food) % | Insufficient Food Intake (One or more in domain 3) % | | |
| Caregiver | Grandparent (n = 24) | 54.6 | 60.9 | 50.0 | 54.2 | 58.3 | 58.3 | 29.2 | 66.7 | 7.04 [sd. 6.28] | 4.96 [sd. 4.69] |
| | Parent (n = 133) | *32.3 (p=0.036) | 60.2 | 30.1 (p=0.049) | 44.4 | 42.9 (p=0.083) | 47.4 | 20.3 | 65.4 | 5.13 [sd. 5.37] | 3.33 [sd. 3.89] (p=0.07) |
| Caregiver Education | No secondary | 37.8 | 67.3 | 40.5 | 62.2 | 53.2 | 59.9 | 26.1 | 74.8 | 6.47 [sd. 5.77] | 4.4 [sd. 4.22] |
| | Some secondary | 30.6 | 53.1 (P = 0.087) | 26.5 (p=0.063) | 40.8 | 30.6 (p=0.008) | 40.8 (p=0.057) | 12.2 (p=0.037) | 55.1 (p=0.012) | 4.69 [sd. 5.78] (p=0.076) | 2.9 [sd. 4.15] (p=0.047) |
| Kin Relations (girls only) | Living in father's home village | 35.2 | 63.0 | 31.5 | 50.0 | 40.7 | 46.3 | 16.7 | 68.5 | | |
| | Living in mother's home village | 35.0 | 50.0 | 35.0 | 25.0 (0.046) | 40.0 | 40.0 | 15.0 | 45.0 (p=0.058) | | |

| Marriage | | | | | | | | | | |
|---|---|---|---|---|---|---|---|---|---|---|
| Yes | 36.4 | 68.2 | 36.4 | 63.6 | 40.9 | 45.5 | 20.5 | 61.0 | 6.0 [sd. 5.81] | 39/1 [sd. 4.28] |
| No | 32.3 | 60.2 | 30.1 | 44.4 (p=0.02) | 42.9 | 47.4 | 20.3 | 69.7 | 5.13 [sd. 5.37] | 3.33 [sd. 3.89] |
| Married boys | 26.1 | 65.2 | 21.6 | 47.8 | 30.4 | 43.5 | 34.8 | 65.2 | 5.7 [sd. 6.01] | 3.74 [sd. 4.51] |
| Married girls | 36.1 | 63.9 | 38.9 | 58.3 | 38.9 | 44.4 | 11.1 (p=0.032) | 58.3 | 5.17 [sd. 5.28] | 3.26 [sd. 3.84] |
| Youth-club Participation | | | | | | | | | | |
| Yes | 35.4 | 71.6 | 40.2 | 62.2 | 50.0 | 57.3 | 29.3 | 76.8 | 6.58 [sd. 5.56] | 4.38 [sd. 4.17] |
| No | 33.6 | 54.1 (p=0.009) | 28.7 (p=0.086) | 42.6 (p= 0.006) | 39.3 | 41.8 (p=0.03) | 17.2 (p=0.042) | 59.0 (p=0.008) | 4.71 [sd. 5.42] (p=0.018) | 3.09 [sd. 3.92] (p=0.026) |

*Note:* *While small numbers make the disaggregation of this question by gender difficult, it is worth noting that over 75% of girls living with their grandparents said they had frequently consumed fewer meals in the past 30 days due to insufficient food, suggesting that while both boys and girls living with grandparents are vulnerable, girls living with their grandparents are more vulnerable to food insecurity than boys for reasons taken up below.

**Table 10.2    Dietary diversity and marriage**

| Girls Only | Dietary Diversity Score (0–14) Mean (t-test) | Percentage with Very Low (0–3) Dietary Diversity % |
|---|---|---|
| Married | 4.08 [sd. 1.40] | 41.7 |
| Unmarried | 4.61 [sd. 1.32] (p=0.057) | 16.7 (p=0.018) |

**Discussion**

Rural youth food security and nutrition are frequently subsumed in household level analyses. In this research, however, by conducting individual-level studies with young people in rural households, we found that the factors influencing household-level food security and child nutrition differed from those affecting youth food security and dietary diversity. In particular, we found that agroecological innovations by participants with the SFHC project, which significantly improved household-level food security and dietary diversity of young children in rural northern Malawi villages (Bonatsos et al. 2009), did not have the same impact on youth food security and nutrition, despite their embeddedness in the social and productive dynamics of participating households. By analysing the quantitative, qualitative and visual data gathered in this research together, we suggest that in northern Malawi an array of processes and changing social relations are critical to understanding the ways in which young people encountered rural spaces, which in turn affected their access and quality of food. The predominance of food insecurity among rural youth was affirmed in many ways throughout this research. The most common story emerging from their photographs[7] of 'what most makes you suffer' was related to inadequate access to food. Some 'suffer' photos which explicitly depicted food insecurity can be found in Figure 10.1.

These photos and the stories accompanying them demonstrate the perceived severity of food insecurity among the young but also hint at the dynamics of food insecurity and youth culture in the rural village today. One person said, (Figure 10.1a) 'The main problem to our family is lack of food. We have a very big field but we yield very little, of which half is consumed while the maize is still in the field and the remaining half doesn't even last for more than three months' (Figure 10.1b). 'As you can see this maize crop is very poor. There are times we spend the day just searching for our supper ... The old ones [grandparents] go out begging for nsima and green vegetables' (Figure 10.1c). 'That which makes me suffer is my family eating only pumpkin because there is no other food'. 'These pigs are what makes me suffer because, just look at their pen is very poor and they do not have enough food'. The pigs in photo (Figure 10.1d) died not long after this photo was taken.

Food insecurity described by these young people is reflective of Malawi's declining rural economy. Malawi was one of the first countries to demonstrate a commitment to neoliberal reform, adopting the Structural Adjustment Program (SAPs) in 1981 (Englund 2006). The

---

7   All photographs shown have the permission of the photographer and everyone featured in the photograph. In cases where permission was not granted, the photographs were staged to replicate the originals using actors.

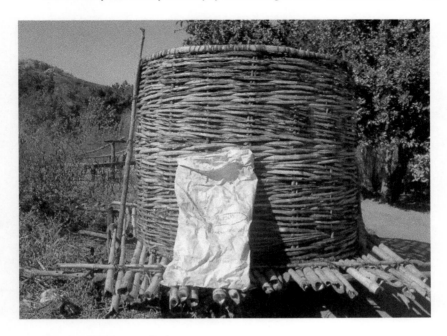

**Figure 10.1a    Hunger is suffering**

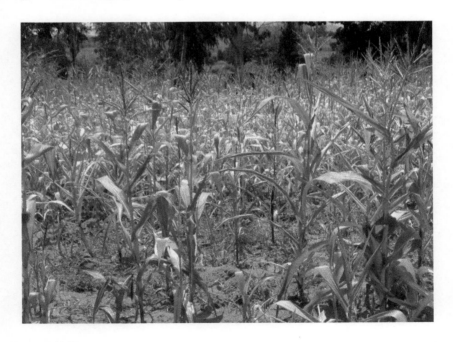

**Figure 10.1b**

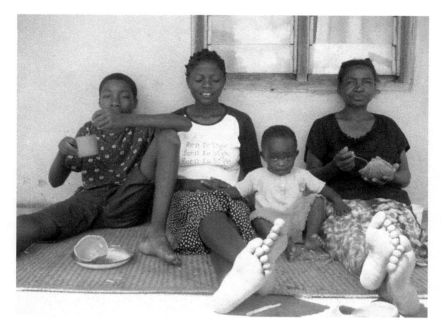

**Figure 10.1c**

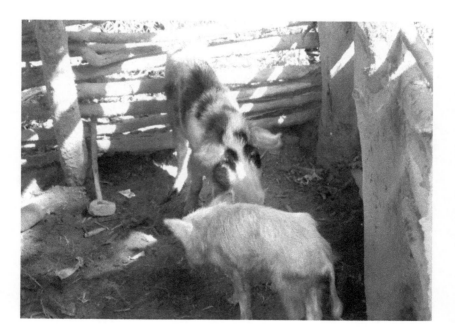

**Figure 10.1d**

SAPs led to promotion of high input hybrid maize and burley tobacco,[8] reduced support for public agricultural research, devalued the Kwacha, reduced strategic grain reserves, agricultural extension programs and public health services (Sahn and Arulpragasam 1991; Frankenburger 2003; Dorward and Kydd 2004). Over the two decades since the first implementation of SAPs, rising seed, food and fertiliser prices led to declining rural economies and increased food insecurity (Sahn and Arulpragasam 1991; Frankenberger 2003; Dorward and Kydd 2004; Englund 2006). Since 2005, the Government of Malawi has been hailed as a 'model' for improved national food security through provision of agricultural input subsidies (Denning et al. 2009). Household food insecurity, however, remains high (NSO 2012a), and the reason the 'maize crop is very poor' one person explained is in part because several groups, including the unmarried, in particular, do not seem to benefit from these subsidies.

Death or divorce, which moves young people to their mother's home village, where access to productive resources are limited (including land, labour, agency to make agricultural decisions and subsidies), has gendered impacts on food security. The survey data indicated that girls tended to be more food secure when living with their mothers. Studies have shown some mothers to dedicate more resources to child feeding than fathers (Kennedy and Peters 1993). Interestingly, young men who lived in their mother's home village reported feeling significantly less secure about their futures, due to precarious access to agricultural land, and unpredictable relations with mother's kin. Many young men in this situation planned to move away from the rural village to find employment rather than stay and farm. Nearly every boy involved in this research who lived under their mother's care in their mother's home village said that they planned to look for employment in town when they grew up. Young people who lived in their father's home village frequently said they would grow tobacco. The story of one 23-year-old boy, told by his sister, explains this:

> Now when I went home, the last time, he [my brother] was there. But just now I found that he has been chased and is not at home. I learned he has built a temporary shelter somewhere … My uncles chased him. He does not have land there and they say this is not his land. He wants to marry this girl but he says he cannot marry for he has nothing [no agricultural resources].

Thus, whereas living in the mother's home village appeared to have a small but significant and positive impact on food security of girls, it places significant stress on young boys about their future livelihoods and well-being.

Reflecting findings elsewhere, caregiver education is also important to the food security of their children. Living with a caregiver with at least some secondary school education was associated with increased food security. Maternal education often has a significant effect on child nutrition. Secondary school education may instill in caregivers the importance of proper nutrition, motivating them to channel more household resources towards food. Education is also a common proxy measure for income. Studies have shown education to be associated with higher agricultural yields, particularly the education of women (Alderman et al. 2003). Rural households with greater income are more able to purchase food when experiencing shortages of agricultural produce. In Malawi, where youth responsibility to procure resources outside of agriculture is higher in more

---

8  Both crops are heavily reliant on chemical inputs and have led to significant soil erosion (Frankenberger 2003).

economically vulnerable households, such as households headed by grandparents, caregiver education may also explain youth food security by way of enabling them to spend more time at home eating in the household.

Young people play a critical role in procuring household resources in the context of this research, most importantly through their participation in household agriculture. Deplorable economic conditions in rural villages combined with an influx of foreign consumer goods in Malawi, however, have increasingly made mixed livelihoods desirable and necessary in rural areas (Bryceson 2002). Rural households commonly subsist off a combination of maize agriculture for household consumption, tobacco production for sale, casual on-farm labour and income from stop-gap employment in town or urban areas – the latter two frequently reliant on the physical capabilities and mobility of the young. High rates of HIV/AIDS have depleted labour resources, exacerbating poverty in rural villages (Frankenberger 2003) and further contributed to youth cyclical migration in and away from the household and thus their reliance on extra-familial and extra-agricultural sources for securing daily food.

Unmarried and married young people who sought opportunities outside of agriculture, within or beyond the village, eat food apart from the family, sourced through individual contacts with friends and/or hunting and gathering of wild foods, which explains, in part, why youth food security and nutrition were not significantly impacted by agricultural innovations which otherwise improved food security and nutrition in rural households. The results of the survey indicated that 51.6 per cent had hunted or gathered wild food during the 24 hours previous to the survey, 30.8 per cent ate food apart from their families that they had received as gifts from friends, and 31.9 per cent ate food they had purchased with their own money. These findings correspond with finding that relatively few reported going a whole day without eating anything because there was not enough food (21.6 per cent compared to 44 per cent who ate smaller meals). Even when they ate very little, they frequently were able to purchase something small like a cassava, a fried donut, bananas, packaged biscuits, or were able to pick wild fruits while they were away from the house during the day.

Compounding their need to look for employment beyond the village, and due, at least in part to the hollowing out of the middle generation by HIV/AIDS, the qualitative data indicated that children and young people were increasingly living with parents who were sick or with grandparents. As one girl said succinctly, living with grandparents, 'is not very fine, just there is no [choice] because old people are the only people we remain with'. This health burden was reflected very strongly in their *suffer* photographs and stories showing grandparents for whom they increasingly feel responsible (Figure 10.2).

About these photos, the photographers said in turn, (Figure 10.2a) 'she is too old to work. She was farming in the [past] but since 2008 she didn't do anything … me and my young sisters we grow maize. One acre, one acre of maize' (boy, 15 years old). '[I took this photo because] it makes me suffer … this is my father's bedroom and it has a single bed which he shares with my brother and he has no blankets or a mat[tress] under the bed … my sisters husband don't want to help my father and we didn't have enough fertiliser and my father has no job' (boy, 19 years old) (Figure 10.2b). One 21-year-old girl, who photographed both of her grandparents (above) said, 'I feel pity with him. It sticks to my heart. When I took this snap, my grandmother was out begging for salt' (figures 10.2c and d). While the role of grandmothers in caring for children in the context of HIV/ AIDS is well-established, through these photos and accompanying stories the young people showed how this dynamic of care was often reversed as grandparents become too elderly

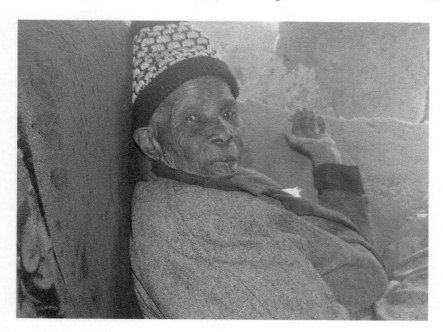

**Figure 10.2a    Caring for grandparents is suffering**

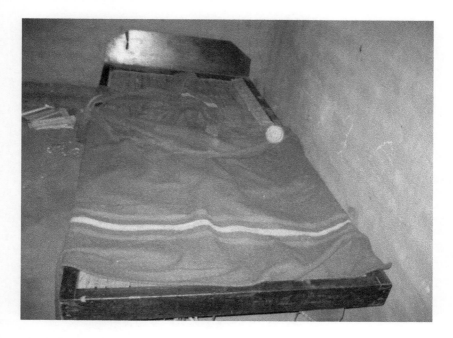

**Figure 10.2b**

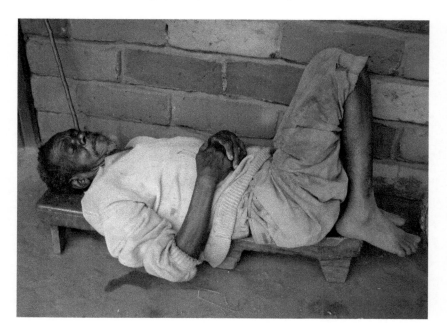

**Figure 10.2c**

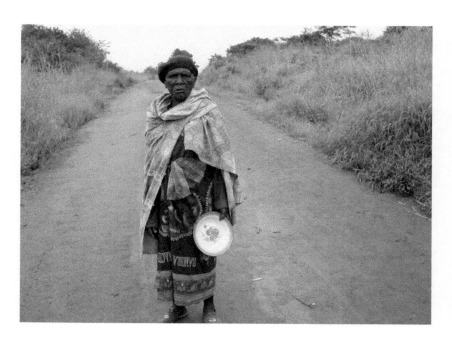

**Figure 10.2d**

to work or provide for themselves and others (Classen et al. 2008). Food insecurity and significant anxiety about securing adequate food were expressed in interviews with those living with grandparents.

Shifts in the social meaning of 'youth' and adulthood in the contemporary context of globalisation, however, also have impacts on youth experiences of place and space in rural villages (Nayak 2003) in this context, which further complicates youth food security and nutrition. Elders, and grandparents in particular, found that they had little authority to prevent young people from being too enamoured with money and thus off-farm employment. They worried that they risked their health and well-being in many ways to access money and 'modern' lifestyles. Whereas it was often necessary for them to seek non-agricultural employment, parents and grandparents worried that some were dangerously lured by money. 'The big deal is money', Mary (78) exclaimed worriedly:

> Many people they love money much more than in the past. [In the past] there was no money. Many people have learned [gone to school] but there is a lack of job opportunities. As a result there are a lot of thieves. [But in the past] we should just say that they had no money. We should give a reason. The reason is that those who had money, even if they give it to the girl child she was not taking it because they were respecting themselves. [They would ask themselves] "Why has he given this to me?" … [Laughing and shaking her head]. Nowadays youth rush at receiving it.

Elders' authority to suggest alternatives, however, was significantly diminished by economic decline, leaving the young with little guidance and dwindling respect for elders. This reduced respect was especially true for grandparents who 'have no right' as some put it, to discipline them. Grandparents effectively became like the young again, when they became partially dependent. 'They are like brothers and sisters to youth.' As a result, elders felt frustrated. Abel, 80 years old, explained, 'When she [his granddaughter] does not listen then we know that even where she will go, there will be problems because … to me as a parent I have failed, I have failed to talk … whatever I say, she doesn't listen'. As young people took on more responsibility for grandparents' care, grandparents relinquished some of their disciplinary rights and authoritative voice.

Marriage was sometimes seen as another strategy employed to fulfil shifting obligations in the changing rural context. Access to productive resources in rural villages was determined by marriage. In this region, men accessed land and social agency to make agricultural decisions upon marriage; women accessed land through their husbands. Some young people, in circumstances where they or their families did not have adequate food and other resources, opted or felt significant pressure to marry. As one girl (21) explained when talking about the photograph of her grandmother,

> My grandmother says, you should go and get married. Yes. But I am not, maybe, [laughs] willing to get married just because early marriages [laughs] I am not prepared [at this age] to get married. If possible when I am prepared then I can get married but just being forced to get married [laughs] it's not good.

Many boys and girls expressed feeling obligated to marry before they felt 'prepared' or 'fit', due to the dire economic situation in which many households found themselves, especially if one or both of their parents had passed away. While girls in such circumstances explained that they married so their grandmothers could receive bride price, boys explained that marriage enabled access to land from the village headman and their ability to take charge of that property. Cane, a young man who had married a few years prior to us meeting and at 21 years old himself was holding his 2-year-old and awaiting the birth of what turned out to be twins, said his own marriage was,

> more like just a forced marriage because I was forced to do that, having seen that my father is having a problem, so what can I do? Then it's what led me to get married and take care of the left young sisters and brothers from the … the other wife who has passed away … but in reality, in real sense, I was suggesting maybe to get married in 2010, but due to this crisis, this situation, I failed. It's really a problem to me that eeeeh, at the stage I am, I am not fit to hold this family. So I am trying my best each and every day.

After one of Cane's father's wives, who had several young children, had passed away, and his father himself become very ill, Cane decided to marry. Upon marrying he received social respect and authority over the land and agricultural resources. Whereas marriage would have marked the transition to social adulthood in the past, Cane did not feel this is accurate today. Despite feeling that marrying was necessary given his responsibility for siblings from the deceased mother, Cane expressed not feeling he was 'at the stage' of marriage, 'not fit' to hold a family; in other words, Cane felt he was not socially prepared to be an 'adult'. Regardless, as noted above, many end up marrying very young (UN 2004; Ueyema and Yamauchi 2009; PRB 2011).

Being 'not fit' as Cane put it, was one of many reasons early marriage was associated with greater food insecurity among rural youth and very low dietary diversity among young girls, though perhaps for reasons other than those commonly noted in the literature. Malawian elders, for instance, frequently lamented the young not knowing how to dry meat and vegetables and prepare foods as was done in the past, preferring 'English/white foods'.[9] Being 'not fit' may be understood as Cane not having had sufficient time to gain the knowledge on food preservation from his elders prior to marrying. A reduction in the transfer of agricultural and food preparation knowledge from elders to younger generations, has been shown to be particularly affected by HIV/AIDS related illness and deaths in several African contexts (Alumira et al. 2005). Being not 'fit', in this context, however, also referred to not having employment that provided income with which to purchase desired foods and other things. Finishing school and finding non-agricultural employment, money and independence – whether from husbands or on kin and village headmen for resources – are increasingly deemed more important markers of adulthood than getting married for girls and boys. Mary, a 78-year-old grandmother who was particularly vocal about her discontent with the changes in the desire for and value of money among the youth of today explained:

> They [youth] want to show themselves, to say, we differ. [This is] because we, your friends, we are not living the way you live. But now, we want to dress properly, we need

---

9   In Malawi, as Charles Piot (2010) has described in the Togolese context, there is a significant shift in desires in the context of this relatively new democracy characterised by liberalised markets and widening socio-economic divides. 'Africanity is rejected and Euro-modernity embraced; futures are replacing the past as cultural reservoir' (Piot 2010, 16). 'Euro-modern' desires, particular to the Malawian context, have come to be known locally as desires for 'umoyo wachizungu' or English/white life. The desire for and consumption of 'English Foods' is seen to be part of this.

to show ourselves. And, when it comes to eating, we want to eat English things at home, taking this kind of relish, taking this kind of relish. But we were just eating vegetables and beans these two things and okra – three things [in the past].

Young people's desire for new lifestyles, characterised by purchased foodstuffs, was also reflected in their agricultural preferences in rural villages. Young men, in particular, took greater interest in producing the cash crop, tobacco than previous generations, rather than staple food production. Steven, 27 years old, for example, said, when outlining what he will grow when he marries and is not restricted by his parents' authority over the land,

> R: I will add [to what my parents already grow] tobacco.
> L: Why?
> R: For income.
> L: I can see many young people want to grow tobacco?
> R: It's the only way of finding income. I want to boost up my family from the level it is now to another level, because right now we are poor and can't be able to provide [school] fees for someone.

Chawanangwa (21), reflecting youthful enthusiasm about the money that can be made planting tobacco, called it 'jackpotting'. Furthermore, if young men do not plant tobacco, he explained, girls will not be interested in them:

> R: [Male youth] don't want to plant what their parents' plant. They, as youth, need to plant tobacco.
> L: Aaaah! And why? Why do you think there is this difference?
> R: Mmm … aaah. Maybe I don't know, maybe they are shy … They are saying maybe that the girls, they will laugh at [them] [laughing].

Young men frequently commented that young women. too, want money and material things and that they will often leave a marriage if they do not feel adequately financially supported. With extremely limited access to agricultural resources, women had little choice but to demand access through men who control these resources. These changes in the social value of money, dietary preference, and cropping patterns compounded the effects of HIV/AIDS to seriously limit the transmission of local knowledge on food provision and preparation, leading to significant vulnerability among the newly married.

The extremely low dietary diversity among newly married girls, however, was also due to significant abuse of women in marriages. When women move to their husband's home village upon marriage, they can face significant abuse, especially if the husband's family was not involved in arranging the marriage. Violence towards women, including physical abuse, infidelity that puts women at risk of HIV/AIDS, poverty and neglect in rural households, however, were the greatest risk factors for poor nutrition among married young women. As Perilla, a 25-year-old young woman who had recently left her husband, said about girls in the village like herself:

Ah, they think that marriages will provide everything for them. But they are just a hassle. They are just a problem. The men are just out there somewhere spending the money on other girls. This is very dangerous. You can be very poor and suffering with your children. And, then there is this disease, you know … [HIV/AIDS].

While the most predominant 'suffer' photograph taken by both boys and girls was of hunger and food insecurity, girls and boys also frequently linked food insecurity to photos of abusive relationships with fathers, husbands, and in-laws.

Both boys and girls spoke about the relationship between alcoholism, neglect and hunger in rural villages. The photo (Figure 10.3) was taken by Marcus, a 14-year-old boy currently in the 7th year of primary school. It shows two men drinking unregulated, locally brewed alcohol from pink plastic cups in a bar demarcated by sparsely thatched walls. Marcus was the youngest and only male among his siblings. He lived with both parents in his father's home village. In his story Marcus started by speaking abstractly about men who drink:

> When [the man in the photo] is drunk and he is going home ... he can shout all the way, and is quarrelling and fighting with people when he gets home. When they are at home, he quarrels with his wife. (Later he spoke about his own father who drinks.) My father was beating me sometime back ... Aaa, it was so painful to me, if I could have been an adult I could have been fighting him back. [Instead] Aaa, I was just running away.

Marcus' joy photo juxtaposed this suffering by showing a man he admired who 'finds for himself – he doesn't even have time to be at somebody's house for begging'. 'Drunk men', he said 'beg, for money and then for food when they run out'. Such stories, however, were much more common from women. Valerie (25 years old), who, after much deliberation and calculation said she married in 2001, at 17 years old, while still attending the nearest primary school in seventh grade. She commented about her husband being

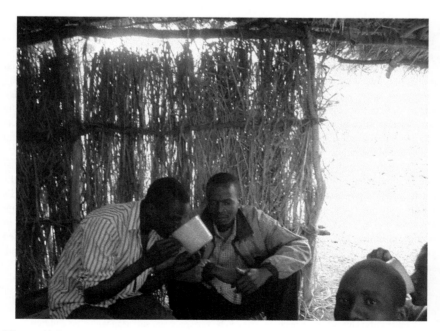

**Figure 10.3      Alcoholism, abuse and hunger**

lazy. 'This is the biggest problem to the children, because as of now when the food is not enough then you will find that children will start to swell.' This swelling Valerie spoke of may be a form of protein malnutrition referred to as kwashiorkor, for which abdominal swelling is a symptom. Valerie connected her husband's alcohol consumption to his laziness as well as to her husband's infidelity, which contributed to the family's hunger since he spent household resources on his new girlfriend/wife. This infidelity also put Valerie at risk of HIV. 'Maybe he does not even know the girl, how she is [her HIV status] and then he comes from there to me. That can make our life short because we don't know each other's movement.'

It appears that youth-targeted programs in the region, while not food security programs per se, attracted those with the highest levels of food insecurity. Many young people travelled significant distances to participate with projects, contributing to dietary consumption outside the household and perhaps explaining, in part, the limited impact household-level agroecological improvements had on youth food security and dietary diversity. Youth programmes, however, also targeted the most vulnerable in rural villages, and frequently provided snacks or stipends for trainings related to reproductive health and HIV/AIDS, the latter of which were used to buy food and soap to meet personal and family needs. Further, narratives about the potential for employment as a result of dedicated volunteerism with youth programs were a persistent rationale for participating. In interviews, young people frequently responded to questions about why they participated with the youth club in their village with: 'Chowa began volunteering in 2003 and now he went to Scotland. Then he will have a job with the hospital.' While volunteering did turn into employment for some, caution must be taken that this does not lead to disillusionment. Many more were never employed by such programs.

## Conclusion

By combining individual youth food security and dietary diversity surveys with youth photos and narratives about the most pressing challenges facing youth who live with their families in rural villages in northern Malawi, the research discussed here captures the complicated factors influencing youth food security and nutrition differently from others in the household. Participants in the study experienced significant food insecurity and extremely low dietary diversity, in part because of their increase in spatial mobility, but also related to gender and age-based social roles. Interestingly, whereas a household food insecurity and dietary diversity survey conducted simultaneously and in the same villages as this survey found improved farming techniques combined with participatory nutrition education and attention to gender relations to be associated with significantly better food security and dietary diversity at both the household level and for children under 5 in the household (Bonatsos et al. 2009; Bezner Kerr et al. 2010), youth food security and dietary diversity was determined by different factors.

Youth food security and nutrition are influenced by several factors unique to this life stage. Food security and dietary diversity among the young were positively associated with care by maternal kin (as opposed to paternal kin) and caregiver education, and negatively associated with having grandparents as primary caregivers, marriage (particularly for girls), and participation with youth clubs. In narratives of the lived experience of food insecurity, young people explained how their reliance on extra-familial relations for access to food outside of the household while working and studying, deeply ingrained gender inequalities and gender-based violence in youth marriages, very limited access to agricultural resources (land, labour, subsidies and agency), their role in providing care for ailing grandparents (rather than the reverse), and unemployment played a role in shaping these different food security and nutrition determinants. We show how shifting agricultural policies led to increasing poverty in rural villages, HIV/AIDS significantly changed the social architecture of rural villages, increasing youth responsibilities for provision of basic needs in rural households, and an influx of foreign goods and ideas influenced desires in rural villages for 'modern' lifestyles with money. Together, all three led some to seek employment beyond the household and others to marry, which provided access to agricultural resources, independence and sometimes money. Regardless of the strategy they employed to meet the changing pressures on their lives, they faced deeply ingrained age and gender inequalities that make it difficult for them to access enough nutritious foods to eat. As noted above, the effects of this could be detrimental; young women in this research frequently expressed deep concern that their young children 'swell' with hunger as a result of their own limited access to quality food. We argue here that understanding the 'friction' (Tsing 2005) among various actors and processes that affect youth access to enough, nutritious foods is critical to beginning to address these challenges.

These findings have important implications for program planning for youth health. First, shifting youth cultures as they interact with changing responsibilities in rural villages in contemporary social and political contexts need be taken into consideration. In Malawi today there is little incentive for young people to work on food production, as access to cash to meet shifting rural desires and perceived responsibility in rural villages make money more important aspects of rural youth livelihoods. Viable and sustainable sources of income from agriculture are critical to youth food and dietary security. Youth-targeted programs may also directly impact their food intake by providing provisions for packed lunches to carry to school, work or volunteer positions. Additionally, recognising the importance of food sharing among them and extra-familial networks in helping secure food, opportunities to facilitate the forming and strengthening of these networks may also be important. Working with village headmen and elders to secure access to land and other productive resources by the unmarried and initiatives that address gender inequalities, violence against women and women's dependence on men in rural villages are critical.

## References

Alderman, H., Hoddinott, J., Haddad, L. and Udry, C. 2003. 'Gender differentials in farm productivity: implicatations for household efficiency and agricultural policy', in *Household Decisions, Gender and Development: A Synthesis of Recent Research*, edited by A. Quisumbing. Washington, DC: IFPRI.

Ansell, N. and van Blerk, L. 2004. Children's migration in household/family strategy: coping with AIDS in Malawi and Lesotho. *Journal of Southern African Studies*, 30, 673–90.

Baro, M. and Deubel, T.F. 2006. Persistent Hunger: Perspectives on Vulnerability, Famine, and Food Security in Sub-Saharan Africa. *Annual Review of Anthropology*, 35, 521–38.

Belachew, T., Lindstrom, D., Abebe, G. et al. 2012. Predictors of chronic food insecurity among adolescents in Southwest Ethiopia: a longitudinal study. *BMC Public Health*, 12(604), 1471–2458.

Bezner Kerr, R. 2012. Lessons from the old Green Revolution for the new: Social, environmental and nutritional issues for agricultural change. *Africa Progress in Development Studies*, 12 (2&3), 213–29.

Bezner Kerr, R., Berti, P.R. and Shumba, L. 2010. Effects of Participatory Agriculture and Nutrition project on Child Growth in Northern Malawi. *Public Health Nutrition*,14(8),1466–72.

Bonatsos, C., Bezner Kerr, R. and Shumba, L. 2009. *SFHC Food Security Status and Crop Diversity, 2007–2009 Survey Results*. Soils, Food and Healthy Communities project, 41 pages.

Brown, L.A., Thurman, T.R., Rice, J.C. and Snider, L.M. 2008. Depressive Symptoms in Youth Heads of Household in Rwanda: Correlates and Implications for Intervention. *Archives of Pediatrics & Adolescent Medicine*, 162, 836–43.

Bryceson, D. 2002. The scramble in Africa: Reorienting rural livelihoods. *World Development*, 30(5), 725–39.

Bull, N.L. 1992. Dietary habits, food consumption, and nutrient intake during adolescence. *Journal of Adolescent Health*, 13, 384–8.

Classen, L., Kamanga, R., Khongolo, C. et al. 2008. Revising Conventional Perceptions of Orphanhood. *Anthropology News: In Focus*, 49(7), 15.

Dehne, K.L. and Riedner, G. 2001. Adolescence – a Dynamic Concept. *Reproductive Health Matters*, 9(17), 11–15.

Denning, G., Kabambe, P., Sanchez, P. et al. 2009. Input Subsidies to Improve Smallholder Maize Productivity in Malawi: Toward an African Green Revolution. *PLoS Biology*, 7, e1000023.

Dorward, A. and Kydd, J. 2004. The Malawi 2002 food crisis: the rural development challenge. *Journal of Modern African Studies*, 42, 343–61.

Durham, D. 2008. Apathy and Agency: The Romance of Agency and Youth in Botswana, in *Figuring the Future: Globalization and the Temporalities of Children and Youth*, edited by J. Cole and D.L. Durham. Santa Fe, NM: School for Advanced Research Press, 151–78.

Englund, H. 2006. *Prisoners of Freedom: Human Rights and the African Poor*. Berkeley: University of California Press.

Evans, B. 2008. Geographies of Youth/Young People. *Geography Compass*, 2(5), 1659–80.

FAO. 2007. *Guidelines for measuring household and individual dietary diversity*. Version 2. FAO Nutrition and Consumer Protection Division. Rome, Italy.

Frankenberger, T., Luther, K., Fox, K., and Mazzeo, J. 2003. *Livelihood Erosion through Time: Macro and Micro Factors that Influenced Livelihood Trends in Malawi over the Last 30 Years*. Malawi: TANGO International, Inc. for CARE Southern and Western Africa Regional Management Unit (SWARMU).

Gibson, R.S., Yeudall, F., Drost, N. et al. 1998. Dietary strategies to prevent zinc deficiency. *American Journal of Clinical Nutrition*, 68(suppl), 484S–7S.

Gillespie, S. and Kadiyala, S. 2005. *HIV/AIDS and Food and Nutrition Security: From Evidence to Action*. Washington, DC: International Food Policy Research Institute (Food Policy Review No. 7).

Government of Malawi (GOM). 2004. *The Malawi Coverage Exercise Report: Providing evidence for youth services coverage*. Ministry of Youth Development and Sports and the National Youth Council of Malawi. Lilongwe, Malawi: Government of Malawi.

GOM and World Bank. 2006. *Malawi Poverty and Vulnerability Assessment: Investing in Our Future*. Lilongwe, Malawi: Government of Malawi.

GOM. 2012. *2012 Global AIDS Response Progress Report: Malawi Country Progress Report for 2010 and 2011*. Lilongwe, Malawi: Government of Malawi.

Hendriksen, E.S., Pettifor, A., Lee, S.J. et al. 2007. Predictors of condom use among young adults in South Africa: the Reproductive Health and HIV Research Unit National Youth Survey. *American Journal of Public Health*, 97(7), 1241–8.

Juma, C. 2010. *The New Harvest: Agricultural Innovation in Africa*. Oxford University Press, New York.

Kennedy, E. and Peters, P. 1993. Household food security and child nutrition: the interaction of income and gender of household head. *World Development*, 20, 1077–85.

Kesby, M. 2007. Editorial: methodological insights on and from Children's Geographies. *Children's Geographies*, 5(3), 193–205.

MDHS. 2004. *Malawi Demographic and Health Survey 2004*. Zomba: National Statistics Office.

MDHS. 2010. *Malawi Demographic and Health Survey 2010*. Zomba: National Statistics Office.

Maleta, K., Virtanen, S.M., Espo, M. et al. 2003. Seasonality of growth and the relationship between weight and height gain in children under three years of age in rural Malawi. *Acta Pediatrica*, 92, 491–7.

Massey, D. 1998. The Spatial Construction of Youth Cultures, in *Cool Places: Geographies of Youth Cultures*, edited by T. Skelton and G. Valentine. London/New York: Routledge, 121–9.

Massey, D. and Allen, J. 1984. *Geography Matters: A Reader*. Cambridge: Cambridge University Press.

McEwan, C. 2001. Postcolonialism, feminism and development: intersections and dilemmas. *Progress in Development Studies*, 1, 93–111.

Msachi, R., Dakishoni, L. and Bezner Kerr, R. 2009. 'Soils, food and healthy communities: working towards food sovereignty in Malawi'. *Journal of Peasant Studies*, 36(3), 700–706.

Munthali, A.C., Chimbiri, A. and Zulu, E. 2004. *Adolescent Sexual and Reproductive Health in Malawi:A Synthesis of Research Evidence. Occasional Report*. New York: The Alan Guttmacher Institute. No. 15.

Nayak, A. 2003. *Race, Place and Globalization: Youth Cultures in a Changing World*. Oxford and New York: Berg, Oxford International Publishers Ltd.

NSO (National Statistical Office). 2005. *Malawi Demographic and Health Survey 2004: Preliminary Report*. National Statistical Office, Zomba, Malawi and ORC Macro, Calverton, Maryland.

NSO. 2012a. *Malawi Demographic and Health Survey 2011: Preliminary Report*. National Statistical Office, Zomba, Malawi and ORC Macro, Calverton, Maryland.

NSO. 2012b. *Malawi Integrated Household Survey 2010–11*. National Statistical Office, Zomba, Malawi.

Oladoja, M. 2008. Contributions of fadama farming to household food security amongst youth in rural communities of Lagos State, Nigeria. *Journal of Food, Agriculture & Environment*, 6(1), 139–44.

Panelli, R., Punch, S. and Robson, E. 2007. *Global Perspectives on Rural Childhood and Youth: Young Rural Lives*. Oxford and New York: Taylor & Francis.

Piot, C. 2010. *Nostalgia for the Future: West Africa after the Cold War*. Chicago: University of Chicago Press.

PRB (Population Reference Bureau). 2011. *The World's Women and Girls: 2011 Data Sheet*. Washington, DC. [Online]. Available at: www.prb.org.

Punch, S. 2007. Negotiating migrant identities: young people in Bolivia and Argentina. *Children's Geographies*, 5(1–2), 95–112.

Ruel, M. 2003. Operationalizing Dietary Diversity: A Review of Measurement Issues and Research Priorities. *Journal of Nutrition*, 133(11, Suppl.2), 3911S–3926S.

Sahn, D. and Arulpragasam, J. 1991. The stagnation of smallholder agriculture in Malawi: a decade of structural adjustment. *Food Policy*, 219–34.

Swindale, A. and Bilinsky, P. 2006. Development of a Universally Applicable Household Food Insecurity Measurement Tool: Process, Current Status, and Outstanding Issues. *Journal of Nutrition*, 136, 1449S–1452S.

Tsing, A. 2005. *Friction: An Ethnography of Global Encounter*. Princeton, NJ: Princeton University Press.

Ueyema, M. and Yamauchi, F. 2009. Marriage Behavior Response to Prime-Age Adult Mortality: Evidence from Malawi. *Demography*, 46(1), 43–63.

UN (United Nations). 2004. *World Fertility Report 2003*. New York: UN Department of Economic and Social Affairs, Population Division.

UNAIDS, World Health Organisation. 2008. Report on the Global AIDS Epidemic. [Online]. Available at: www.unaids.org/en/KnowledgeCentre/HIVData/GlobalReport/2008/2008_Global_report.asp.

Van Blerk, L. and Ansell, N. 2006. Imagining migration: Placing children's understanding of 'moving house' in Malawi and Lesotho. *Geoforum*, 37(2), 256–72.

Van Blerk, L. and Kesby, M. 2008. *Doing Children's Geographies*. London: Routledge.

Varga, C.A. 1997. Sexual decision-making and negotiation in the midst of AIDS: youth in KwaZulu-Natal, South Africa. *Supplement 3 to Health Transition Review*, 7.

WHO. 2005. *Nutrition in Adolescence – Issues and Challenges for the Health Sector: Issues in Adolescent Health and Development*. WHO, Geneva.

World Bank. 2011. Country level data. [Online]. Available at: http://data.worldbank.org/country/malawi [accessed: October 1 2012].

# Chapter 11

# Resource Depletion, Peak Oil, and Public Health: Planning for a Slow Growth Future

Michael Pennock, Blake Poland and Trevor Hancock

The scale, speed and complexity of twenty-first century challenges suggest that responses based on marginal changes to the current trajectory of the human enterprise – "fiddling at the edges" – risk the collapse of large segments of the human population or of globalised contemporary society as whole. (Steffen et al. 2011, 752)

Many of the consequences of peak petroleum will fall disproportionately on at-risk populations, especially those who are poor. Rising fuel prices will place a special burden on poor drivers; this may be compounded by long commutes for those who cannot find affordable housing near where they work, and by aging vehicles with poor fuel efficiency. (Frumkin, Hess and Vindigni 2009, 4)

## Introduction

The purpose of this chapter is to consider the public health implications of rising energy prices and growing energy insecurity associated with a tightening of global oil supplies, and to consider what 'peak oil' might mean for the future of globalisation, 'development', and discourses of economic growth and 'progress'. Society's deep dependency on cheap oil reveals a number of key vulnerabilities that require urgent attention. But such a dependency needs to be considered alongside three other emerging challenges to population health: climate change; ecosystem degradation (including pollution, eco-toxicity, and loss of habitat species and biodiversity); and growing socioeconomic inequality. Since these emerging threats have been well described elsewhere (Harrison 2006; Homer-Dixon 2006) and to a lesser extent and more recently within the public health literature (Frumkin et al. 2007; Hanlon and McCartney, 2008; Parker and Schwartz 2010; Hancock 2011; Neff et al. 2011; Nisbet et al. 2011; Poland et al. 2011; Schwartz et al. 2011; Winch and Stepnitz 2011), and a full explication is beyond the scope of this chapter, we focus our attention here more pointedly on the health implications of the end of cheap oil. Nevertheless, we argue against viewing this issue in isolation, and therefore begin with a brief review of the larger context.

The dilemma of focusing on one expression of this problem and ignoring other dimensions and the many interactions between these dimensions has been summarised by MO Andreae of the Max Planck Institute for Chemistry:

In the public mind, "global change" has become almost synonymous with "global warming" or "climate change", a narrow reduction of the original meaning. Although there is no doubt that the possibility of climate change is of great concern to the Earth"s population, we must not forget that we are living in a period when almost all components of the Earth system are undergoing change. The chemical composition of the atmosphere is being perturbed at a vast scale by human activities. The terrestrial biota are modified by land use change, biomass burning, deforestation, and species extinction. Marine life is impacted by overfishing, eutrophication and pollution. There is a tendency to see these issues as independent environmental problems, each grabbing the public"s attention for some time, and each demanding a specific solution.

This approach obscures the fact that all these phenomena are occurring simultaneously, and within the same "Earth system". As a result, they interact with one another, reinforcing or damping each other, or changing each other's temporal evolution. (Andreae 2001)

One of the earliest attempts to model this complexity was the World3 computer simulation model of the Massachusetts Institute of Technology (MIT). This model was used by the Club of Rome in the late 1960s to develop a comprehensive forecast of key global trends (Meadows et al. 1972). It is instructive to look back upon the projections which this model produced.

**The Club of Rome Revisited**

In 1968 an international think-tank of industrialists, scientists and politicians called the Club of Rome asked a group at the MIT to model the effects of major global trends on the health of the planet. The MIT group built a world computer model to investigate five major trends of global concern – accelerating industrialisation, rapid population growth, widespread malnutrition, depletion of nonrenewable resources, and a deteriorating environment. The results were published in the 1972 book entitled *Limits to Growth* (Meadows et al. 1972). Three general conclusions arose from the projections:

1.  If the present growth trends in world population, industrialisation, pollution, food production, and resource depletion continue unchanged, the limits to growth on this planet will be reached sometime within the next 100 years. The most probable result will be a sudden and uncontrollable decline in both population and industrial capacity.
2.  It is possible to alter these growth trends and to establish a condition of ecological and economic stability that is sustainable far into the future. The state of global equilibrium could be designed so that the basic material needs of each person on earth are satisfied and each person has an equal opportunity to realise his or her individual human potential.
3.  If the world's people decide to strive for this second outcome rather than the first, the sooner they begin working to attain it, the greater will be their chances of success (Meadows et al. 1972).

In 1992, the modellers published an update of their original projections and found the trends relatively unchanged (Meadows 2004). They stated that they would re-write the three basic conclusions as follows:

1.  Human use of many essential resources and generation of many kinds of pollutants have already surpassed rates that are physically sustainable. Without significant reductions in material and energy flows, there will be in the coming decades an uncontrolled decline in per capita food output, energy use, and industrial production.

2. This decline is not inevitable. To avoid it two changes are necessary. The first is a comprehensive revision of policies and practices that perpetuate growth in material consumption and in population. The second is a rapid, drastic increase in the efficiency with which materials and energy are used.

3. A sustainable society is still technically and economically possible. It could be much more desirable than a society that tries to solve its problems by constant expansion. The transition to a sustainable society requires a careful balance between long-term and short-term goals and an emphasis on sufficiency, equity, and quality of life rather than on quantity of output. It requires more than productivity and more than technology; it also requires maturity, compassion, and wisdom.

In 2008 Graham Turner at the Commonwealth Scientific and Industrial Research Organisation in Australia published a paper called 'A Comparison of 'The Limits to Growth' with Thirty Years of Reality' (Turner 2008). It examined the extent to which the trends of the past 30 years were consistent with the *Limits to Growth* forecasts and concluded that changes in industrial production, food production and pollution are all in line with the book's predictions of economic and societal collapse by the middle of the twenty-first century.

In summary, the original forecasts produced by the MIT group which predicted a substantial collapse of the global ecosystem and economy during the mid-century period appear to be on track 30 years after they were generated.

One of the key trends included in the MIT/Club of Rome analysis involved a sharp tightening of global energy supplies and this is the topic of the remainder of this chapter. Peak oil is a compelling and imminent example of a resource depletion issue that has profound environmental, economic and social implications. Although some effects will be potentially positive, many will be negative. As we argue below, the likely effects will include a reversal of historic post-industrial trends in globalisation, economic growth, travel, and availability and cost of both staples and luxury goods, a worsening of income inequalities, and negative impacts upon the social determinants of health. Although many of the scenarios which are sketched around peak oil are described by some in almost 'doomsday' overtones, a successful adaptation to the new reality of scarce and expensive oil could create a future which is also consistent with many of the characteristics of a healthy community: cleaner air, healthier lifestyles, improved food security, greater conviviality/ social capital and, possibly, improved economic security.

The chapter will conclude with a brief discussion of the role that public health can play in facilitating a successful adaptation to this new world of resource scarcity.

**What is Peak Oil?**

The term 'peak oil' refers to the expectation that global oil production will reach a maximum or 'peak' at some point and then decline in subsequent years. This is not about the 'end of oil' but rather the point at which it cannot be extracted any faster. This usually happens when roughly half of the available reserve has been exploited, necessitating additional measures (e.g. injection of high pressure steam) to continue expected extraction rates. Since most of the largest oil fields in current production have already peaked, and they decline at a documented rate of 4–12 per cent (a rate that may increase over time) (Hook et al. 2009; UKERC 2009), this has necessitated chasing after more remote (and expensive) sources (deep water, oil sands etc.). This cost issue is often expressed in terms of the amount of energy (expressed in barrels of oil) that is required to extract each barrel of oil, also known as 'energy return on investment' (EROI). Mature Saudi oil fields had an EROI of 1:100 for most of their pre-peak years. As the surface levels of those sources were extracted, the energy requirements increased to extract deeper reserves. By 1999 world production averaged out at 35 barrels produced for each barrel invested and the numbers continued to fall as new sources such as the tar sands produce only two to four barrels and shale production average five barrels for each barrel invested (Murphy and Hall 2010). The majority of new oil discoveries are in deep sea locations and the estimated cost of developing those sites is between $60 and $85 a barrel, compared to $20 for Saudi Arabian oil (Murphy and Hall 2011).

## History of Peak Oil

In the mid-1950s, an American geologist named M. King H Hubbert developed a model which predicted that production from US oil fields would peak in the early 1970s (Bridges 2010; Hubbert 1956). Although his projections were widely rejected by his colleagues in the petroleum industry, his projection turned out to be remarkably accurate. This midway point became known as Hubbert's Peak. Discussion about when the global Hubberts Peak would occur have been numerous and passionate. The estimated dates, from various sources are presented in Table 11.1 (Based on Frumkin, Hess and Vindigni, 2009, with more recent sources added).

The more recent estimates seem to cluster around 2015–2020 or out to 2030, although some suggest there will be no peak.

Fatih Birol, the Chief Economist of the International Energy Agency, stated in an April 2011 interview on the Australia Broadcasting Corporation that the IEA believed that world oil production had peaked in 2006:

> On the one hand we have this pressure on the demand side, but when we look at the production side the prospects are a little bleak. We think that the crude oil production has already peaked in 2006, but we expect oil to come from the natural gas liquids, the type of liquid we have through the production of gas, and also a bit from the oil sands. But in any case it will be very challenging to see an increase in the production to meet the growth in the demand, and as a result of that one of the major conclusions we have from our recent work in the energy outlook is that the age of cheap oil is over. We all have to prepare ourselves, as governments, as industry, or as a private car driver, for higher oil prices. (Birol 2011)

The concept, reality, and timing of peak oil have been hotly debated since Hubbard's first formulation, and understandably so given the centrality of cheap oil to the global economy and the ramifications that the end of cheap oil would have on globalisation. Accurate projections of remaining supplies are complicated by uncertainties in estimating the size of reserves, economic and political pressures to over-estimate the size of known reserves (e.g. OPEC production quotas are tied to reserve size, as are oil company share values), and the sheer complexity of the field. Moreover, production rates depend not only on underlying geology but also drilling techniques, production quotas, and political developments (insurgency, local unrest, sanctions). More recently, it has been suggested

**Table 11.1    Forecasted Dates for World Peak Petroleum Production**

| Forecasted Date of Peak Petroleum Production | Source and background | Date of Forecast |
|---|---|---|
| 2005 | K.S Deffeyes (oil company geologist and Princeton professor) | 2005 |
| Ca. 2006 | C.J. Campbell (oil company geologist) | 2004 |
| 2006 | Energy Watch Group (Germany) | 2007 |
| 2006–2007 | A.M.S. Bakhtiari (Iranian oil executive) | 2004 |
| 2007–2009 | M.R. Simmons (investment banker) | 2005 |
| Before 2010 | D. Goodstein (California Institute of Technology Vice Provost) | 2004 |
| 2013 | UK Industry Taskforce on Peak Oil and Energy Security | 2008 |
| 2014 | Kuwait University study | 2010 |
| Before 2015 | Oxford University researchers in the journal Energy Policy | 2010 |
| Before 2016 | OPEC | 2006 |
| 2003–2020 | US Geological Survey | 2000 |
| 2020–2030 | US Department of Energy (Oak Ridge National Laboratory) | 2003 |
| 2020 - 2030 | International Energy Agency | 2008, 2009 |
| 2006 | International Energy Agency | 2010 |
| 2020 –2030 | UK Energy Research Centre | 2009 |
| 2021–2112 | US Department of Energy (Energy Information Administration) | 2004 |
| After 2025 | Shell Oil | 2003 |
| After 2030 | Cambridge Energy Research Associates (consulting firm) | 2006 |
| After 2030 | International Energy Agency | 2006 |
| No foreseeable peak | M.C. Lynch (energy consultant) | 2003 |
| No foreseeable peak | Leonardo Maugeri | 2004 and also 2012 |
| No foreseeable peak | Abdullah S Juma'ah, President, Director and CEO, Saudi Aramco | 2008 |

that new developments in 'fracking' for shale oil has altered the picture significantly, with some claims being made that peak oil is postponed indefinitely or that the US will soon emerge as a global energy superpower and net exporter (Ungar 2012; McClanahan 2012; Cohen 2013). On the other hand, detailed analysis of existing fracking wells reveal high annual depletion rates- with observed rates between 33 per cent (Biermann 2012) and 52 per cent (Hughes 2012) – well above the 4–10 per cent reported for conventional oil fields, such that growth in production can only be achieved with exponential increases in drilling rates (Whipple 2012). With these more recent developments in mind, then, we make two crucial observations.

On balance, it seems that most analysts accept that there will be a peak to oil production, and that it will come in the next 10–15 years. But that may not be – indeed probably is not – the key issue. There are two other aspects of the argument that are more important than deciding when/if peak oil will arrive.

- First, peak oil is not so much a peaking of supply or production as it is the end of the era of cheap oil. Since globalisation requires not just oil but cheap oil, the ramifications are significant, regardless of when peak production (which will only be evident in hindsight) occurs. The development of deepwater, arctic and tar sands sources despite a weak economy suggests the end of cheap oil is upon us, as many of these new sources are only economical at $80+/barrel. The implications for the global economy are profound.
- Second, as McKibben (2012) and others have made clear, even if there was no peak oil, we are fast approaching – and may already be past – the peak of oil production (and fossil fuel production more generally) that the planet can tolerate. It has been estimated that we cannot burn more than another 565 gigatons of carbon dioxide if we are to stay below the 2°C of warming that is the target upper limit for global warming, but it is also estimated that the fossil fuel corporations now have 2,795 gigatons in their reserves, or five times the allowable upper limit (Carbon Tracker Initiative 2012). And they have no intention of leaving it unburned.

Put simply, we're beyond the era of cheap or limitless oil and other fossil fuels, because even if oil, coal and gas were limitless, we need peak oil, because we can no longer afford (environmentally) to exploit remaining known reserves. However, as Hopkins (2008) points out in *The Transition Handbook*, although we might 'need' peak oil, the likelihood is that without a clear societal commitment and plan to transition to a low-carbon future, the response to peak oil is likely to be to chase whatever alternative fossil fuel reserves we can get – and many of these, like coal, are going to exacerbate climate change.

Thus so-called 'solutions' to peak oil can exacerbate climate change and so the response must be a coordinated one on both fronts, one that deals with the economic, political, social, and distributive impacts of a fossil-fuel-constrained future alongside the ecological impacts of the damage we've already wrought – and will continue to wreak, because it will take us decades of continued fossil fuel use to make the transition.

### The Health-related Implications of Rising World Oil Prices

The debate about the actual date of the global Hubbert's Peak, although interesting, is less important than the implications for energy prices. Regardless of when the actual peak takes place, it is expected that prices will rise and, in the short term, become more volatile as the peak is approached and continue to rise thereafter. As reflected in the figure below, world oil prices have behaved in recent years in a way that is consistent with the peak oil theory.

Prices rose dramatically after 2005 as a result of increased costs of production coupled with the impact of increasing demand from China and India. They reached a peak of $140 a barrel at the start of the current recession, and it has been suggested that these prices were the underlying cause of the recession (Rubin 2009). Further, it is suggested that in this close relationship between energy prices and economic performance, the spare capacity required to fuel a global economic 'recovery' no longer exists, and that globalisation (itself highly dependent on cheap oil) is in question (ibid.). It's unlikely that we can continue to fill Dollar

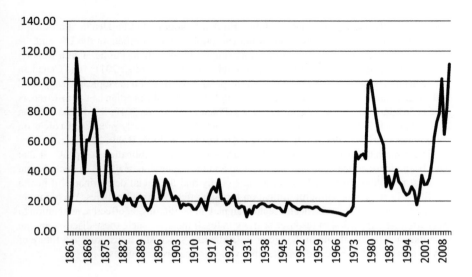

**Figure 11.1    Crude Oil Prices 1861–2011 (2011 US Dollars)**
*Source:* BP Statistical Review of World Energy June 1012; http://www.bp.com/statisticalreview.

Stores and Walmarts in North America with items produced in China when shipping costs outweigh the actual dollar value of the items themselves.

The effects of these rising prices are expected to be widespread and profound given the widespread use of petroleum as both an energy source and an input into the many products of the petrochemical industry, such as plastics and fertilisers. Widespread inflation is anticipated, particularly in food prices, heating, transportation, fertilisers and all plastic products. Some industries, such as tourism and airlines will be particularly hard hit and some analysts, such as former CIBC world markets chief analyst Jeff Rubin have argued that the world economy will be in danger of entering a long period of stagflation (ongoing recession accompanied by high levels of inflation) (Rubin 2009).

Not all of the consequences will be negative. An era of high energy prices could decrease the quantity of $CO_2$ produced into the atmosphere as individuals are forced to reduce their consumption. In essence, Peak Oil will accomplish the goals of a carbon tax by decreasing the supply of energy (and thus increasing its price) to the point where individuals are forced to conserve. Rubin (2009) has argued that rising energy prices will bring an end to globalisation by dramatically increasing the transportation costs of bringing goods to market, but that this will also boost local production. However, none of this is a foregone conclusion. It's just as possible that rising oil prices will press more coal into production, not only for electricity production, but also in terms of large-scale coal 'gasification' projects, and/or make oil extraction from tar sands or through fracking more economical. The potential for a catastrophic increase in Greenhouse Gas emissions from coal at a time when we are already perilously close to major climatic tipping points, should not be underestimated.

In recent years the implications of increasing energy prices on health has received increased attention from within the public health community. In March 2008, the US

Centers for Disease Control and the Johns Hopkin School of Public Health sponsored a symposium on the subject, and three prominent public health journals in the UK and the US have devoted special issues to the topic (Public Health 2008, Public Health Reports Jan–Feb 2008; and the American Journal of Public Health September 2011). The Canadian public health community has been slower to respond. No articles on the topic have appeared in the Canadian Journal of Public Health, although a number of Canadian health researchers have been addressing peak oil in other venues (Poland and Dooris 2010; Spady and Gagnon 2010; Hancock 2011; Poland et al. 2011) and Canadians were early prominent voices on these issues outside of the health sector (e.g. Homer-Dixon 2006; Rubin 2009).

The remainder of this chapter will discuss some of the implications of peak oil that have been identified for the health care system and for population health. We conclude that the most profound effects will be on income equity and the social determinants of health and that will require meaningful mitigation through effective social policies. We highlight potential roles that the public health sector can play in facilitating an effective adaptation to this particular expression of resource scarcity in fossil fuels. As such, these discussions can illuminate the potential role of the sector in facilitating successful transitions to a future of slower growth and diminished supplies of a variety of natural resources.

## Peak Oil and Environmentally Responsible Health Care

As large-scale consumers of fossil-fuel energy for uses such as heating, transportation and electrical equipment, lighting etc., health care providers will experience the inflationary impact of peak oil. The sector is also a major consumer of plastics, as the majority of modern anti-septic practices have come to rely on disposable plastic materials, including tubing, syringes and gloves. In addition, many medications are developed from petroleum-based products, including aspirin, many antihistamines, antibiotics, antineoplastics, and psychoactive drugs. Petroleum-based products are also used for tablet binders and pill-coatings. Hospitals are substantial users of energy. A Natural Resources Canada study in 2003 concluded that Canadian hospitals consumed as much energy as 450,000 households (Natural Resources Canada 2003). The upward pressure on health care costs which will result from escalating energy prices will occur at a time when governments are facing other revenue and expenditure challenges which are associated with the cost increases and an economy in decline. Based on past performance in the US, Hess, Bednarz, Bae and Pierce (2011), estimated that a 1 per cent increase in monthly fuel oil prices would result in a 0.03 per cent increase in monthly medical care prices with an 8 month time lag. Thus a doubling in fuel prices would result in a 3 per cent increase in medical costs.

The good news is that the past decade has seen the emergence of a growing global movement to encourage and support environmentally responsible health care. Starting in the USA, Health Care Without Harm (HCWH) has grown to be 'an international coalition of more than 470 organisations in 52 countries working to transform the health care sector so it is no longer a source of harm to people and the environment', with regional groupings and national affiliates in the USA, Canada, Europe, South East Asia and Latin America. The Coalition and its members are focused on issues such as waste management, climate change, reducing the use of toxic materials, and promoting 'green' approaches such as green buildings and energy, the use of safer chemicals and the development of healthy food systems (Health Care Without Harm 2012).

## Peak Oil and a Healthy Built Environment

Kaza et al. (2011) employed land use, economic and development models to study the potential impact of peak oil on the urban form of the Baltimore-Washington area. Their modeling concluded that peak oil would have some effect on increased densities in downtown areas, increased public transit and non-automobile travel modes, increased rates of communicable diseases, injuries and assaults. However, their projections did not highlight an 'end of suburbia' outcome of escalating commuting costs that others (e.g. Kunstler 2005; Greene 2008; Brown 2011) have projected because, in their view:

- Fuel consumption related to commuting has changed relatively little in the past due to price changes because consumers tend to cut back in other expenditure areas.
- A nation's housing stock changes relatively little on an annual basis and a wholesale shift from the suburbs to urban cores would take a long time to occur.

It is more likely, then, that many suburban commuters would remain in the suburbs, and reduce expenditures in other areas, *if their incomes are sufficient to support this shift* (note that a disproportionate percentage of US home mortgage foreclosures since 2008 have been in the 'drive to qualify' 'distant suburbs'). The primary negative impacts would fall on individuals and families who are already using their full incomes to support basic consumption of food and shelter. Kaza et al. (2011) make this point succinctly-

Although it is not the focus of this paper, we believe that the loss of purchasing power, the loss of economic productivity, and a redistribution of wealth are probably the most important means by which peak oil could affect public health (1600).

It should be noted that relatively few jurisdictions have addressed the implications of rising energy prices on social inequity, which suggests the need for an explicit use of an 'energy justice' lens to examine the uneven impacts of rising energy costs on the urban poor, who tend to inhabit substandard and energy-inefficient rental units (Teelucksingh and Poland 2011).

There are several potential upsides in the long run that are worth highlighting here: even in the context of car-dependent suburban sprawl, an increase in public transit use (where densities allow such services to be economically viable), walking and cycling is likely as fuel prices increase; coupled with increased participation in gardening (as food prices soar). The result is likely to go beyond the kind of hardships outlined above to also include increased physical activity, healthier food (see below), stronger connections between producers and consumers, and increased community conviviality and mutual aid (Hopkins 2008; Schwartz et al. 2011). More broadly, the positive associations between healthy and sustainable communities have been recognised for several decades (Hancock 1994, 1996, 1997, 2000; Brown et al. 2005).

## Peak Oil and Food Security

The potential negative impacts of peak oil on the food system are significant and related to increases in food costs across the board, particularly foods which require intensive farming, heavy fertiliser use or long distance transportation. Notwithstanding recent interest in local food, most people have become accustomed to having a wide variety of foods available regardless of season or travel distance. The 2008 peak in oil prices was accompanied by a dramatic spike in food prices that resulted in riots in 40 major cities around the world.

However, some of the news concerning Peak Oil and the food system might be positive. For example, among the foods that require the greatest energy use for their production are foods that fall into the low-nutrient and 'junk food' category – prepared snacks, alcoholic beverages, bottled water, soft drinks, baking products, and sugar/ sweets (Neff et al. 2011). Given the relatively high energy intensity of intensive meat production (Pelletier et al. 2011), a shift to a lower meat diet might also result in both health and environmental benefits. Some healthier alternatives, such as fish, eggs, fresh fruit and fresh dairy fall at the less energy-intensive end of the continuum, but there are noteworthy exceptions there too: lettuce grown in California and shipped to Canada for off-season consumption takes more than 10 times as many calories of oil to produce as it offers in nutritional value. It is likely that peak oil would significantly increase the price and reduce the consumption of leafy greens in the winter months in the North American northeast, much as we already see in the far North, until such a time as practices such as geothermal-heated greenhouses, root cellaring, solar drying, preserving and canning become widespread enough to make these more widely available and inexpensive in the off-season. In addition, increased local food production and consumption, including through community-shared agriculture, community gardens, growing food on municipal land (Nordahl 2009), foraging (Henderson 2000), 'urban homesteading' (Coyne and Knutzen 2008; Hess 2012), and even 'guerilla gardening' (Tracey 2007) might be expected to lead to increased conviviality and social capital.

## Population Health and Equity Considerations of Peak Oil

The experiences of the former Soviet Union nations and the growing research literature on the health effects of economic decline demonstrated the immediate and marked effects that economic collapse can have on health status indicators such as life-expectancy, suicide rates, alcohol use, and mental health (Walberg et al. 1998; Catalano et al. 2011). Even less extreme impacts, however, could have substantial and severe implications for health equity. Frumkin, Hess and Vindigni (2009) summarised some of the issues as follows:

> many of the consequences of peak petroleum will fall disproportionately on at-risk populations, especially those who are poor. Rising fuel prices will place a special burden on poor drivers; this may be compounded by long commutes for those who cannot find affordable housing near where they work, and by aging vehicles with poor fuel efficiency. (14)

Poor individuals and families will also be affected disproportionately by rising food prices as food expenditures account for a larger proportion of their household budgets. This will be particularly true of fresh fruit and vegetable prices in the off-season, when higher transport costs will increase the price of imports. They will also face rising prices in clothing, medications and other consumer goods for which petroleum is a major input.

Central to this argument is the notion of the 'growth paradox' – when oil prices reach a certain level they cause a reduction in economic growth and the onset of recessions. Oil consumption falls, prices decrease and economic growth restarts. In an age of peak oil, however, prices do not fall far enough to bring about sustained growth because the costs of production in deep ocean sites or the Canadian Oil Sands is so high. And every time economic growth restarts (which all our politicians claim as their 'Job 1'), it bumps its head up against constraints in oil production. As in the case of the most recent slowdown, prices fell dramatically after the July 2008 peak at over $140 a barrel but very quickly rose to the $80 a barrel level, and higher. By 2011 and 2012 they were vacillating around the $100 mark – back at historically high levels. At this level, oil is too expensive to fuel an expansion in economic growth (Murphy and Hall 2011). The 'growth paradox' states that a return of economic growth will rapidly send oil prices to a level that snuffs out economic growth. For this reason, some analysts believe that the end of cheap oil also means the end of the kind of economic growth that we have come to believe represents a normal state of affairs (Rubin 2009; Murphy and Hall 2011). While this may be seen as a calamity for some, it may be a relief to those who have been warning of dire consequences of unfettered growth and consumption for climate change and environmental degradation (Meadows 2004; Hopkins 2008; Speth 2008; Victor 2008; Poland, Dooris and Haluza-Delay 2011).

Within the broader economic downturn, low-wage workers may be at disproportionate risk for job loss, and loss of benefits as employers cut back. An analysis of the impacts of the 2008 recession by Statistics Canada reported that employment losses were concentrated at the lower end of the pay scale and the most substantial losses were found among recent immigrants, young workers, and workers with lower levels of education (LaRochelle-Cote and Gilmore 2009).

## Planning for an Era of High Cost Energy

The future cannot be forecasted with much certainty. In risk analysis terms, however, there appears to be growing consensus that the probability of escalating energy prices in the near future, due to Peak Oil, is high, and the potential population health consequences are also substantial, especially among many already disadvantaged and marginalised groups. Peak Oil should be understood as an emerging threat to public health, and in particular an emerging threat to health equity. The literature, to date, suggests that the direct impacts upon health care supply and labour costs will be measurable, though moderate. There will be some impacts upon urban form but these changes will occur over a longer period of time. Food costs will be affected but there may also be positive impacts on local food production.

The most dramatic impacts are likely to be felt through the social determinants of health. The most vulnerable populations will be those who have been traditionally impacted by economic downturns – the young, persons with limited education and skills, persons with low income, and immigrants. Similar impacts are expected at the international level. Increased costs of fuels, food and fertilisers will have the greatest impact upon the poorer developing countries (Klare, Levy and Sidel 2011). The public health sector can respond to this issue through three primary routes – surveillance, mitigation/adaptation, and supporting new ways of measuring 'progress' and new development paradigms.

### Surveillance

Traditional public health surveillance and community health assessment could incorporate fuel prices, food and travel data for the purposes of monitoring trends and identifying areas and groups that are most at risk from increased energy prices. In the United Kingdom, the national statistics office has begun producing an annual report on fuel poverty for the Department of Energy and Climate Change (DECC 2011). Households are classified as 'fuel poor' if they spend more than 10 per cent of their income on heating fuel. In Canada, Statistics Canada maintains price indices for energy and the annual Survey of Household Spending yields estimates of expenditures on fuel as a percentage of total household expenditures.

*Mitigation and Adaptation*

A number of communities have developed peak oil task forces to develop community-based mitigation and adaptation strategies. Many have joined the Transition Towns movement that developed out of Totnes, England in 2005 as a creative grassroots response to peak oil and climate change. It is noteworthy that many of the mitigation and adaptation strategies that have been recommended are entirely consistent with current public health approaches to the promotion of healthy built environments – issues such as food security, local employment and production, walkability, urban transportation, higher density development and lower carbon emissions. The agendas of peak oil adaptation/ mitigation and healthy built environments appear entirely consistent. Public health also needs to argue for the protection of vulnerable groups during the transition to a low-carbon future.

In 2006, the Portland City Council established a 12-person Peak Oil Task Force and charged them with the responsibility for '… developing recommendations to mitigate the impacts of rising energy costs and declining supplies'. The key recommendations of the Task Force were:

1.  Reduce total oil and natural gas consumption by 50 per cent over the next 25 years.
2.  Inform citizens about peak oil and foster community and community-based solutions.
3.  Engage business, government and community leaders to initiate planning and policy change.
4.  Support land use patterns that reduce transportation needs, promote walkability and provide easy access to services and transportation options.
5.  Design infrastructure to promote transportation options and facilitate efficient movement of freight, and prevent infrastructure investments that would not be prudent given fuel shortages and higher prices.
6.  Encourage energy-efficient and renewable transportation choices.
7.  Expand energy-efficiency programs and incentives for all new and existing structures.
8.  Preserve farmland and expand local food production and processing.
9.  Identify and promote sustainable business opportunities.
10. Redesign the safety net and protect vulnerable and marginalised populations.
11. Prepare emergency plans for sudden and severe shortages (City of Portland 2007).

To the extent that these actions have health implications – and many of them do – public health organisations and professionals clearly need to play a role in understanding and making clear the public health and health equity implications of the implementation of these recommendations.

*Rethinking Progress: New Paradigms Emerging*

Traditional notions of progress have relied heavily on economic growth rates that have been dependent on cheap oil, using measures such as GDP that actually 'benefit' from oil spills and the ensuing clean-up, for example. There has been an increased recognition internationally of the need to develop more comprehensive models and indicators of progress that support sustainable development and the promotion of human wellbeing. In 2007, the Organisation for Economic Cooperation and Development launched a major initiative entitled 'Measuring and Fostering the Progress of Societies' which called for the development of broader measures that incorporate social and ecological dimensions of development (OECD 2007). In 2008 French President Nicolas Sarkozy established a Commission on the Measurement of Economic Performance and Social Progress that resulted in an influential report that recommended the incorporation of social and ecological dimensions into new measures of progress in France (Stiglitz, Sen and Fitoussi 2009). In July 2011, the United Nations passed a motion that supported the establishment of a Task Force to articulate a new holistic paradigm for development. This initiative is being led by the nation of Bhutan that pioneered the measurement of 'Gross National Happiness' as a holistic paradigm for its development (Pennock and Ura 2010).

As discussion once again focuses on the 'limits to growth' (Meadows, 2004), a growing chorus of authors have called for Western governments to rethink the deep-seated commitment to 'progress' narratives that emphasise consumerism and economic growth (Daly 1997; Szreter 1999; Victor 2008; Heinber 2011; Jackson, McKibben and Robinson 2011) and we have seen the emergence of a global 'Degrowth' movement with it's own conferences and intellectual leaders. Indigenous perspectives on 'buen vivir' (Gudynas, 2011; Thomson, 2011), living in sacred balance (Jacobs 1998; Harding 2006), Earth rights (Earth Charter 2000; Universal Declaration on the Rights of Mother Earth 2010), but also the nature of the transition we are going through globally (Hill 2009), take these ideas further and are instructive examples of the need for a radical paradigm shift from industrial growth society to something more life-sustaining (Macy 2009; Poland, Dooris and Haluza-Delay 2011). Clearly there are important public health implications – many of them positive – of such a transformation, and public health organisations and professionals need to be part of the discussion and part of the solution.

The need for a fundamental paradigm shift is underscored by Bierman and Bernstein (2012) who argue that

> The need for action hardly needs rehearsing. To put it bluntly, humanity is demanding more of the Earth than it can supply, sending us toward tipping points beyond which the planet's air, water and other natural systems can't recover. ... *Tinkering won't be enough. The situation requires a fundamental transformation of existing practices.* (emphasis added)

Particularly noteworthy, in the context of this book, is the way in which a theoretically-grounded and practice-based 'sociology of creative transformation' highlights the importance of groundedness in place, the capacities of local 'communities of practice' to innovate new ways of sustainable living where widespread education and risk management approaches have failed, and the potential for relatively rapid social change (Poland, Dooris and Haluza-Delay 2011). These themes are increasingly echoed in the Transition Town literature (Bailey et al. 2010; Hopkins 2008), relocalisation movement (North 2010; DeYoung and Princen 2012), and emerging understandings of the nature of social change informed by complexity science and other perspectives (Gunderson and Holling 2001; Scharmer 2009; Senge et al. 2004; Westley et al. 2006, 2011).

Through initiatives such as the Portland Peak Oil Task Force, many of the early responses to develop mitigation and adaptation strategies have occurred at the local level. These initiatives will ultimately need to be supported by enabling legislation at higher jurisdictions. Equally, as the momentum continues to build, it is important that the tools and measures that result from the international activities described above are adapted and applied to communities. Local communities will also require new approaches to monitoring progress that incorporate themes of adaptation and wellbeing, rather than relying on traditional approaches of measuring building permit and construction activity.

### Conclusions

Many of the discussions surrounding peak oil are of a 'doomsday' nature. There is no denying the potential for considerable disruption and damage as the world leaves behind a century of cheap energy. But as also noted, the successful transition to lower-carbon communities, which may be necessitated by peak oil (and also climate change and environmental degradation), could create healthier, more vibrant and sustainable communities which are consistent with public health's vision of healthier built environments. The challenge was summarised by Rubin (2009)-

> Here's the question; will we decide to reinvest in a global economy and an infrastructure that keeps us bound to oil consumption ... If so, we are committing ourselves to a damaging cycle of recessions and recoveries that keeps repeating itself as the economy keeps banging its head on oil prices. If we go this route, peak oil will soon lead to peak GDP. Or we can change ... and don't be surprised if the new smaller world that emerges isn't a lot more livable and enjoyable than the one we are about to leave behind. (23–4)

As we have noted several times, the public health community can and should play a critical role in supporting a healthy and equitable transition to sustainability.

### References

Andreae, M.O. 2001. Feedbacks and Interactions between Global Change, Atmospheric Chemistry and the Biosphere. Chapter 2 in Bengtsson, Lennart and Hammer, Claus, *Geosphere-Biosphere Interactions and Climate*. Cambridge: Cambridge University Press.

Bailey, I., Hopkins, R. and Wilson, G. 2010. Some things old, some things new: The spatial representations and politics of change of the peak oil relocalisation movement. *Geoforum*, 41(4), 595–605.

Berman, A. 2012. *Oil-Prone Shale Plays: The Illusion of Energy Independence*. Proceedings from ASPO-USA Annual Conference, November 30–December 1, Austin, Texas.

Biermann, F., Abbott, K., Andresen, S. et al. 2012. Navigating the Anthropocene: Improving Earth system governance. *Science*, 335(6074), 1306–7.

Birol, Fatih. 2011. Peak Oil: Just Around the Corner. *The Science Show, Australian Broadcasting Corporation*, April 23, 2011. [Online]. Available at: http://www.abc.net. au/radionational/programs/scienceshow/peak-oil-just-around-the-corner/3010606.

Bridge, G. 2010. Geographies of peak oil: the other carbon problem. *Geoforum*, 41(4), 523–30.

Brown, W. 2011. *Surviving the Apocalypse in the Suburbs: The Thrivalist's Guide to Life Without Oil*. New Society Publishers.

Brown, V.A., Grootjans, J., Ritchie, J. et al. 2005. *Sustainability and Health: Supporting Ecological Integrity in Public Health*. Sydney, Australia: Allen and Unwin.

Carbon Tracker Initiative. 2012. *Unburnable Carbon – Are the World's Financial Markets Carrying a Carbon Bubble?* London: Carbon Tracker Initiative

Catalano, R., Goldman-Mellor, S., Saxton, K. et al. 2011. The health effects of economic decline. *Annual Review of Public Health*, 32, 431–50

City of Portland Peak Oil Task Force. 2007. *Descending The Oil Peak: Navigating the Transition from Oil and Natural Gas*. [Online]. Available at: http://www.portlandonline.com/bps/index.cfm?c=42894&a=145732.

Cohen, M. 2013. A renaissance in US production: light tight oil. *IEA Energy: The Journal of the International Energy Agency*, January 3, http://www.iea.org/newsroomandevents/ieajournal/iea-journal-issue-3/name,34049,en.html.

Coyne, K., and Knutzen, E. 2008. *The Urban Homestead: Your Guide to Self-Sufficient Living in the Heart of the City*. Port Townsend, WA: Process Media.

Daly, H. 1997. *Beyond Growth: The Economics of Sustainable Development*. Boston: Beacon Press.

De Young, R. and Princen, T. 2012. *The Localization Reader: Adapting to the Coming Downshift*. Cumberland, RI: MIT Press.

Department of Energy and Climate Change. 2011. *Annual report on fuel poverty statistics 2011*.

Earth Charter . 2000. [Online]. Available at: http://www.earthcharterinaction.org/content/pages/What-is-the-Earth-Charter%3F.html.

Frumkin, H., Hess, J. and Vindigni, S. 2007. Peak petroleum and public health. *JAMA*, 298(14), 1688–90.

Frumkin, H., Hess, J. and Vindigni, S. 2009. Energy and public health: the challenge of peak petroleum. *Public Health Reports*, (January–February), 5–19

Greene, G. 2008. *End of Suburbia* (film).

Gudynas, E. 2011. Buen vivir: today's tomorrow. *Development*, 54(4), 441–7.

Gunderson, L.H. and Holling, C.S. 2001. *Panarchy: Understanding Transformations in Human and Natural Systems*. Washington, DC: Island Press.

Hancock, T. 1994. 'A healthy and sustainable community: the view from 2020', in *The Ecological Public Health: From Vision to Practice*, edited by C. Chu and R. Simpson. Brisbane: Griffith University and Toronto: Centre for Health Promotion.

Hancock, T. 1996. 'Planning and creating healthy and sustainable cities: the challenge for the 21st century', in *Our Cities, Our Future: Policies and Action for Health and Sustainable Development*, edited by C. Price and A. Tsouros. Copenhagen: WHO Healthy Cities Project Office.

Hancock, T. 1997. 'Healthy, sustainable communities: concept, fledgling practice and implications for governance', in *Eco-City Dimensions: Healthy Communities, Healthy Planet*, edited by M. Roseland. Gabriola Island, BC: New Society Press

Hancock, T. 2000. 'Healthy Communities Must Be Sustainable Communities Too'. *Public Health Reports*, 115(2 and 3), 151–6.

Hancock, T. 2011. It's the environment stupid! Declining ecosystem health is THE threat to health in the 21st century. *Health Promotion International*, 26(supp 2), ii168–ii172.

Hanlon, P. and McCartney, G. 2008. Peak oil: will it be public health's greatest challenge? *Public Health*, 122(7), 647–52.

Harding, S. 2006. *Animate Earth: Science, Intuition and Gaia*. White River Jt, VT: Chelsea Green.

Harrison, D. 2006. Peak oil, climate change, public health and well-being. *Journal of the Royal Society for the Promotion of Health*, 126(2), 62–3.

Health Care Without Harm. 2012. [Online]. Available at: www.noharm.org [accessed: May 2012].

Heinberg, R. 2011. *The End of Growth: Adapting to Our New Economic Reality*. New Society.

Hess, A. 2012. *The Weekend Homesteader: A Twelve-Month Guide to Self-Sufficiency*. New York: Skyhorse Publishing.

Hess, J., Bednarz, D., Bae, J. and Pierce, J. 2011. Petroleum and health care: Evaluating and managing health care's vulnerability to petroleum supply shifts. *American Journal of Public Health*, 101(9), 1568–79.

Hill, W. 2009. *Understanding Life: What My Ancestors Taught Me Through My Dreams*. Pittsburgh, PA: Red Lead Press.

Homer-Dixon, T. 2006. *The Upside of Down: Catastrophe, Creativity, and the Renewal of Civilization*. Toronto, ON: Alfred A Knopf Canada.

Hook, M., Hirsch, R. and Aleklett, K. 2009. Giant oil field decline rates and their influence on world oil production. *Energy Policy*, 37(6), 2262–72.

Hopkins, R. 2008. *The Transition Handbook: From Oil Dependency to Local Resilience*. Totnes: Green Books.

Hopkins, R. 2011. *The Transition Companion: Making Your Community More Resilient in Uncertain Times*. White River Jt, VT: Chelsea Green.

Hubbert, HK. 1956. *Nuclear energy and the fossil fuels*. Paper presented to the Southern District Division of Production, American Petroleum Institue. March 1956. [Online]. Available at: www.hubbertpeak.com.

Hughes, D. 2012. *Will Natural Gas Forestall a U.S. Oil Crisis?* Proceedings from ASPO-USA Annual Conference, November 30–December 1, Austin, Texas.

IEA. 2010. *World Energy Outlook 2010*. Paris, France: International Energy Agency.

Jackson, T., McKibben, B. and Robinson, M. 2011. *Prosperity without Growth: Economics for a Finite Planet*. EarthScan.

Jacobs, D.T. 1998. *Primal Awareness*. Rochester, Vermont: Inner Traditions.

Kaza, N., Knaap, G-J., Knaap, I. and Lewis, R. 2011. Peak oil, urban form, and public health: Exploring the connections. *American Journal of Public Health*, 101(9), 1598–606.

Klare, M.T., Levy, B.C. and Sidel, V.W. 2011. The Public health implications of resource wars. *American Journal of Public Health*, 101(9), 1615–19.

Kunstler, J.H. 2005. *The Long Emergency: Surviving the End of Oil, Climate Change, and Other Converging Catastrophes of the 21st Century*. New York, NY: Grove Press.

LaRochelle-Cote, S. and Gilmore, J. 2009. Canada's employment downturn. *Perspectives*, Dec (5–11) Statistics Canada Cat# 75-001-X

Macy, J. 2009. The greening of the self, in *Ecotherapy: Healing with Nature in Mind*, edited by L. Buzzell and C. Chalquist. San Francisco: Sierra Club Books, 238–45.

Macy, J., and Johnstone, C. 2012. *Active Hope: How to Face the Mess We're in without Going Crazy*. Novato, CA: New World Library.

McClanahan, E.T. 2012. The United States, future energy superpower. *The Kansas City Star*, November 17, http://www.kansascity.com/2012/11/17/3921780/the-united-states-future-energy.html.

McKibben, Bill. 2012. Global Warming's Terrifying New Math. *Rolling Stone*, August 2nd

Meadows, D.H. 2004. *Limits to Growth: The 30-Year Update*. White River Junction, VT: Chelsea Green.

Meadows, D.H., Meadows, D.L., Randers, J. and Behrens III, W.W. 1972. *The Limits to Growth*. London, UK: Pan.

Meadows, D. and Randers, D. 1993. Beyond the limits of growth. *Context, A Quarterly Journal of Human Sustainable Culture*, Summer, 10.

Murphy, D.J. and Hall, C.A.S. 2010. Year in review-EROI or energy return on (energy) invested. *Annals of the New York Academy of Sciences*, 1185, 102–19

Murphy, D.J. and Hall, C.A.S. 2011. Energy return on investment, peak oil, and the end of economic growth. *Annals of the New York Academy of Sciences*, 1219, 52–72.

Natural Resources Canada. 2003. *Consumption of energy survey for universities, colleges and hospitals*. Office of Energy Efficiency 2005. [Online]. Available at: http://oee.nrcan.gc.ca/corporate/statistics/neud/dpa/data_e/consumption03/pdf/consumption.pdf.

Neff, R.A., Parker, C.L., Kirschenmann, F.L., 2011. Peak oil, food systems, and public health. *American Journal of Public Health*, 101(9), 1587–97.

Nisbet, M.C., Maibach, E., and Leiserowitz, A. 2011. Framing peak petroleum as a public health problem: Audience research and participatory engagement in the United States. *American Journal of Public Health*, 101(9), 1620–26.

Nordahl, D. 2009. *Public Produce: The New Urban Agriculture*. Washington, DC: Island Press.

North, P. 2010. Eco-localisation as a progressive response to peak oil and climate change: A sympathetic critique. *Geoforum*, 41(4), 585–94.

OECD Measuring the Progress of Societies. [Online]. Available at: http://www.oecd.org/site/0,3407,en_21571361_31938349_1_1_1_1_1,00.html.

Parker, C.L. and Schwartz, B.S. 2010. Human health and well-being in an era of energy scarcity and climate change, in *The Post-Carbon Reader: Managing the 21st Century's Sustainability Crises*, edited by R. Heinberg and D. Lerch. University of California Press.

Pelletier, N., Audsley, E., Brodt, S. et al. 2011. Energy intensity of agriculture and food systems. *Annual Review of Environment and Resources*, 36, 223–46.

Pennock, M. and Ura, K. 2011. Gross national happiness as a framework for health impact assessment. *Environmental Impact Assessment Review*, 31(1), 61–5.

Poland, B. and Dooris, M. 2010. A green and healthy future: the settings approach to building health, equity and sustainability. *Critical Public Health*, 20(3), 281–98.

Poland, B., Dooris, M. and Haluza-DeLay, R. 2011. Securing 'supportive environments' for health in the face of ecosystem collapse: Meeting the triple threat with a sociology of creative transformation. *Health Promotion International*, 26(S2), ii202–ii215.

Rubin J. 2009. *Why Your World Is About To Get a Whole Lot Smaller*. Toronto: Random House Canada

Scharmer, C.O. 2009a. *Seven Acupuncture Points for Shifting Capitalism to Create a Regenerative Ecosystem Economy*. Proceedings from Roundtable on Transforming Capitalism to Create a Regenerative Economy, MIT.

Scharmer, C.O. 2009b. *Theory U: Leading From the Future as It Emerges*. San Francisco: Berrett-Koehler.

Schwartz, B.S., Parker, C.L., Hess, J. and Frumkin, H. 2011. Public health and medicine in an age of energy scarcity: The case of petroleum. *American Journal of Public Health*, 101(9), 1560–67.

Senge, P., Scharmer, C.O., Jaworski, J. and Flowers, B.S. 2004. *Presence: An Exploration of Profound Change in People, Organisations, and Society.* New York, NY: Currency/ Doubleday/Random House.

Spady, G. and Gagnon, F. 2010. *Public Health in the Era of Peak Oil: An Interview with Dr. Donald Spady.* Ottawa: National Collaborating Centre for Healthy Public Policy (PHAC)/Institut national de santé publique du Québec.

Speth, J.G. 2008. *The Bridge at the End of the World: Capitalism, the Environment, and Crossing From Crisis to Sustainability.* New Haven, CT: Yale University Press.

Steffen, W., Persson, A., Deutsch, L. et al. 2011. The Anthropocene: From global change to planetary stewardship. *Ambio: A Journal of the Human Environment*, 40(7), 739–61.

Stiglitz, J.E., Sen, A. and Fitoussi, J-P. 2009. *Report by the Commission on Measurement of Economic Performance and Social Progress.* [Online]. Available at: http://www. stiglitz-sen-fitoussi.fr/en/index.htm.

Szreter, S. 1999. Rapid economic growth and 'the four Ds' of disruption, deprivation, disease and death: public health lessons from nineteenth century Britain for twenty first century China?. *Tropical Medicine & International Health*, 4(2), 146–52.

Teelucksingh, C. and Poland, B. 2011. Energy solutions, neo-liberalism, and social diversity in Toronto, Canada. *International Journal of Environmental Research and Public Health*, 8, 185–202.

Thomson, B. 2011. Pachakuti: Indigenous perspectives, buen vivir, sumaq kawsay and degrowth. *Development*, 54(4), 448–54.

Tracey, D. 2007. *Guerrilla Gardening: A Manualfesto.* Gabriola Island, BC: New Society Publishers.

Turner, G. 2008. *A Comparison of the Limits of Growth With Thirty Years of Reality.* CSIRO Working Paper series 2008–2009. Canberra: CSIRO Sustainable Ecosystems. [Online]. Available at: http://www.csiro.au/files/files/plje.pdf.

UKERC. 2009. The Global Oil Depletion Report. London, UK, Energy Research Centre. http://www.ukerc.ac.uk/support/Global%20Oil%20Depletion.

Ungar, R. 2012. IEA Report: USA set to become number one oil producer by 2020 – energy independent by 2035. *Forbes Magazine*, November 12, http://www.forbes.com/sites/ rickungar/2012/11/12/iea-report-usa-set-to-become-number-one-oil-producer-by-2020- energy-independent-by-2035/.

Universal Declaration on the Rights of Mother Earth. [Online]. Available at: http:// motherearthrights.org/universal-declaration/.

Victor, P.A. 2008. *Managing Without Growth: Slower by Design, Not Disaster.* Northampton, MA: Edward Elgar.

Walberg, P., McKee, M., Shkolnokov, V. et al. 1998. Economic change, crime and mortality crisis in Russia: regional analysis. *BMJ*, August 1, 317(7154), 312–18.

Westley, F., Olsson, P., Folke, C. et al. 2011. Tipping toward sustainability: Emerging pathways of transformation. *Ambio: A Journal of the Human Environment*, 40(7), 762–80.

Westley, F., Zimmerman, B. and Patton, M.Q. 2006. *Getting To Maybe: How the World is Changed.* Toronto: Random House Canada.

Whipple, T. 2012. The peak oil crisis: deep in the heart of Texas. *Falls Church News-Press*, December 12, http://fcnp.com/2012/12/12/the-peak-oil-crisis-deep-in-the-heart-of-texas/.
Winch, P. and Stepnitz, R. 2011. Peak oil and health in low- and middle-income countries: impacts and potential responses. *American Journal of Public Health*, 101(9), 1607–14.

# Chapter 12
# The Water-Health Nexus

Corinne J. Schuster-Wallace, Susan J. Elliott and Elijah Bisung

## Introduction

Improving access to safe water and adequate sanitation has been part of the global development agenda for decades. The obvious social inequities around the world, including access to safe water and sanitation, were addressed globally in 2000 through the creation and recognition of the Millennium Development Goals (MDGs).[1] The MDGs were established to help target disparities and create a shared vision of the world for 2015, but progress has not always kept up with intention, and many of the issues addressed by the MDG targets are dealt with separately (in 'silos') rather than within a holistic framework. Water and sanitation are worthy targets in and of themselves but are part of the solution for achieving other targets, especially reducing maternal, infant and child morbidity and mortality.

In 2012, it was estimated that more than 800,000 deaths, or 1.5% of the global disease burden in low- and middle-income countries were water and sanitation related (Prüss Üstün et al. 2014). Further, those experiencing the greatest impacts from poor water access are the world's most vulnerable; those with the least amount of resilience to cope. It is also widely recognised that the situation will only worsen, as we continue to experience the increasingly serious impacts of global environmental change (i.e., population growth, migration pressures, climate change). While water is essential for life, close to 750 million people still do not have access to safe water; adequate sanitation continues to elude 2.5 billion (JMP 2014). This deadly combination results in unacceptable mortality rates from diarrhoea in young children (approximately 360,000 deaths in 2012 could have been prevented) (Prüss Üstün et al. 2014). This tragic human price is exacerbated by the social and economic burden water-related illnesses pose: to healthcare systems, caregivers, education, local economies and society in general as people are unable to maximise their physical, social and economic potential. Furthermore, water is a cornerstone of economic activity and fundamental for ecosystem integrity; agriculture and industry require large amounts of water and we depend on ecosystems for food and services such as water purification, soil fertility and mitigation of weather-related hazards.

This chapter explores the linkages between water, environment and human health framed within the water-health nexus itself, as represented by the intersection between the bio-physical system, the hydrosocial system,[2] and human health. These linkages are illustrated in two sections – Water and Health, and Water-Health and Development – using a range of global examples highlighting the burden of illness, and the facilitators and

---

1 See http://www.un.org/millenniumgoals/for more information regarding the various goals and targets.

2 The hydrosocial cycle is a useful heuristic for describing flows of water through human (as opposed to hydrologic) systems (i.e., political, cultural, economic) and their inherent power imbalances.

barriers to both ownership and sustained management of water resources for health. In our conclusions, we draw attention to the imperatives of research and development at the water-health nexus.

## Linkages: Water and Health

Since John Snow established the link between cholera and contaminated water in the middle of the nineteenth century, understanding the relationships between health and safe water, adequate sanitation and hygiene has been a central focus of global public health (Gatrell and Elliott 2009). Water-related diseases can be transmitted in a variety of ways (e.g., Black et al. 2010), the most common of which are ingestion (waterborne) or through another animal (vector-borne).Many pathogens spend at least part of their lifecycle in water, or depend upon vectors that do. In general, the diseases that result from these pathogens are collectively referred to as water-related. Other transmission pathways include water-washed infections such as trachoma, a leading cause of preventable blindness in low and middle income countries (LMICs), which are exacerbated under poor hygiene conditions that increase under conditions of water shortage. Lack of hygiene facilitates the faecal-oral route of many waterborne diseases, through contamination of foods during preparation (use of contaminated water) or handling (lack of handwashing with soap) or simply use of dirty utensils.

Among the many diseases associated with water, diarrhoea cases attributable to unsafe water, inadequate sanitation and poor hygiene contribute a significant share to the disease burden. Estimates indicate that diarrhoea results in about 1.4 million child deaths around the world each year, the majority of which occur in developing countries (Prüss-Üstün et al. 2008). While it has long been established that short periods of diarrhoea can be fatal through dehydration (e.g., cholera) and that some waterborne diseases can be toxic (e.g., vtec and etec strains of *E. coli*), there is increasing evidence of health impacts as a result of chronic diarrhoea (i.e., regular or systemic infections). One such impact is upon cognitive development. In Brazilian shanty towns, a cohort study demonstrated a significant relationship between diarrhoea under the age of two and manifestations of reduced cognitive functioning between the ages of six and 12 (Oriá et al. 2009). This outcome is a consequence of nutritional disorders resulting from lack of absorption of nutrients during diarrhoea episodes. Related health impacts for young children include growth retardation and increased susceptibility to secondary infection. However, these impairments could be avoided through appropriate water, sanitation and hygiene interventions (Esrey et al. 1991; Fewtrel et al. 2005; Waddington and Snilstveit 2009). Aside from diarrhoeal diseases, studies have also identified schistosomiasis and other intestinal helminth diseases like hookwarm, trichuriasis, ascariasis to be important barriers to child development and performance in schools (WHO 2002). For example, a study conducted by Ezeamama et al. (2005) in the Philippines found that children with trichuriasis had almost 4.5 times greater odds of performing poorly in verbal fluency tests. They also found evidence of association between ascariasis and poor performance in cognitive memory tests.

These water-related health impacts start affecting children even before they are born. Pregnant mothers infected with malaria (a vectorborne disease) can become severely anaemic (Brabin et al. 1990), resulting in increased likelihood of infant and maternal death through preterm births and low birth weights (Kalaivani 2009). Schistosomiasis, an infection that results from a snailborne nematode, can result in low birth weights and therefore babies already more susceptible to infections and more likely to experience stunted growth (Kurtis et al. 2011). Another issue with lack of access to drinking water is caloric expenditure, which has been raised as an issue within the context of pregnant and breastfeeding women by Sorenson et al. (2011). This lack of water and sanitation facilities at birth is a further risk factor for infections, for both mother and baby. In the area of newborn and maternal care, there have been concerns that 'expectations of improved neonatal outcomes are being subverted by hospital-acquired infections and their associated morbidity, mortality, and cost' in many developing countries (Zaidi et al. 2005, 1175). The lack of hygiene facilities such as sinks, running water or waste disposal facilities are some of the problems that hinder many of the infection-control programmes in hospital nurseries (Zaidi et al. 2005). People might not seek treatment in facilities because of fear of infections or inadequate care due to unavailability of water in the facility. For deliveries that occur at home, infections due to inadequate water for handwashing and other hygiene practices are a risk to both newborns and mothers; newborns are especially susceptible to life-threatening infections when bathed with unclean water. Moreover, if a mother dies before the baby is six months old, her child is 25 times more likely to die before the age of 10 (Anderson et al. 2007). In many schools in Kenya around the Lake Victoria area, nematode infection incidence can be as high as 90 per cent (personal communication); school food programmes are unlikely to improve nutrition within this context. Thus poor water, sanitation and hygiene conditions have widespread implications not only for individuals but for the social fabric of communities.

Given that two thirds of the world population will be living in water-stressed regions by 2030 (UNESCO 2011), food security and nutrition, hygiene practices and water-related diseases will only continue to increase in significance. According to Cheng et al. (2012), there were statistically significant findings that for every quartile improvement in access to water and sanitation, under-five mortality and infant mortality decrease by 1.17 and 1.66 per 1,000, respectively. A similar significant relationship holds for maternal mortality and improved water and sanitation access. Other findings in the larger study include statistically significant relationships between the prevalence of underweight children under five years of age and improved water access as well as the ratio of girls to boys in primary education (Cheng et al. 2011). Indeed, the only MDG indicator evaluated that did not demonstrate a statistically significant relationship with access to improved water and/or sanitation was school enrolment. Arguably, this speaks to the nature of the indicator, rather than that of the relationship, as enrolment levels are above 90 per cent in almost all countries that make these data available. In this case, school attendance would be a far more telling indicator.

Given evidence of the wide reaching impacts of lack of water and sanitation, it is not difficult to recognise the significant burden placed on individuals, communities and society as a whole. Indeed, recent estimates suggest global economic losses of US$260 billion per year resulting from lack of access to water and sanitation (Hutton 2012). These losses vary by region, for example India and Indonesia, which respectively lost 6.4 per cent and 2.3 per cent of GDP in 2006 due to poor sanitation and hygiene (Water and Sanitation Program 2008; 2011)

Specifically, the benefit to cost ratio on money spent for universal access to improved drinking water ranges between 0 to 3.7 for East Asia, with a global average rate of return of US$2 per dollar invested (Hutton 2012). For sanitation, the returns are higher and range from just under three to eight for East Asia, with a global average rate of return of US$5.5 per dollar invested (Hutton 2012).

**Linkages: Water-Health and Development**

Despite the commitment[3] and general consensus on the importance of safe drinking water and adequate sanitation to population health and poverty reduction, about 605 million people will still lack access to improved drinking water and more than 2.4 million of the world's population will be without improved sanitation facilities by 2015 if the current trend in progress continues (WHO/UNICEF 2012). This will have negative implications for achieving other MDGs, as previously discussed, as well as in addressing issues of poverty especially in LMICs given that water is a 'key element of the development equation' (Schuster-Wallace et al. 2008, 8). This section addresses the impacts and implications of the water-health nexus on individual wellbeing, poverty reduction and national development.

As early childhood diarrhoea affects cognitive development and attendance, it impacts children's performance in school and could further lead to low economic potential and the inability to effectively compete in the job market. In the absence of basic sanitation in schools, the impact of practicing open defecation also affects girls' attendance and enrolment; because dignity and privacy is not assured, girls do not attend school during menstruation or drop out entirely once they reach adolescence (Elliott 2011). This has direct consequences for achieving gender-parity in basic education as targeted in MDG 3, further leading to the inability of girls to participate in many sectors of the economy in later years. Investment in water and sanitation infrastructure not only generates immediate health benefits but also secures the well being of future generations to engage in economic activities.

Time spent and distance travelled to collect water are important elements in defining 'reasonable access' to improved drinking water and sanitation (WHO/UNICEF 2010), and have important implications for the health of women. Data from 25 sub-Saharan African countries show that an average of 30 minutes is required for a round-trip of water for households without water on their premises and several trips may be required in a day depending on the household size and needs (UNICEF/WHO 2012).Women, who mostly bear the task of providing water for households in most developing countries are exposed to diseases including typhoid fever, malaria, dengue fever, yellow fever and schistosomiasis during water collection (Watt and Chamberlain 2011) and usually report declining health status during periods of water scarcity (Bour 2004). Aside from these health risks, women and girls are sometimes targets of assault and abuse when walking long distances between communities in search of water (Sorenso, Morssink and Campos 2011). They are equally vulnerable to sexual assaults and abuse when searching for privacy in bushes and in the dark to practice open defecation due to lack of sanitation facilities (Elliott 2011). Providing safe water and adequate sanitation within the household or within reasonable distance has other significant health and social gains. For example, aside from evidence of reduced risk of contamination through transportation, shorter distance and time travelled is more likely to result in collection of sufficient water for household consumption and personal hygiene needs (Howard and Bertram 2003; Clasen et al. 2006). Further, less time spent in water collection affords women the opportunity to save time and engage in other productive ventures and housekeeping activities, as does improved health of their children. Children, especially girls, are also able to save time to participate in educational activities.

---

3 The United Nations declared 2005–2015 the second decade for water and sanitation with commitment on action towards achieving internationally agreed water-related goals contained in the MDGs (WHO/UNICEF 2005).

Within the household, water use can be categorised into consumption, hygiene, amenity and productive uses (Thompson et al. 2001). Productive uses of water include backyard gardening, livestock, food production and household construction. In many poor households, productive use of water is essential for wealth creation and poverty reduction through small household businesses and agricultural activities. The availability of piped water encourages backyard gardening which is beneficial for household nutrition requirements and food security (Howard and Bertram 2003). In many rural areas in sub-Saharan Africa, households spend long hours in search of water for their herds of livestock. Engaging in other productive activities becomes impossible during periods of water scarcity. Without appropriate water interventions, such conditions are likely to worsen and further lead to worsening poverty conditions for such vulnerable households in the face of global climate change.

In efforts to reduce poverty, households and government can make significant savings from reduced water-borne and water-related disease burden. Aside from the cost of treatment and drugs, significant household income is lost through an inability to work during sick periods. Poverty becomes self-perpetuating in already poor households without safe water and sanitation as they are more prone to water-borne diseases, unable to work due to sickness, and could spend their little household savings on treatment, if care is indeed available. Further, with improved public and population health through adequate provision of safe water, governments are able to make significant savings on the public health sector which could be invested in other sectors of the economy. Indeed, (partial) financing water and sanitation access through health ministries makes economic sense, as seen by the returns on investment, the large proportion of which accrues to the health sector. Though developing countries will make significant savings in this regard, the outbreak of *cryptosporidiosis* and *Escherichia coli O157* in Canada, the United States and the United Kingdom in recent years shows that developed nations also stand to make some savings through further improvement in their water, sanitation and hygiene conditions (Prüss Üstün et al. 2004) with returns on investment in these countries estimated at just under two (Hutton 2012).

The effects of global climate change – which include changes in the water cycle with increasingly unpredictable rainfall, increase in uncertainty and frequency of droughts and rainfalls, rise in sea-levels with increased risk of the salinity of groundwater and rivers (WHO 2009) – are a threat to human health and well-being across the globe. Water-related health impacts are forecasted to include a reduction in the availability of water, human injury and disruption in medical service resulting from floods, malnutrition due to decreasing crop yield and increase and/or spread of vector-borne and water-borne diseases (WHO 2009). Other indirect health impacts include increased food insecurity, disruption in livelihoods and damage to infrastructure resulting from extreme climate events. The impacts and health risks may vary depending on where and how people live; communities in coastal regions, megacities, those in tropical regions, polar regions and mountain populations are particularly vulnerable in different ways (IPCC 2007). Whether measures are taken at the community and/or global level to mitigate climate change or not, strategies are needed to protect human health and well-being in vulnerable communities. Building and maintaining public health infrastructure such as public water systems, sanitation facilities, and wastewater treatment systems are significant in building resilience and adaptive capacity at the community level. In order to effectively respond to the risks and build greater community resilience in water and sanitation, there is an urgent need to promote resilient technologies, enhance management of services and update technical and regulatory guidelines at all levels (Howard et al. 2010).

For example, though flooding can be a risk for pit latrines in many communities, simple adaptation strategies could include using raised latrines, constructing low-cost temporary sanitation facilities that can be moved in highly vulnerable communities and changes in design to vault latrines (Howard and Bartram 2010).

In some peri-urban poor areas and rural communities in LMICs, many people rely on water vendors and other informal providers to meet their needs; often more expensive than the formal utility providers (Hofman 2011). Households spend a significant share of their income on water and this leaves little savings available to meet other educational, food and health needs. For example, in Nairobi, 64 per cent of slum residents pay 18 times more the price charged by utility providers because they rely on kiosk[4] operators for their daily water needs. (Gulyani et al., 2005; Gulyani and Talukdar 2008). Similarly, close to a quarter of peri-urban poor household income is spent on paying for water in Dar es Salaam, Tanzania (Hofman 2011). In Usoma, a rural community in Kenya, much of the population use water from the lake – regardless of the known health effects – partly because they cannot afford water from vendors (Levison et al. 2011). In many places, the poor who buy water from informal providers pay more for a litre than the rich who are connected to public water systems (Gulyani et al., 2005). These examples indicate that with the appropriate supply mechanism, especially the upfront capital investment, they will be willing and able to pay for water supplied by formal utility providers. On the other hand, the informal water sector creates business opportunities for local entrepreneurs to generate income for their household. It creates jobs especially for unemployed youth in both urban and rural communities. In a study of independent water and sanitation providers in 10 sub-Saharan African cities, Collignon and Vezina (2000) found between 70–90 per cent of the total workforce in the water sector were employed as independent service providers with a majority using hand carts, animal traction and bicycles to transport water around neighbourhoods for sale. In such countries, central governments can create an enabling environment through regulation, recognition and investments in the informal water sector and encourage local governments or municipal service providers to partner with local entrepreneurs in providing safe water through more standardised, effective and technologically efficient ways.

Further, in terms of community mobilisation to solve poverty-related issues, community-driven initiatives and activities aimed at securing safe water and sanitation can be used to facilitate other community development projects and economic programmes. Communities are sometimes driven by their water and sanitation needs to mobilise resources and undertake appropriate self-help projects like construction of boreholes and building of pit latrines. This activity can act as a catalyst for community development more broadly through investment of community profits in education, community commercial activities and/or expansion of services. One such community is that of West Kagan, Kenya, a very dry region of Nyanza Province where the nearest surface water is a minimum of 3 km away and significantly contaminated; cholera outbreaks used to be regular reports in the local newspaper. The community drilled a 45m borehole in 2002 under the Abala Women's Group with the support of the Lake Victoria Environmental Management Programme. However, with the repercussions of the HIV/AIDS epidemic leaving grandmothers to care for their grandchildren, it was physically very difficult for these women to use a manual footpump to obtain enough water for the daily needs of each family. As a result, the United Nations University Institute for Water, Environment and Health implemented a project in 2007 in

---

4    In Kenya, a water kiosk or standpipe is often managed by private individuals or nongovernmental organisations, rather than the public utility (Gulyani, Talukdar and Kariuki 2005).

partnership with the Lake Victoria Basin Commission to replace the manual footpump with a solar powered pump and additional elevated storage for wider distribution. Since then, the community response has been significant. Over 4,000 people use the borehole within a radius of 2 km. Women bring their cattle with them so that they do not have to collect so much water and local households are taking advantage of the water to irrigate cash crops. While the Water Management Committee has experienced some problems with the type of pipe initially installed and with establishing appropriate rates and payment schedules, this small investment of less than US$15,000 has provided the impetus for expanding the network to a local school and clinic with maternity ward. The next stage of development, subject to pumping capacity, is a larger storage tank at the top of the Abala Hill, which would facilitate water delivery to both sides of the community.

In some peri-urban areas success in solving water and sanitation problems partly depends on the level of trust and ability of residents to mobilise through informal structures like neighbourhood associations, women's groups and other civic organisations (Cariola and Lacabana 2004). In some developing countries, these initiatives have been integrated into the formal water supply programme in urban areas to ensure sustainability and quality in service delivery and prevent illegal connections of municipal piped systems (Cariola and Lacabana 2004; Hofman 2011). With the needed support from governments and donor agencies, such social structures and the culture of responsibility, trust, accountability and leadership skills developed through community mobilisation to solve water and sanitation problems could be extended to solve problems in other sectors like education, health care and agriculture.

Access to safe water and sanitation follows a predictable socio-economic and geographical pattern (Rheingans, Dreibelbis and Freeman 2006). At the global level, there are significant differences in access between developed and developing countries. The majority of the global population without access to safe water live in developing regions, specifically in sub-Saharan Africa, Oceania, Southern Asia and South Eastern Asia (WHO/ UNICEF 2012). Similarly, disparities are found within these countries – between high-income and low-income households and between people living in urban areas and those in rural areas (WHO/UNICEF 2012). These disparities in water and sanitation between urban and rural areas are likely to be reflected in health, poverty and income. In terms of development policy, agendas and partnerships that seek to address global, regional and local inequalities through economic and social opportunities should consider the fundamental role of water and sanitation in social and economic development. Further, such development frameworks should take into account the structural challenges that hinder the ability of developing nations, the urban poor and otherwise marginalised rural communities in getting access to basic social services.

## Conclusions

Water directly and indirectly impacts many facets of health and wellbeing, through diseases that temporarily or permanently incapacitate, through requirements for economic productivity and nutrition, as well as through societal development. The total cost to achieve universal coverage by 2015 is estimated to be over US$500 million (Hutton 2012). While not an insignificant amount, this figure pales in comparison to the economic bailouts, while achieving a net benefit, not only in terms of individual health and dignity, but in terms of economic and broader societal benefits. It is time that water and sanitation were afforded the recognition of being a pillar of public health, as established in the Alma Ata declaration (1978). Primary health care, particularly in rural and marginalised communities, must incorporate upstream public health; preventing disease in the community reduces the burden on already stressed rural clinics.

More specifically, in the public health sector, policy should address water both as a determinant of health and a prerequisite in safe health care delivery. Goals in the public health sector cannot be achieved without due consideration to water, sanitation and hygiene in both health facilities and in community health care delivery. The example of maternal and newborn health used above is to highlight the need for policies that seek to strengthen public health in developing countries to address issues of adequate supply of water and proper sanitation within health facilities. Water and sanitation is fundamental to public health policy and it is important to engage the health sector in water policy setting and implementation whether at the local or national level in order to assure maximum health benefits of water projects in both disease prevention and medical care. New partnership models have to be developed and examined within this context.

Historically, emphasis has been placed on large scale engineering projects for supplying water, treating water and wastewater and ensuring sanitation. Projects such as that in West Kagan demonstrate that small investments made in partnership with the community to ensure that real needs are being met, can result in large changes, both in infrastructure and the subsequent health of the community, but additionally in social capital and so-called soft skills within the community. This can be enhanced through demonstration sites and local networks of communities. These latter benefits can be translated into concomitant causes, such as education and economic activity. They further contribute to empowerment of individuals and communities, giving voices to the marginalised. Overall, individuals and especially decision-makers at all levels must be engaged in identifying issues and planning and operationalising solutions; they must be empowered through knowledge to minimise power differentials and enhance informed decision-making; and, they must be enlightened, because understanding problems and solutions can only take you so far – bridging to sustained action is the key.

Finally, the water-health nexus is one of the most important paths to achieving the MDGs in developing countries. This requires adequate commitments and investments by both donor agencies and governments in water, sanitation and hygiene for the poor and underserved. It also requires recognition of the different roles of both men and women in water-related activities at the household and community level and adequate understanding of the social, economic, political and cultural circumstances within which people live and work. Further, local interventions should aim at community mobilisation and actions to solve water and sanitation problems and should further encourage community ownership of water projects.

**References**

Anderson, F., Morton, S., Naik, S. and Gebrian, B. 2007. Maternal Mortality and the Consequences on Infant and Child Survival in Rural Haiti. *Maternal and Child Health Journal*, 11(4), 395–401.

Bartram, J., Lewis, K., Lenton, R. and Wright, A. 2005. Focusing on improved water and sanitation for health. *Lancet*, 365, 810–12.

Berkman, D.S., Lescano, A.G., Gilman, R.H. et al. 2002. Effects of stunting, diarrhoeal diseases and parasitic infections during infancy on cognitive functioning in later childhood; a follow-up study. *Lancet*, 357, 564–671.

Black, R.E., Cousens, S., Johnson, L. et al. 2010. Global, regional, and national causes of child mortality in 2008: a systematic analysis. *The Lancet*, 375(9730), 1969–87.

Bour, D. 2004. Water needs and women health in Kumasi metropolitan area of Ghana. *Health and Place*, 10, 85–103.

Brabin, B.J., Ginny, M., Sapau, J. et al. 1990. Consequences of maternal anaemia on outcome of pregnancy in a malaria endemic area in Papua New Guinea, *Ann Trop Med Parasitol*, 84(1), 11–24.

Cariola, C. and Lacabana, M. 2004. *WSS practices and living conditions in the peri-urban poor interface of metropolital Caracas. The Cases of Bachaquero and Paso Real. Report Prepared for the Service Provision Governance in the Peri-urban Interface of Metropolitan Areas Research Project. Development Planning Unit, University College of London.* UK. [Online] Available at: http://www.envirobase.info/PDF/R81372.pdf [accessed: October 2014].

Cheng, J.J., Schuster-Wallace, C.J., Watt, S. et al. 2011. Summary Analysis: Quantifying Water Supply, Sanitation and the Millennium Development Goals. [Online]. Available at: http://inweh.unu.edu/wp-content/uploads/2013/05/SummaryAnalysis_QuantifyingWaterSupplySanitationandMDGs.pdf [accessed: October 2014].

Cheng, J.J., Schuster-Wallace, C.J., Watt, S. et al. 2012. An Ecological Quantification of the Relationships Between Water, Sanitation and Infant, Child, and Maternal Mortality. *Journal Env. Health*, 11(4). Available at: doi:10.1186/1476–069X-11–4.

Clasen T., Roberts I., Rabie, T. et al. 2006. Interventions to improve water quality for preventing diarrhoea. (A Cochrane Review). *The Cochrane Library* [Online], 3. Available at: http://onlinelibrary.wiley.com/doi/10.1002/14651858.CD004794.pub2/abstract;jsessionid=3C80E64FC02F179538CAAE028BB32D54.d03t03?systemMessage=Wiley+Online+Library+will+be+disrupted+on+4+August+from+10%3A00–12%3A00+BST+%2805%3A00–07%3A00+EDT%29+for+essential+maintenance [accessed: October 2014].

Collignon, B. and Vezina, M. 2000. *Independent water and sanitation providers in African cities: full report of a ten-country study.* The World Bank. Washington. [Online]. Available at: https://www.wsp.org/wsp/sites/wsp.org/files/publications/af_providers.pdf [accessed: October 2014].

Elliott, S.J. 2011. The transdisciplinary knowledge journey: a suggested framework for research at the water-health nexus. *Current Opinion in Environmental Sustainability*, 3, 257–530.

Esrey, S.A., Potash, J.B., Roberts, L. and Shiff, C. 1991. Effects of improved water supply and sanitation on ascariasis, diarrhoea, dracunculiasis, hookworm infection, schistosomiasis, and tracoma. *Bulleting of World Health Organization*, 69, 609–21.

Ezeamama, E.A., Friedman, F.J., Acosta, P.L. et al. 2005. Helminth infection and cognitive impairment among Filipino children. *The American Society of Tropical Medicine*, 72(50), 540–48.

Fewtrell, L., Kaufmann, R., Kay, D. et al. 2005. Water, sanitation, and hygiene interventions to reduce diarrhoea in less developed countries: a systematic review and meta-analysis. *Lancet Infectious Diseases*, 5, 42–52.

Gatrell, C.A. and Elliot, J.S. 2009. *Geographies of Health: An Introduction.* 2nd Edition. Blackwall Publishing, Oxford.

Guerrant, R.L., Kosek, M., Moore, S. et al. 2002. Magnitude and impact of diarrhoeal diseases. *Archives of Medical Research*, 33, 351–5.

Gulyani, S. and Talukdar, D. 2008. Slum real estate; the low-income high price puzzle in Nairobi's slum rental market and its implication for theory and practice. *World Development*, 36(10), 1919–37.

Gulyani, S., Talukdar, D. and Kariuki, R.M. 2005. *Water for the urban poor: Water markets, household demand, and service preferences in Kenya*. Water Supply and Sanitation Sector Board Discussion Series. Paper No. 5. The World Bank. Washington. [Online]. Available at: http://documents.worldbank.org/curated/en/2005/01/5730972/water-urban-poor-water-markets-household-demand-service-preferences-kenya [accessed: October 2014].

Hofman, P. 2011. Falling through the net: access to urban water and sanitation by the urban poor. *International Journal of Urban Sustainable Development*, 3(1), 40–55.

Howard, G. and Bertram, J. 2003. *Domestic Water Quantity, Service Level and Health*. WHO. Geneva. [Online]. Available at: http://www.who.int/water_sanitation_health/diseases/wsh0302/en/ [accessed: October 2014].

Howard, G. and Bartram, J. 2010. *Vision 2030.The resilience of water supply and sanitation in the face of climate change*. Technical Report. WHO. Geneva. [Online]. Available at: http://www.who.int/water_sanitation_health/publications/9789241598422/en/ [accessed: October 2014].

Howard, G., Charles, K., Pond, K. et al. 2010. Securing 2020 vision for 2030: climate change and ensuring resilience in water and sanitation services. *Journal of Water and Sanitation*. IWA Publishing. [Online]. Available at: http://www.iwaponline.com/jwc/001/0002/0010002.pdf [accessed: October 2014].

Hutton, G. 2012. *Global Costs and Benefits of Drinking-water Supply and Sanitation Interventions to Reach the MDG Target and Universal Coverage*. WHO. WHO/HSE/WSH/12.01. [Online]. Available at: http://www.who.int/water_sanitation_health/publications/2012/globalcosts.pdf [accessed: October 2014].

Kalaivani, K. 2009. Prevalence and Consequences of Anaemia in Pregnancy. *Indian J. Med. Res.*, 130, 627–33.

Kurtis, J.D., Higashi, A., Wu, H-W. et al. 2011. Maternal Schistosomiasis Japonica Is Associated with Maternal, Placental, and Fetal Inflammation. *Infection and Immunity*, 79(3), 1254–61.

Levison, M.M., Elliott, S.J., Karanja, S.M.D. et al. 2011. You cannot prevent a disease; you only treat diseases when they occur: knowledge, attitudes and practices to water-health in a rural Kenyan community. *East African Journal of Public Health*, 8(2), 103–11.

Oriá, R.B., Costa, C.M.C., Lima, A.A.M. et al. 2009. Semantic fluency: A sensitive marker for cognitive impairment in children with heavy diarrhoea burdens? *Medical Hypotheses*, 73, 682–6.

Parry, M.L., Canziani, O.F., Palutifok, J.P. et al. 2007. *Climate Change 2007: Impacts, Adaptation and Vulnerability*. Contribution of Working Group II to the Fourth Assessment. Report of the Intergovernmental Panel on Climate Change, Cambridge University Press, Cambridge, UK. [Online]. Available at: http://www.ipcc.ch/publications_and_data/publications_ipcc_fourth_assessment_report_wg2_report_impacts_adaptation_and_vulnerability.htm [accessed: October 2014].

Patrick, D.P., Oria, B.R., Madhavan, M. et al. 2005. Limitations in verbal fluency following heavy burdens of early childhood diarrhoea in Brazillian Shantytown children. *Child Neuropsychology*, 11, 233–44.

Prüss-Üstün, A., Bartram, J., Clasen T. et al. 2014. Burden of disease from inadequate water, sanitation and hygiene in low- and middle-income country settings: a retrospective analysis of data from 145 coutnries. Tropical Medicine and International Health. 19, 894–905. [Online]. Available at: http://onlinelibrary.wiley.com/doi/10.1111/tmi.12329/ pdf [accessed: October 2014].

Prüss-Üstün, A., Kay, D., Fewtrell, L. 2004. Unsafe water, sanitation and hygiene, in *Comparative quantification of health risks: global and regional burden of disease*, edited by M. Ezzati, D.A. Lopez, A. Rodgers and J.L.C. Murray. World Health Organization, Geneva. [Online]. Available at: http://www.who.int/healthinfo/global_ burden_disease/cra/en/ [accessed: October 2014].

Rheingans, R., Dreibelbis, R., and Freeman, M.C. 2006. Beyond the Millennium Development Goals: public health challenges in water and sanitation. *Global Public Health*, 1(1), 31–48

Schuster-Wallace, C.J., Grover, I.V., Adeel, Z. et al. 2008. *Safe Water as the Key to Global Health*. UNU-INWEH, Hamilton. [Online]. Available at: http://inweh.unu.edu/wp-content/uploads/2013/05/SafeWater_Web_version.pdf [accessed: October 2014].

Sorenson, B.S., Morssink, C. and Campos, P.A. 2011. Safe access to safe water in low income countries: water fetching in current time. *Social Science and Medicine*, 72, 1522–6.

Thompson, J., Porras, I.T., Tumwine, J.K. et al. 2001. *Drawers of Water II; 30 years of change in domestic water use and environmental health in East Africa*, IIED, London, UK. [Online]. Available at: http://pubs.iied.org/pdfs/9049IIED.pdf [accessed: October 2014].

UNESCO. 2011. The Impacts of Global Change on Water Resources: The Response of UNESCO's International Hydrological Programme. SC/HYD/2011/PI/H/1. International Hydrological Programme UNESCO/Division of Water Science, Paris. [Online]. Available at: http://unesdoc.unesco.org/images/0019/001922/192216e.pdf [accessed: October 2014].

United Nations. 1977. *Report of the United Nations Water Conference, Mar del Plata, 14–25 March 1977*. United Nations publication, Sales No. E.77.II.A.12.

Waddington, H. and Snilstveit, B. 2009. Effectiveness and sustainability of water, sanitation, and hygiene interventions in combating diarrhoea. *Journal of Development Effectiveness*, 1(3), 295–335.

Water and Sanitation Program. 2008. *Economic Impacts of Sanitation in Indonesia. A five-country study conducted in Cambodia, Indonesia, Lao PDR, the Philippines, and Vietnam under the Economics of Sanitation Initiative (ESI)*. Water and Sanitation Program East Asia and the Pacific, World Bank Office, Jakarta. [Online]. Available at: https://www.wsp.org/wsp/sites/wsp.org/files/publications/esi_indonesia.pdf [accessed: October 2014].

Water and Sanitation Program. 2011. *Flagship Report: Economic Impacts of Inadequate Sanitation in India*. Water and Sanitation Program. New Delhi, India. [Online]. Available at: http://water.worldbank.org/publications/economic-impacts-inadequate-sanitation-india-inadequate-sanitation-costs-india-rs-24-tr [accessed: October 2014].

Watt S. And Chamberlain J. 2011. Water, climate change and maternal and newborn health. *Current Opinion in Environmental Sustainability*, 3, 491–8.

WHO. 2002. *Prevention and Control of Schistosomiasis and Soil-Transmitted Helminthiasis*. Report of a WHO Expert Committee. Geneva, World Health Organization, 2002 (WHO

Technical Report Series, No. 912). [Online]. Available at: http://whqlibdoc.who.int/trs/WHO_TRS_912.pdf [accessed: October 2014].

WHO. 2003. *Climate Change and Human Health: Risks and Responses.* Summary. WHO, Geneva. [Online]. Available at: http://www.who.int/globalchange/publications/cchhsummary/en/ [accessed: October 2014].

WHO/UNICEF Joint Monitoring Programme for Water Supply and Sanitation. 2005. *Water For Life: Making It Happen.* WHO, Geneva. [Online]. Available at: http://www.wssinfo.org/fileadmin/user_upload/resources/1198249448-JMP_05_en.pdf [accessed: October 2014].

WHO/UNICEF Joint Monitoring Programme for Water Supply and Sanitation. 2010. *Progress on Drinking Water and Sanitation: 2010 Update.* UNICEF. New York. [Online]. Available at: http://www.wssinfo.org/fileadmin/user_upload/resources/1278061137-JMP_report_2010_en.pdf [accessed: October 2014].

WHO/UNICEF Joint Monitoring Programme for Water Supply and Sanitation. 2012. *Progress on Drinking Water and Sanitation: 2012 Update.* UNICEF. New York. [Online]. Available at: http://www.wssinfo.org/fileadmin/user_upload/resources/JMP-report-2012-en.pdf [accessed: October 2014].

WHO/UNICEF Joint Monitoring Programme for Water Supply and Sanitation. 2014. *Progress on Sanitation and Drinking Water: 2014 Update.* UNICEF. New York. [Online]. Available at: http://www.wssinfo.org/fileadmin/user_upload/resources/JMP_report_2014_webEng.pdf [accessed: October 2014].

Zaidi, M.K., Huskins, C.W., Thaver, D. et al. 2005. Hospital-acquired neonatal infections in developing countries. *Lancet*, 365, 1175–88.

# Chapter 13

# Groundwater Arsenic Contamination and its Health and Social Impacts in Rural Bangladesh

Bimal Kanti Paul

## Introduction

Arsenic contamination of tube well (TW) water, which constitutes the primary source of drinking water, has emerged as a serious health and social problem in rural Bangladesh (Caldwell et al. 2003a and 2003b). Although estimates differ substantially by source, the Health Effects of Arsenic Longitudinal Study (HEALS) conducted from 2000–2009 claims that between 35 and 77 million people in this South Asian country drink contaminated well water (Argos et al. 2010a; 2010b; 2011; UNICEF 2011). According to this cohort study, more than 55 per cent of the sample consumed drinking water contaminated with arsenic in excess of 50 parts per billion (ppb), the current Bangladesh standard, and more than 75 per cent of those in the study consumed water with arsenic levels above the World Health Organisation's (WHO) recommended level of 10 ppb (Ahsan and Argos 2007; Argos et al. 2010a; UNICEF 2011).

Adverse health effects resulting from continuous consumption of arsenic contaminated water for 10–20 years range from gangrene of the peripheral organs to skin cancer and cancer of internal organs such as the lung, liver, kidney and bladder, as well as cardiovascular and neurological disorders (Table 13.1). There have also been reports of increased risk of stillbirths and pregnancy complications from arsenic contamination (Argos et al. 2011; Hasnat 2004). Arsenic poisoning also creates an economic burden on families. It affects the productivity of arsenic victims and many become liabilities for their families (Paul and De 2000). A large part of the population who suffers from illnesses caused by long-term arsenic ingestion lose their ability to participate in economic life. Additionally, the cost of treatment places further burdens on families as the illness is chronic in nature, tests are numerous, and remedies uncertain.

The symptoms of arsenic poisoning include intense stomach pain, vomiting, weight loss, low-grade fever, and delirium. It has been reported that there are at least two million cases of skin lesions (i.e., melanosis, leucomelanosis, and keratosis) in the country caused by drinking arsenic-contaminated water. Such lesions still attract widespread social stigma in Bangladesh, with many people until recently believing they were the result of a curse (Buncombe 2010). Argos and colleagues (2010a) claim that one in five deaths in Bangladesh is caused by consumption of arsenic-contaminated drinking water (also see UNICEF 2011). No treatment has yet been proven effective in treating arsenic victims. Even 10 years after the detection of arsenic in groundwater, most hospital doctors – outside the specialist arsenic units – have limited understanding of the diagnosis and pathophysiology of arsenic poisoning and have not received training in treating this condition.

**Table 13.1** **Long-term health effects of exposure to arsenic**

| Skin lesions | Melanosis |
|---|---|
| | Leucomelanosis |
| | Keratosis |
| Skin cancer | |
| Internal cancers | Bladder |
| | Kindney |
| | Lung |
| Neurological effects | |
| Hypertension and cardiovascular disease | |
| Pulmonary disease | |
| Peripheral vascular disease | |
| Diabetes mellitus | |

*Source:* Compiled from Ahsan and Argos (2007) and Smith et al. (2000).

The objective of this chapter is to provide a critical overview of health effects and social consequences of arsenic contamination of groundwater in Bangladesh. To provide necessary information, a brief background of arsenic poisoning along with its spatial extent in Bangladesh is presented in the next section. This is followed by a section focusing on arsenic mitigation measures currently implemented by both public and private agencies. Health effects and social consequences of arsenic poisoning are then presented along with a description of alternative sources of drinking water in rural Bangladesh. This overview will provide evidence of how development programmes in Bangladesh (similar to many other reported cases in other countries) often have negative implications for human health.

**Background**

Bangladesh's arsenic crisis dates back to the 1970s. Between 1970 and 1990, TW water was heavily promoted and developed in Bangladesh as a safe and environmentally-acceptable alternative to microbiologically unsafe surface water (Hossain 2002; Rammelt et al. 2011). Before national independence in 1971, most people in rural Bangladesh used untreated bacteria-infested surface water from dug wells (DWs), or from ponds, rivers, and lakes. This caused rampant diarrheal and other water-borne diseases throughout the country, primarily affecting children ages one to four (WHO 2000). It was believed that diarrheal diseases caused by consumption of dirty and unsafe surface water was killing up to 250,000 children a year during the 1970s (Buncombe 2010; Rammelt et al. 2011). Reducing the incidence of these diseases required the supply of safe water as well as sanitation and good hygiene practices (Caldwell et al. 2006). While all three efforts are ideal, in Bangladesh the main focus has been on supplying safe water through the introduction of tube wells.

Supplying safe TW water was cheaper than providing both adequate sanitation facilities and programmes aimed at improving hygiene. Additionally, tube well installation is easy; TWs require minimum maintenance, and provide microbiologically pure groundwater directly to the households in plentiful quantities (Caldwell et al. 2006). Thus, the Bangladesh government began installing TWs that tapped into pathogen-free aquifers as an alternative water source in 1971. Installation was facilitated by generous financial assistance from the international aid agencies including the United Nation's Children Fund (UNICEF), the World Bank, and the United Nations Development Programme (UNDP). An estimated 6 to 11 million TWs were drilled throughout the country since 1971. Although checks were carried out for certain contaminants in the newly sourced water, it was never tested for arsenic, which seems to occur naturally in the Ganges and Brahmaputra deltas. Nation-wide surveys have now established that up to half of the country's tube wells are contaminated with arsenic (Buncombe 2010).

It was a source of national pride for Bangladesh that it had brought 97 per cent of the rural population under the coverage of 'safe' TW water by the 1990s (Paul 2004). Country-wide installation of TWs saved the lives of millions of people, and mortality and morbidity rates attributed to water-borne diseases plunged after their use (Caldwell et al. 2006; UNICEF 1998). However, the significant achievement of providing safe drinking water through TWs was overshadowed by the detection of arsenic in groundwater by the Department of Public Health and Engineering (DPHE) of the Bangladesh government in 1993. The following year only eight people were identified who had been suffering from manifestations of arsenic toxicity (Hossain et al. 2005). In early 1995 when arsenic contamination was shown to be present across central and southwestern Bangladesh, this issue received serious government attention (Khatun 2000; Paul and De 2000; Fazal et al. 2001).

Subsequently, health problems associated with elevated arsenic levels began appearing in rural Bangladesh, specifically noticeable were skin lesions on the hands and feet. Because the arsenic problem was relatively new in the 1990s, and it takes up to 20 years for chronic arsenic poisoning to cause cancer, the worst impacts of drinking arsenic contaminated drinking water were yet to come. WHO predicts that between 2003 and 2013, skin and internal cancers are likely to become the principal human health concern arising from arsenic and other experts believe that one in 10 adult deaths in Bangladesh could be due to some form of cancer caused by arsenic poisoning (Chaudhuri 2004).

## Spatial Extent and Causes of Arsenic Contamination

Since the mid-1990s many national and international organisations have been involved in identifying arsenic contaminated tube wells in Bangladesh. However, only four of these organisations (the Dhaka Community Hospital (DCH), the School of Environmental Studies (SOES) of Jadavpur University, Calcutta, India, the British Geological Survey (BGS), and the DPHE) engaged themselves in such activities nation-wide (Paul 2004). The first two organisations jointly collected relevant data during 1995–2000, while the latter two studies were conducted in 1998–1999. Other organisations tested tube well water locally and/or regionally. The survey conducted by the DCH and SOES was biased in that arsenic victims were first identified and then tube well water used by those victims was tested for arsenic contamination (Paul 2004).

The BGS/DPHE survey applied stratified random sampling throughout Bangladesh with the exception of three hilly districts (i.e., Rangamati, Khagrachhari and Banderban) in the southeast. A district is the second largest administrative unit in Bangladesh with an average population of slightly over two million. The three hilly districts were not included in the survey because no primary symptoms of arsenic poisoning were found there. The BGS and DPHE survey revealed that arsenic concentrations ranged from less than 0.25 ppb to over 1,600 ppb; the mean concentration was about 55 ppb (Hossain 2002). Ten of the

61 sampled districts had an arsenic concentration below the WHO standard (10 ppb) and arsenic levels range between the WHO standard and the Bangladesh standard (50 ppb) in 27 districts. The remaining 20 districts had arsenic level exceeding the Bangladesh standard (Paul 2004).

Spatial patterns of arsenic contamination should be viewed carefully because there is considerable short-range variation in arsenic concentration from well to well. Even in areas of generally low arsenic concentrations, there are occasionally 'hot spots' where a cluster of wells with unusually high concentrations of arsenic can be found. Another reason for exercising caution stems from the need for retesting TWs that have previously been reported as being safe (Paul 2004). Arsenic contamination is believed to vary by season and from year to year and thus several researchers have suggested that all arsenic interventions must be guided by repeated testing of TW water for arsenic contamination (Calwell et al. 2003a).

A recent UNICEF survey revealed that 57 per cent of TWs in Bangladesh were contaminated by arsenic in 2009. A household drinking water quality survey conducted by UNICEF in the same year found that 12.6 per cent of drinking water samples still do not meet the Bangladesh Government drinking water standard for arsenic and 23.1 per cent do not meet the WHO standard (UNICEF 2010). These represent approximately 20 and 40 million people at risk of arsenic exposure. UNICEF has been monitoring TW water for the last several years.

Current consensus expert opinion is that arsenic found in the groundwater of Bangladesh is naturally-occurring from arsenic-rich material in the region's river systems, deposited over thousands of years along with the sands and gravels which make up the land of Bangladesh. In contrast to initial assumptions, arsenic contamination is not caused by TWs, irrigation or the application of chemical fertilisers for cultivating crops. Initially, some researchers even claimed that the diversion of surface water from the river Ganga by India was the cause of this arsenic problem. However, other explanations offered include the use of arsenic compound as preservatives in wooden electric utility poles by the Rural Electrification Board, and the coating of tube well filters with arsenic compound (BGS/DPHE 1999). In groundwater, arsenic occurs primarily in two forms: arsenite and arsenate. Arsenic may change chemical form in the natural environment, but it does not degrade (Mahmood and Halder 2011).

**Arsenic Mitigation Measures**

Since 1995, the national government, non-governmental organisations (NGOs), as well as foreign and international aid agencies have become involved in arsenic mitigation and prevention activities in Bangladesh (Khatun 2000). One important component of these activities is the identification of arsenic contaminated TWs. The Bangladesh Arsenic Mitigation and Water Supply Project (BAMWSP), for example, conducts extensive testing of wells and encourages the use of arsenic-free water sources (Caldwell et al. 2006). TW waters are tested for arsenic contamination and contaminated wells are labelled with red markings that signify the water in them should not be used for drinking or cooking. Similarly, 'safe' wells are painted green. Like the Bangladesh government, NGOs are also involved in training villagers to test their well water and mobilising community resources to combat arsenic contamination. Local authorities have been provided with field kits for testing TW water (Paul and De 2000).

In addition, several NGOs, such as the DCH and the SOES, have helped identify and treat arsenic-related symptoms in rural areas. Under the supervision of the DPHE, several NGOs (e.g., CARE International) conducted screening programmes in the late 1990s in selected rural areas severely affected by arsenic pollution. With assistance from UNICEF and the World Bank, arsenic awareness and health education programmes among affected villages has also been initiated by NGOs (Paul and De 2000). Making people in rural areas aware of the arsenic contamination problem in the late 1990s – as well as the symptoms associated with arsenic poisoning – was definitely an important step toward saving many lives.

Most scientific attention in the early part of arsenic poisoning in Bangladesh has focused on identifying the sources and causes of arsenic poisoning and in developing cost-effective procedures to remove arsenic from ground water. These activities were essential in combating the contamination. Several agencies, however, such as UNICEF, have led efforts to develop and provide alternative sources of drinking water, including collecting rainwater and filtering surface water. In 2004 the Government of Bangladesh established the National Policy for Arsenic Mitigation (NPAM) in order to provide guidelines for mitigating the effect of arsenic poisoning on people and the environment in a holistic and sustainable way. The NPAM supplements the 1998 National Water Policy, and the 1998 National Policy for Safe Water Supply and Sanitation in fulfilling the national goals of poverty alleviation, public health, and food security. Subsequent to NPAM, an Arsenic Policy Support Unit (APSU) and a National Committee for the Implementation Plan for Arsenic Mitigation (IPAM) was established. As of 2014 the APSU no longer exists and the IPAM committee is inactive (Rummelt et al. 2011).

The 2004 NPAM incorporates programmes to provide access to safe drinking water through screening and regular monitoring of all TWs to identify the wells that have arsenic above the national levels permissible. These programmes include implementation of alternative water supply options in all arsenic affected areas. NPAM has also outlined a programme to diagnose and manage illnesses associated with arsenic poisoning. Unfortunately, there is little actual integration of these policies; local government agencies in the water and health sectors still operate largely in isolation (Rammelt et al. 2011). Each sector has been facing its own challenges with little dialogue or collaboration between them.

Arsenic-related activities in the public health sector are undertaken by the Ministry of Health and Family Welfare (MHFW). Its activities include the development of education materials, raising awareness regarding the impact of ingestion of arsenic contaminated water, training health professionals, treatment protocols, and identification of persons suffering from arsenicosis. A person with excessive arsenic in his or her body is said to be suffering from arsenicosis. A general weakness is the sector's limited capacity at the local level. There is a tremendous need to learn from local experiences and scale up potentially successful approaches for treating arsenicosis patients while simultaneously continuing activities that result in the provision of safe drinking water.

Cooperation is not only a problem among government organisations with regard to arsenic mitigation efforts in Bangladesh. As noted, the arsenic problem there has attracted the attention of a diverse group of stakeholders. Both domestic and foreign academics and researchers, NGOs, and bilateral/multi-national development partner agencies have been pursuing separate programmes with little and often no coordination. This situation has resulted in duplication among activities and conflicting strategies that inhibit potential synergy and the optimal use of scarce resources.

**Health Effects of Arsenic Poisoning**

As noted, adverse health effects resulting from the consumption of arsenic contaminated water range from skin abnormalities to lung, liver, kidney, and bladder cancers. Not only are millions of Bangladeshis already suffering symptoms from arsenic-related illnesses, the incidence of arsenicosis has been increasing at an alarming rate (Hossain et al. 2005). Arsenic poisoning results from long-term exposure to this heavy metal. Early symptoms include various skin lesions that develop over an incubation period of 5–10 years after continuous exposure. After 10–20 years of prolonged exposure, affected people often develop arsenic-related cancers (Paul and Brock 2006). Chronic arsenic poisoning has four recognised stages (Table 13.2). In the first or pre-clinical stage, patients show no symptoms, but arsenic can be detected in urine or body tissue samples. In the second stage, visual symptoms begin to appear which include a general darkening of skin on the palms, and dark spots on the chest, back, limbs, or gums. Dark spots on the body are medically termed spotted melanosis, and are generally a precursor of skin cancer (Paul and De, 2000). In the third stage, clinical manifestations become more pronounced and the internal organs are affected. In the final stage, affected people may develop skin, lung, or bladder cancer. The first two stages occur before the condition becomes irreversible and clinical manifestations become pronounced. The transition from one stage to another occurs due to continued exposure to arsenic contaminated water. Studies (e.g., Paul 2006) reported either improvement in health or halting further degradation when use of contaminated water is discontinued in the early stages of the arsenicosis. It is therefore imperative that people suffering from arsenic poisoning recognise the early symptoms and completely stop consumption of arsenic contaminated drinking water. No specific treatment has yet been proven effective in treating arsenicosis victims.

Many manifestations of arsenicosis are visible, but there are some which are not visible or only visible when an individual suffers extensive internal damage. There may also be symptoms of internal inflammation of the body associated with long term exposure to low levels of arsenic. The resulting burning is often associated with other common disorders suffered by many Bangladeshis such as gastrointestinal disorders, anaemia, and general weakness (Rahman et al. 2000). Not surprisingly then, the presence of any one of these

**Table 13.2    Stages of chronic arsenic poisoning**

| Stage | Symptom | Length of Exposure (in years) |
|---|---|---|
| I | Shows no symptom | 1–5 |
| II | Darkening of skin on palm, dark spots on the body (spotted melanosis), keratosis, and gangrenous ulcer | 5–10 |
| III | Enlargement of liver, kidneys, and spleen; gastrointestinal, neurological, cardiovascular, and respiratory disorder | 10–15 |
| IV | Skin, lung, or bladder cancer | 10–20 |

*Source:* Paul and De (2000).

symptoms is never diagnostic for arsenicosis. Any confusion can be justified by laboratory tests. The most common parameters for diagnosis are blood, urine, hair, and nail samples. Skin changes in the form of melanosis and keratosis together with urinary concentrations of total and speciated arsenic are important diagnostic criteria for chronic arsenicosis in Bangladesh. Determination of hair and nail contents of arsenic would further substantiate these diagnostic criteria (Rabbani et al. 2002).

*Identification of Symptoms of Arsenicosis*

Although the identification of symptoms of arsenicosis is problematic in itself, it is essential for treatment of this illness. Changes in skin colour and the thickening of skin on the palms and soles are possible markers of arsenic poisoning, but may also be normal characteristics of a hard working rural population (Caldwell et al. 2003b). Available studies (e.g., Paul 2006; Rammelt et al. 2011) indicate that victims used one or more sources to identify their symptoms of arsenicosis. These sources include: self, friends/relatives/family members, neighbours, local physicians, foreign physicians, members of mobile arsenic teams and staff of NGOs. Self-identification seems to be the most popular source. A study conducted by Paul (2006) reported that 37 per cent of all respondents identified arsenicosis symptoms by themselves followed by relatives (19 per cent), physicians of all types (17 per cent), and NGO workers (13 per cent). Foreign physicians, who attended arsenic-related seminars in Bangladesh, diagnosed symptoms of 7 per cent of all respondents. As a part of the seminar, many of these physicians visited arsenic-affected areas in rural Bangladesh. While they were on site, they identified individuals suffering symptoms of arsenicosis.

Many mobile arsenic teams were, and still are dispatched by various organisations to arsenic-impacted rural areas to identify arsenicosis victims by clinical examination. Samples of blood, urine, hair, and fingernails are obtained to determine arsenic concentration in temporary medical camps (Paul 2006; Rabbani et al. 2002). In addition to foreign and domestic physicians, these teams consist of both local and foreign experts and researchers. Rahman et al. (2000) reported that mobile medical teams identified more than 7,000 individuals with arsenicosis from about 300 villages by 1999. Although many NGOs have been involved in arsenic mitigation and prevention activities, several NGOs trained personnel to specifically identify arsenic contaminated TWs and to identify arsenicosis sufferers.

Available studies (e.g., Paul 2006; Rammelt et al. 2011) further suggest that physicians generally diagnose arsenicosis by clinical examinations, while others identified arsenicosis in individuals by an assessment of the visible symptoms. In highly contaminated areas, people without manifested visual symptoms might still have internal problems. In these areas, a full diagnosis may sometime require clinical pathology tests from hair and nail samples. A biopsy may also be needed for the examination of tissue and suspected tumours. Unfortunately, such costs cannot be borne by the vast majority of rural residents (Rammelt et al. 2011).

A study conducted among 1,482 arsenicosis patients living in six (of 496) upzilas (sub-districts) of Bangladesh reveals that 1,437 (97 per cent) of these individuals had melanosis symptoms, 1,018 (68.7 per cent) had keratosis symptoms, and 572 (38.6 per cent) had been suffering from arsenicosis for more than three (median) years (Hossain et al. 2005). These patients were identified through household screening and then confirmed by a trained medical team headed by a medical officer. The average age of arsenicosis patients was 36 years and average duration of arsenic symptoms was three (median) years. About

50 per cent of the patients had been drinking TW water more than 24 years. Melanosis was significantly associated with younger patients and keratosis with older age. Further, the duration of arsenic symptoms was significantly associated with older males, married persons, habitual smokers, and those that had consumed TW water contaminated with arsenic for a longer period of time (Hossain et al. 2005).

Hossain and his colleagues (2005) further reported that nearly 61 per cent of the arsenicosis victims had installed their TW within the last 10 years. They also found that 767 (51.8 per cent) victims indicated that the depth of their TW was less than 75 (median) feet. Mean and Standard Deviation (SD) of TW depth was 85 feet and 42 feet, respectively. A total of 1,181 (79.7 per cent) patients mentioned their TWs were tested for arsenic and out of them 1,139 (96.4 per cent) were found not safe. Seven hundred and thirty-seven (49.6 per cent) patients had been drinking TW water for more than 24 (mean/median) years. Duration of arsenic symptoms was significantly associated with longer duration of contaminated TW water consumption (Hossain et al. 2005). Many studies (e.g., Hossain et al. 2005; Paul 2006) mentioned that cancer manifestations among arsenicosis patients were very low in Bangladesh. This might simply be due to the fact that arsenic contamination of groundwater was first identified in Bangladesh in 1993.

*Arsenicosis Treatment and Treatment Choice*

To date, iterature on arsenicosis treatment and treatment choice is very limited. Based on a field survey, Paul (2006) reported that immediately after the identification of arsenicosis symptoms, nearly 60 per cent of all respondents did nothing. The remaining 40 per cent discussed their symptoms with family members, friends, relatives, and neighbours. They also sought their advice regarding treatment options. An overwhelming majority of these respondents finally sought treatment from practitioners of different medical systems that exist in rural Bangladesh. This clearly supports the contention that the process of seeking medical intervention is a complex one where the victim is not always alone involved in the decision-making process. Family members, relatives, and members of social network also actively participate in this process.

Paul (2006) further reported that nearly 35 per cent of all respondents who had arsenicosis (230 out of 663) consulted physicians regarding their illness. This rate of physician utilisation can be considered relatively high, which suggests that arsenicosis has become a serious health concern in the affected study region. In general, people in rural Bangladesh avoid treatment until an illness causes a serious physical disability or becomes life-threatening (Paul 1992; Paul 2006). Information regarding types of physicians consulted by respondents who sought medical intervention for their arsenicosis problem is presented in Table 13.3. The table shows that nearly 60 per cent of the respondents sought treatment from physicians with a formal degree in Western medicine (M.B.B.S.), nearly 26 per cent from paraprofessionals, 20 per cent from physicians without a formal degree in Western medicine, 16 per cent from homeopaths, and slightly over 9 per cent from traditional healers, such as Kabiraj (practitioners of *Ayurvedic* medicine) and Hakim (practitioners of *Unani* medicine). The 'paraprofessional' category consists of consultation with: *Palli Chikishoks* (village doctors who receive a year of training in diagnosing and treating the most common local ailments), medical assistants (who complete a comprehensive three-year medical training programme), and government and nongovernment community health workers who receive only very basic

**Table 13.3     Types of physician consulted (N=230)1**

| Type | Number | Percentage |
|------|--------|------------|
| M.B.B.S. | 135 | 58.70 |
| Paraprofessionals | 59 | 25.65 |
| Unqualified allopaths | 46 | 20.00 |
| Homeopaths | 36 | 15.65 |
| Traditional healers | 18 | 9.23 |

*Source:* Compiled from Paul (2006).

preventive and curative health training and provide treatment primarily with allopathic drugs (Paul 2006).

Information provided in Table 13.3 also suggests that respondents were not generally relying on traditional healers for treating their illness. The primary reason for this is that respondents consider arsenicosis a new disease caused by consuming arsenic contaminated TW water. Further, they believe that this illness is an outcome of Western technology used to extract water from underground, so it should be treated by practitioners of Western medicine. It became clear from field observations that people in the study area widely believed that there is no effective traditional treatment for a disease considered of recent origin (Paul 2006).

Respondents were asked why they consulted a physician of a specific type. Faith in a physician of a particular type appeared to be the leading cause for consultation followed by other reasons such as proximity and affordability. Nearly 20 per cent of respondents consulted M.B.B.S. doctors free of cost. These physicians were visiting the study area on behalf of several NGOs interested on providing free care for arsenic patients. In addition, victims of arsenicosis also went to the nearest large city to seek care from M.B.B.S. doctors (Paul 2006).

Data provided by Paul (2006) show that nearly one-third of the respondents consulted more than one type of physician. These respondents either switched from one type of physician to another or utilised more than one type concurrently – probably either with the hope of a fast cure from arsenicosis or perhaps they were not completely satisfied with the treatment they received. Switching occurred usually from the care of M.B.B.S. doctors and paraprofessionals to other physicians of Western medicine and to traditional healers. Some respondents used two different physicians of the same medical system, but from different places. Respondents who sought treatment from more than one source did not frequently change their treatment modes. These respondents were under the same physician's care for a relatively long time before switching to another physician. Switching generally occurred to the same type of physician, i.e., from one M.B.B.S. doctor to another M.B.B.S. doctor (Paul 2006).

Interestingly, Paul's 2006 study suggests that severity of illness and utilisation of more than one practitioner were not closely related to each other. Variation in the extent of availability of and accessibility to medical care seems to be more closely associated with utilisation of more than one physician (Paul 2006a). Rammelt et al. (2011) claim that arsenicosis treatment consists of providing medicine such as antioxidant multivitamins (vitamin A, C, and E), folic acid, anti-histamines for itching and salicylates to treat skin lesions. Arsenicosis clinics run by several NGOs distribute these medicines among arsenic victims free of cost on a weekly basis to avoid patients sell the medicine rather than taking it (Rammelt et al. 2011). In some cases, regular treatment is insufficient and serious patients are referred by the clinics to a nearby hospital. Arsenicosis patients who are in the advanced stages (three and four) may require amputation of their legs and/or hands.

However, it is revealed from Paul's (2006) study that a considerable proportion of arsenicosis sufferers in the study area were under self-care when interviewed. These respondents did not seek treatment from existing health care professionals for several reasons. It appears they were observing the progression of their illness while at the same time collecting information on arsenicosis symptoms and treatment options. Some could not decide what treatment options to select for this new disease and were inquiring of others in an attempt to find out more information from someone who had received treatment and how they rated this treatment. Usually the search for medical intervention begins in rural Bangladesh after the failure of home treatment and/or self-medication (Paul 1992).

It is important to note that some of the respondents who did not consult a physician of any type were found to be continuing self-medication or that they had used medicine prescribed by a physician for another individual diagnosed with arsenicosis. In the latter instance, respondent perception was that all of them were suffering from the same illness. They argued that if some of them had consulted a physician and received a prescription then everyone with arsenicosis symptoms could use it (Paul 2006). In fact, when buying medicine in Bangladesh, one does not need a prescription; all that is needed is the name of the medicine. Available studies (e.g., Shafie 2000; Paul 2006) found that arsenicosis patients who practice self-medication for their illness use home-made herbal medicine.

Women affected with arsenicosis use *Mehedi* (Lawsonia Inermis L.) leaf ointment on their palms if they are swollen and have become rough. Since most people associate visual symptoms of arsenicosis with skin disease, they apply bark of the *Chita* (Plumbago Zeylanica L.) tree and its juice to affected areas of their body. In addition to herbal medicine, many patients who practice self-medication for arsenicosis symptoms avoid the consumption of certain types of foods. Such foods include several types of fishes (e.g., prawn, lobster, *hilsha*, *boal*, *taki*, and *gojar*), beef and several vegetables such as *puisak* and eggplant. They also take antioxidant vitamins. Some patients who can afford the costs also eat eggs, milk, and other protein-rich foods such as beans, peas, pulse, wheat, fresh fruits and vegetables (Paul 2006). Consumption of these foods and vitamins tends to delay the onset of asenicosis and can reduce the aggravation of arsenic poisoning in the human body.

In order to identify the determinants of health-seeking behavior of people with arsenicosis in rural Bangladesh, Paul (2006) performed logistic regression analysis and found that illness stage, perceived threat, symptoms identification time and education level were significant for explaining respondents probability of seeking care for arsenicosis symptoms. Thus, this study clearly suggests that cognitive and symptom-appraisal are more important determinants of treatment–seeking behaviour than are social and economic factors. He found an inverse relationship between landholding size and annual household income with respondent health-seeking behaviour. This seemingly paradoxical relationship might, however, be explained in the context of the healthcare services provided by members of medical teams frequently sent by both NGOs and government agencies to the study area. As indicated, these teams provided medical care either free of charge or at minimal cost to individuals with arsenic-related symptoms (Paul 2006).

## Social Consequences of Arsenic Poisoning

In addition to health effects, the arsenic contamination problem has also triggered social problems in rural Bangladesh (Hassan et al. 2005; Paul 2009). Despite the concerted efforts made by both public and private agencies to educate the general public and raise awareness, many people do not make any distinction between arsenic-related skin lesions and leprosy. Since leprosy is an infectious disease, unaffected people often avoid those afflicted with it. Additionally, the disease is often attributed to sins in the current or past lifetimes. Therefore, people affected by arsenicosis are frequently refused water from neighbouring TWs or are discouraged from appearing in public venues (Mannan 2006).

Arsenicosis victims often lose their jobs and even qualified candidates called for interview are usually not offered jobs if skin manifestations are observed. Affected children are often barred from attending school and playing with other kids (Paul and De 2000). Social activities of arsenic victims with outwardly visible manifestation not only come to an end, but people from outside the affected villages often avoid any contact with inhabitants of affected villages. Some parents neglect and/or isolate their children afflicted with arsenicosis (Hassan et al. 2005). There are even suggestions that the social stigma for those suffering from arsenicosis can result in mental health problems (Hanchett 2006).

Although both men and women suffer from arsenicosis, empirical studies (e.g., Hanchett et al. 2002; Hanchett 2006) suggest that arsenic poisoning has led to greater ostracisation of afflicted women and girls. Social stigmatisation is thus disproportionately felt by women and girls in most arsenic-affected areas (Hanchett 2006). Since physical appearance is so important in Bangladeshi culture, parents are often unable to find grooms for their afflicted unmarried daughters. Even if parents do manage to arrange a marriage, it usually entails offering a huge dowry. Married women who are in the latter stages of arsenic poisoning, are often rejected by their husbands and sent back to their parents. Husbands with a spouse suffering arsenic-related skin lesions may also take a second wife (Sultana 2006). There have been reports of divorce and maltreatment of afflicted married women by their husbands; there are even occasional reports of young women committing suicide when they hear that no one is willing to marry them (Hanchett 2006).

Food cooked by afflicted women has also often been refused by non-afflicted family members, neighbours, or relatives. The low status of women and inequitable power relations in patriarchal Bangladeshi society mean women have little control over their situation and fewer resources relative to men in responding to and coping with arsenicosis. Further, they are less likely to get attention for health manifestations of arsenic poisoning (Sultana 2006). Even if a male member of a family becomes a victim of arsenic poisoning, women in the family bear the additional burden of caring for the victims (Paul and De 2000). With increasing knowledge and awareness, the widespread negative attitudes toward arsenic afflicted people has decreased in recent years.

## Alternative Drinking Water Sources

Considering the magnitude of arsenic contamination of TW water and the eventual lethal impacts of long-term arsenic ingestion on human health and society, the Bangladesh government, with support from foreign public and private agencies, has initiated arsenic mitigation and prevention programmes throughout the country. Since arsenic poisoning has no immediate cure, supplying arsenic-free, safe drinking water to people of affected areas has received top priority in government-sponsored arsenic mitigation programmes. The government of Bangladesh has identified and promoted at least 11 alternative sources of drinking water, which can be divided into two broad categories: groundwater and surface water sources (WHO 2000).

The simplest and most immediately achievable groundwater option is the sharing of TWs that currently have low levels or are free from arsenic contamination. Arsenic-contaminated wells may still be used safely for some purposes, for example, for doing laundry. However, in the most highly contaminated areas no TW will contain 'safe' levels of arsenic. Another alternative for groundwater supply is the installation of deep tube wells (DTWs), which is nine times costlier than to install TWs. It should be noted that arsenic contamination is generally confined to shallow aquifers, or generally 33–230 feet below the surface. Most TWs operate within these depths (BGS 2000). However, DTWs may not always be feasible in an area depending on the hydrogeology and water chemistry. Groundwater with high levels of iron, manganese, or sulfide may also discourage use of DTWs. In areas where DTWs are a feasible option, multiple connections to a single TW can provide increased safe water options for a larger community at a fraction of the cost of installing multiple DTWs (UNICEF 2011).

Another alternative option for groundwater supply is treatment of arsenic contaminated TW water to make it safe for consumption by using different types of filters, such as a three pitchers filter (TPF) or an Alcan filter (Ahmed and Halder 2011; Hasant 2004), or by chemical removal methods. An Alcan filter runs water through an activated alumina medium which efficiently removes arsenic. ALUFLOC is a sachet containing chemicals that are added to a bucket of arsenic contaminated TW water. Typically, after about one hour of treatment, the water is safe for human consumption (Mahmood and Halder 2011).

Surface waters (rivers, lakes, ponds, and rainwater) are typically low in arsenic and therefore, constitute potentially alternative drinking water sources in arsenic-impacted areas. However, surface waters are frequently contaminated with human and animal faecal matter as well as other undesirable materials and are unsafe for this reason. Treatment of surface water can be achieved by several means (Mahmood and Halder 2011). The Pond Sand Filter (PSF) is one such method. It encompasses a manually operated filtration unit built by the side of a pond. Water passes slowly through a large tank filled with sand and gravel. Fine particles are filtered out and microorganisms are inactivated by a thin layer formed on the surface of the bed (WHO 2006).

Since 1994, UNICEF has promoted the use of rainwater as an alternative option for safe drinking water (Mahmood and Halder 2011). This option is in use in many developing countries. In a country with a mean annual rainfall in excess of 80 inches, rainwater is a good alternative water source, particularly in the summer season. Rainwater is arsenic-free and it requires little maintenance to harvest. A variety of cost-effective rainwater collection tanks have been developed in Bangladesh by different organisations. Water is not collected during the first few minutes of a rain to avoid contamination by dust, insects, bird droppings, and the like. Rainwater harvesting is largely capital intensive and is dependent on the availability of suitable roofing materials for guttering and storage tanks (Table 13.4). In southwestern coastal Bangladesh, the rainwater harvesting system (RWHS) has proven to be successful.

The above and other alternative sources (e.g., pipeline water supply at the household or collection point level from any safe aquifer) of safe drinking water have both advantages and disadvantages. The production capacity and efficiency of these sources differ greatly. Some of the recommended drinking water options are cost-effective, while others are not.

**Table 13.4    The cost of different alternative drinking water sources**

| Alternative Option | # People Served | Capital Cost (US$) | Cost/Capita (US$) |
|---|---|---|---|
| Deep Tube Well (DTW) | 50 | 745 | 16.14 |
| DTW – Multiple Connection | 200 | 1,344 | 7.97 |
| Rainwater Harvest | 50 | 855 | 21.45 |
| Pond Sand Filter (PSF) | 50 | 559 | 24.80 |
| PSF (30 Households) | 150 | 559 | 7.06 |
| Dug Well (DW) | 50 | 773 | 29.07 |

*Source:* Compiled from UNICEF (2011), 21.

Similarly, some sources, such as the TPF, use indigenous technology and materials that are familiar to rural people. The PSF and rainwater harvesting system have been in existence (on a limited scale) for quite some time as alternative options for potable water supply in coastal areas of Bangladesh, most of which have high salinity problems. A number of the alternative sources are modifications of existing sources and require little or no skill to operate and maintain, like the TW. To operate and maintain several water options (e.g., PSF), there is a need for community involvement, while others (e.g., TPF) can be adopted at the household level.

Available studies (e.g., Rammelt et al. 2011) suggest that among all alternative sources, DTWs are the most popular among people in arsenic-impacted areas. However, because of their high cost, there is a need to build community-based institutions to install DTWs. This is needed not only to look after the operation and maintenance of DTWs, but also to encourage activities in other sectors of development, such as sanitation, education, and/or village infrastructure. People in affected areas have started building such institutions. Still, experts express concerns regarding the long-term uncertainties surrounding water supplies based on pumping water from deep aquifers and of the possible need to switch to other alternative sources (Rammelt et al. 2008).

## Conclusion

Contamination of TW water with arsenic surfaced, and ultimately challenged efforts to provide safe drinking water to rural households. Continuous consumption of arsenic contaminated well water for several years causes serious adverse health effects. Chronic arsenic poisoning can only be reversed by the provision of arsenic free drinking water. With the hope of reducing or arresting the adverse health effects and social impacts of arsenic poisoning, the government of Bangladesh has introduced several interventions assuring the provision of safe drinking water in arsenic-impacted areas.

Along with providing safe drinking water, the Bangladesh government should also continue testing well water for arsenic contamination as well as identifying and marking 'safe' water wells, and it should simply seal the most contaminated wells. Diagnosing people with arsenicosis or arsenic-associated cancers may be useful in highlighting and prioritising areas of intended intervention. Since poor families are suffering more from the arsenic problem, the government should pay special attention to their access to alternative safe drinking water sources. It is important to assess the future health and socioeconomic impacts of alternative mitigation methods so that policy-makers in Bangladesh can take the appropriate measures to combat widespread arsenic contamination of TW water.

## References

Ahsan, H.A. and Argos, M. 2007. Arsenic and Cancer: A Crisis in Bangladesh. *Cancer Prevention*, 9, 1–3.

Argos, M., Kalra, T., Pierce, B.L., Chen, Y. et al. 2011. A Prospective Study of arsenic Exposure from Drinking Water and Incidence of Skin Lesions in Bangladesh. *American Journal of Epidemiology*, 174(2), 185–94.

Argos, M., Kalra, T., Rathouz, P.J. et al. 2010a. Arsenic Exposure from Drinking Water, and All-cause and Chronic-Disease Mortalities in Bangladesh (HEALS): A Prospective Cohort Study. *Lancet*, 376(9737), 252–8.

Argos, M., Rathouz, P.J., Kalra, T., Pierce, B.L. et al. 2010b. Dietary B Vitamin Intakes and Urinary Total Arsenic Concentration in the Health Effects of Arsenic Longitudinal Study (HEALS) Cohort, Bangladesh. *European Journal of Nutrition*, 49, 473–81.

BGS (British Geological Survey)/DPHE (Department of Public Health Engineering). 1999. *Arsenic Contamination of Groundwater in Bangladesh.* Volume 1. Summary. Dhaka: DPHE.

Buncombe, A. 2010. How the West Poisoned Bangladesh. *Independent*, 21 March.

Caldwell, B.K., Cadwell, J.C., Mitra, S.N. and Smith, W. 2003a. Tubewells and Arsenic in Bangladesh: Challenging a Public Health Success Story. *International Journal of Population Geography*, 9, 23–38.

Caldwell, B.K., Smith, W.T., Lokuge, K. et al. 2006. Access to Drinking-water and Arsenicosis in Bangladesh. *Journal of Health and Population Nutrition*, 24(3), 336–45.

Caldwell, B.K. Cadwell, J.C., Mitra, S.N. and Smith, W.. 2003b. Searching for an Optimum Solution to the Bangladesh Arsenic Crisis. *Social Science & Medicine*, 56, 2089–96.

Chaudhuri, A. 2004. Dealing with Arsenic Contamination in Bangladesh. *MIT Undergraduate Research Journal*, 10, 25–30.

Fazal, M.A., Kawachi, T. and Ichion, E. 2001. Extent and Severity of Groundwater Arsenic Contamination in Bangladesh. *Water International*, 26, 370–79.

Hanchett, S. 2006. Social Aspects of the Arsenic Contamination of Drinking Water: A Revew of Knowledge and Practice in Bangladesh and West Bengal, in *Selected Papers on the Social Aspects of Arsenic and Arsenic Mitigation in Bangladesh*, edited by Arsenic Policy Support Unit (APSU). Dhaka: APSU, 1–55.

Hanchett, S. Nahar, Q., Van Agthoven, A. et al. 2002. Increasing Awareness of Arsenic in Bangladesh: Lessons from a Public Education Programme. *Health Policy and Planning*, 17, 393–401.

Hasnat, M.A. 2004. Assessment of arsenic mitigation options; adverse pregnancy outcomes due to chronic arsenic exposure; and the impact of nutritional status on development of arsenicosis, in *Bangladesh. A PhD Dissertation*. The Centre for epidemiology and Population Health, the Australian National University.

Hassan, M.M., Atkins, P. and Dunn, C.E. 2005. Social Implications of Arsenic Poisoning in Bangladesh. *Social Science & Medicine*, 61, 2201–11.

Hossain, M.A. 2002. Arsenic Contamination in Drinking Water and Environmental Threats: Mitigation Perspectives in Bangladesh. *Regional Development Dialogue*, 298, 1602–6.

Hossain, M.K., Khan, M.M., Alam, M.A. et al. 2005. Manifestation of Arsenicosis Patients and Factors Determining the Duration of Arsenic Symptoms in Bangladesh. *Toxicology and Applied Pharmacology*, 208(1), 78–86.

Khatun, K. 2000. Arsenic Contamination in Ground Water of Bangladesh: A Study of Measure of Knowledge and Awareness of People in Selected Villages of Bangladesh. *Social Science Review*, 17, 83–98.

Mahmood, S.A.I. and Halder, A.K. 2011. The Socioeconomic Impact of arsenic Poisoning in Bangladesh. *Journal of Toxicology and Environmental Health Sciences*, 3(3), 65–73.

Mannan, F. 2006. The Arsenic Crisis in Bangladesh and Human Rights Issues, in *Selected Papers on the Social Aspects of Arsenic and Arsenic Mitigation in Bangladesh*, edited by Arsenic Policy Support Unit (APSU). Dhaka: APSU, 85–94.

Murshed, R., Douglas, R.M., Rammuthugala, G., Cadwell, B. 2004. Clinicians' Roles in Management of Arsenicosis in Bangladesh: Interview Study. *BMJ*, 328, 493–4.

Paul, B.K. 1992. Health Search Behavior of Parents in Rural Bangladesh: An Empirical Study.*Environment and Planning A*, 24, 963–73.

Paul, B.K. 2004. Arsenic Contamination Awareness among the Rural Residents in Bangladesh. *Social Science and Medicine*, 59, 1741–55.

Paul, B.K. 2006. Health Seeking Behaviour of People with Arsenicosis in Rural Bangladesh. *World Health and Population*, 8(4), 1–18.

Paul, B.K. 2009. Attitudes Toward Arsenicosis Victims in Rural Bangladesh: An Empirical Study. *Papers of the Applied Geography Conferences*, 32, 115–23.

Paul, B.K. and Brock, T.V.L. 2006. Treatment Delay Period: The Case of Arsenicosis in Rural Bangladesh. *Health and Place*, 12(4), 580–93.

Paul, B.K. and De, S. 2000. Arsenic Poisoning in Bangladesh: A Geographical Analysis. *Journal of the American Water Resources Association*, 36, 799–809.

Rabbani, G.H., Nasir, M., Saha, S.K. et al.. 2002. Clinical and Biochemical Profiles of Chronic Arsenicosis Patients, in *Bangladesh Environment 2002*, edited by M.F. Ahmed. Dhaka: BPA, 361–71.

Rahman, M., Quamruzzaman, Q., Das, R. et al. 2000. Health Hazards of Arsenic Poisoning, in *Bangladesh Environment 2001*, edited by M.F. Ahmed et al. Dhaka: BPA, 135–50.

Rammelt, C.F., Boes, J., Bruining, H., Ahmed, K.M. et al. 2008. *Technical and Social Feasibility of Deep Tube Wells for Arsenic Free Drinking Water in Bangladesh*. Delft: Delft University of Technology.

Rammelt, C.F., Masud, Z.M., Boes, J. and Masud, F.. 2011. Beyond Medical Treatment, Arsenic Poisoning in Rural Bangladesh. *Social Medicine*, 6(1), 22–30.

Shafie, H. 2000. Health Seeking Behavior of the Arsenic Contaminated People in Rural Bangladesh. *Social Science Review*, 17(1), 140–47.

Smith, A.H., Lingas, E.O. and Rahman, M. 2000. Contamination of Drinking-Water by Arsenic in Bangladesh: A Public Health Emergency. *Bulletin of the World Health Organisation*, 78(9), 1093–103.

Sultana, F. 2006. Gender Concerns in Arsenic Mitigation in Bangladesh: Trends and Challenges, in *Selected Papers on the Social Aspects of Arsenic and Arsenic Mitigation in Bangladesh*, edited by Arsenic Policy Support Unit (APSU). Dhaka: APSU, 53–84.

UNICEF, Bangladesh. 2011. *Making Economic Sense for Arsenic Mitigation: A Case Study of Comilla District, Bangladesh*. Dhaka: UNNICEF, Bangladesh.

UNICEF. Bangladesh. 2010. *Arsenic Mitigation in Bangladesh*. Dhaka: UNICEF, Bangladesh.

WHO (World Health Organisation). 2000. *Towards an Assessment of the Socioeconomic Impact of Arsenic Poisoning in Bangladesh.* Geneva: World Health Organization.

WHO (World Health Organisation). 2006. *Towards an Assessment of the Socioeconomic Impact of Arsenic Poisoning in Bangladesh.* [Online]. Available at: http://www.who.int/water_sanitation_health/dwq/Arsenic2/en/index.html.

# PART IV
# Globalisation and Urbanisation: Global Policy Consequences on Local Health Problems

# Chapter 14

# Tuberculosis: A Scourge for Development?

Jana Fried and John Eyles

## Introduction

In this chapter, we will examine the case of tuberculosis (TB), focusing on the TB epidemics current global spread, its drivers and health sector responses. Along with the epidemiological transition in many richer parts of the world, TB had moved out of the general public's awareness and become a 'forgotten plague' (Farmer 2001; Barnes 1995). Attention only recently renewed somewhat with the increasing co-occurrence of HIV and TB and media headlines on drug-resistant TB (e.g., Boseley 2011; Tackling TB better 2011). However, in her book on the public perception of TB in the United States, Ott (1996) notes that TB is not actually an emerging or re-emerging disease and that such labelling obscures its persistently high global prevalence levels over decades. In the decades since the 1980s, there has been a threefold increase in reported cases to 2005 but some decline since then (WHO 2011; 2012b). Benatar and Upshur (2010) argue that TB has passed through four eras, the first two seeing the disease and its successful treatment in Europe and North America. The third phase may be regarded as a time of denial and social failure, marked by the development of drug-resistant strains – a dimension already recognised as a possibility when the therapies were initially started. The present era is seeing an increase of global TB burden, frequent co-infection with HIV and a growing anxiety about drug-resistant strains of TB that are more complicated and up to 50 times more costly to treat (Grimard and Harling 2004). In fact, in 2009 and 2012, the globally first two clusters of totally drug resistant TB cases were reported in Iran and India, respectively (Velayati et al. 2009; Udwadia et al. 2012). In 2011, 8.7 million people newly developed active TB and 1.4 million died of the disease. Why should this be the case as TB, like several other infectious diseases, is both preventable and curable (see WHO 2012b)?

In fact, TB reduction is one of the three infectious disease-related Millennium Development Goals (MDG 6) (together with HIV/AIDS and malaria) that aim to decrease disease burden and mortality rates. It is also one of the goals of the Global Fund to Fight AIDS, TB and Malaria (The Global Fund 2012). Some progress toward these goals has been made, however, it is challenged by the resource-limited environments of many developing countries and in those experiencing abrupt economic and political change.

In this chapter we argue that TB remains problematic largely because of societal failure, stemming from the ways in which human societies are structured and operate with massive inequities in resources among and between social groups. As Farmer (2001) puts it, the forgotten plague was forgotten largely because it had stopped bothering the wealthy. In fact, the British playwright Arnold Wesker asked 'Whatever happened to the good old days: you know, dirty attics, tuberculosis and general all-round suffering?' With improved living conditions and available medical interventions, it seemed a problem of the past.

Yet nearly 20 years ago, Porter and McAdam (1994, 303) reaffirmed that 'tuberculosis is a disease of poverty ... it spreads readily in crowded conditions and among the malnourished'. Thus, TB in today's developing countries is similar to the situation in Europe and North America in the 1930s, exacerbated by frequent co-infection with HIV. It is telling that Farmer (2001) regards TB as 'the consumption of the poor'. This economic link between TB incidence and poverty has been identified in many studies (see WHO 2005; Harling et al. 2008; De Alencar Ximenes et al. 2009) and reviewed by Dye et al. (2009) and Lonnroth et al. (2010). The demonstration of an economic gradient and the area effects of deprivation add pessimism to attempts to control TB. Rasathan et al. (2011) point to intermediate risk factors which may worsen the risk to succumb to TB among the disadvantaged, such as crowding and thus heightened exposure to those already infected, poorly ventilated dwellings with indoor burning of biomass, and increased vulnerability due to poor nutrition and to HIV infection. All these factors indicate a close link between TB epidemiology and development, as both the spread of TB impacts (economic) development and vice versa. Thus it is important to note that – due to TB's dynamic relationship with productive capacity (see Delfino and Simmons 2005) – the illness has a draining effect on economies with an estimated 0.2 to 0.4 lower growth for every 10 per cent higher incidence of TB (Grimard and Harling 2004). We will examine these individual and societal impacts globally and then at different geographic scales in the contexts of the former Soviet Union and South Africa.

### Why Is Tuberculosis Important?

Tuberculosis is a contagious disease, spread through the air. It is caused by the bacteria *Mycobacterium tuberculosis* that predominantly affects the lungs of a person (pulmonary tuberculosis). While an estimated third of the global population are carriers of the bacteria, only people having active TB, i.e. those that are sick with TB in their lungs, are infectious (WHO 2012a). TB's importance is partly determined by its scale and the ease of its transmission as 5–10 per cent of people who are infected with TB bacilli (but who are not infected with HIV) become sick or infectious at some time during their life. People with HIV and TB infection are much more likely to develop active TB. Left untreated, a person with active TB disease will infect on average between 10 and 15 people every year. People infected with TB bacilli will not necessarily become sick with the disease but it becomes a killer when immune systems are compromised. It is a disease of poverty affecting mostly young adults in their most productive years (WHO 2012a; 2012b).

The vast majority of TB deaths are in the developing world. The 22 countries with the highest disease burden carry more than 80 per cent of the global TB disease load (WHO 2012b). As mentioned above, nearly one and half million people died annually from TB in both 2010 and 2011 (WHO 2011, 2012). But the TB death rate has fallen by 41 per cent since 1990, and the absolute number of deaths is also declining. In addition, the global incidence of TB has started to decrease since 2001, reaching a decline of 2.2 per cent between 2010 and 2012. This is a promising indication of achieving some of MDG 6 sub-targets. Yet there were 8.7 million new TB cases in 2011, of which 2.9 million were women and 1.1 million were co-infected with HIV (WHO 2012). In order to understand these numbers, it is important that it is not just the poverty of individuals but the resource limitations of many countries that remain problematic.

Drug therapies are available and are helping to save numerous lives, but resistance can occur when therapies are misused or mismanaged. Examples include patients that do not complete their full course of treatment; health-care providers who prescribe the wrong treatment, the wrong dose, or length of time for taking the drugs; drug supplies that get interrupted; or drugs that are of poor quality (CDC 2011). All these have contributed to the development of multidrug-resistant (MDR)-TB, currently still underlined by the fact that MDR most commonly develops in the course of TB treatment. Multidrug-resistance describes a situation where a mycobacterium is unresponsive to two at least the two most effective first line drugs (WHO 2012a). Such outbreaks occur more readily in people with weakened immune systems (e.g., patients with HIV). Outbreaks among not immuno-compromised, healthy people do occur, but are less common. Complicating things further is the rise in extensively drug-resistant TB (XDR-TB), strains that are resistant to isoniazid and rifampin, and resistant to any fluoroquinolone and at least one of three injectable second-line drugs (i.e., amikacin, kanamycin, or capreomycin) as well.

Remaining treatment options are few and, as underlined by the above mentioned first clusters of totally drug-resistant TB, are increasingly under threat. WHO estimates that there were 310,000 MDR-TB cases in 2011, up from 65,000 estimated cases in 2010 (WHO 2011; 2012b). In 2010, the largest WHO MDR-TB survey reported the highest rates of MDR-TB thus far, with peaks of up to 28 per cent of new TB cases in parts of the former Soviet Union (WHO 2011). XDR-TB has been found in 84 countries in 2011. This development is particularly problematic considering that XDR-TB has an extraordinarily high mortality rate. A study in a sentinel case area in KwaZulu-Natal (South Africa) showed that from 2005 to 2007, 272 MDR TB and 382 XDR TB cases were diagnosed with HIV co-infection rates of 90 and 98 per cent, respectively. One-year mortality was 71 per cent for patients with MDR-TB and 83 per cent for those with XDR-TB. Forty per cent of MDR TB and 51 per cent of XDR TB patients died within 30 days of the first diagnosis attempt (sputum collection). Hence, one-year and 30-day mortality rates were worse with increased drug resistance (Gandhi et al. 2010). One-year mortality among both MDR and XDR TB patients improved from 2005 to 2007, but the majority of deaths still occurred within the first 30 days. The lack of treatment success is not only lamentable for the individual lives lost, it also raises the dread of a transmitted (rather than treatment-acquired) multi-drug resistant strain.

In order to address some of the challenges around lack of treatment-adherence, treatment-success and development of drug-resistancies, WHO has been recommending the adoption of the Directly-Observed Therapy, short-course (DOTS) since 1995. This control strategy involves five key components, including political and financial commitment; early case detection and diagnosis; standardised treatment with patient supervision and support; effective drug supply systems; and adequate monitoring and performance management (WHO 2012b). Since its introduction, WHO (2012a) estimates that more than '51 million people have been successfully treated and an estimated 20 million lives saved through use of DOTS and the Stop TB Strategy'. Nonetheless, TB remains to present challenges to medical science but also to public health, civil rights and economic development. These challenges will emerge in the following sections.

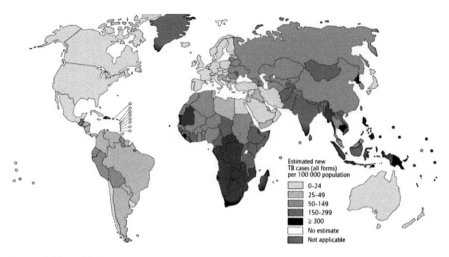

**Figure 14.2    Estimated TB incidence rates, 2011 (WHO 2012)**

### Tuberculosis: The Global Picture

In 2011, the estimated per capita TB incidence rates were falling in all six WHO regions. Between 2010 and 2011, the decline in incidence rates per capita was for the first time big enough to offset population growth, hence the absolute number of new cases arising each year was finally falling, although slowly (WHO 2012b). WHO (2012b) estimates that the largest burden of TB disease in 2012 occurred in the South-East Asia and Western Pacific Regions, with India and China alone accounting for 40 per cent of global prevalence cases. However, the African Region carries 24 per cent of the global TB disease burden and has the highest prevalence and mortality rates. Globally, the highest number of deaths was in the Africa Region. Crucially, in terms of future productive capacity, 10 million children have been orphaned because of parental deaths from TB. Many of these cases are now associated with HIV.

### Tuberculosis: A Regional Picture

*Economic Decline and MDR-TB*

We now examine the regional scale. The countries of the former Soviet Union are facing a serious and widespread epidemic with the highest prevalence of MDR-tuberculosis ever reported. Almost half of all TB cases in countries of the former Soviet Union are resistant to at least one drug in one in eight new cases. As well, one in three retreatment cases are MDR (WHO 2011). In this region, MDR-tuberculosis cases have more extensive resistance patterns and the highest prevalence of XDR tuberculosis (WHO 2011). Trend data from the Baltic countries probably represent the best situation within this region, with the prevalence of MDR tuberculosis in new cases remaining stable and tuberculosis notification rates declining. This may be an indication of political commitment and long-term investment in tuberculosis control, optimum management of susceptible and drug-resistant tuberculosis cases, and an improving socioeconomic situation. By contrast, the data reported from two Russian oblasts with well-performing tuberculosis control programmes (implementing the WHO recommended strategy to control TB and with decreasing tuberculosis notification rates) show increases in both absolute number and prevalence of MDR tuberculosis in new cases and a slowly declining tuberculosis notification rate (Wright et al. 2009). The increasing rate of MDR-TB in this region is related to TB's common associations – poverty, crowding and ineffective treatment, including environmental, structural, and operational factors that place adherence to treatment beyond a patient's control. The existence of selective environmental pressures on *M. tuberculosis* that cause it to acquire drug resistance – thought to be the result of patients receiving wrong prescriptions or taking anti-TB medications irregularly – are directly linked to broader social, economic, and political determinants that affect a patient's access to appropriate medications and appropriate care. TB thus increased in Eastern European countries because of economic decline and the general failure of TB control and other health services since 1991 (Shilova and Dye 2001). Drug resistance is likely not the primary cause but a by-product of the events that led to TB resurgence in these countries. First, resistance is generated initially by inadequate treatment caused, for example, by interruption of the treatment schedule or use of low-quality drugs. Second, resistance levels tend to build up over many years, and yet TB incidence increased suddenly in Eastern European countries after 1991. Third, although formal calculations have not been done, resistance rates are probably too low to attribute all of the increase in caseload to excess transmission from treatment failures (Dye and Floyd 2006).

Russia is not a poor country but the social and economic upheaval after the collapse of the Soviet Union resulted in profound wealth disparity and greater poverty among already marginalised populations. The abrupt economic and political transformation in the 1990s was associated with increases in alcohol consumption, a breakdown of health and social services, and socioeconomic instability. Differences in mortality by socioeconomic status (e.g. income, educational level, and type of employment) widened in the 1990s, especially among alcohol-related deaths and those due to infectious causes. As social cohesion became increasingly fragmented in Russian society, individuals living in relative poverty became further isolated and unable to access formal and informal resources, including health services and social support. It is in this context that the Russian Federation witnessed the reversal of 30 years of successful TB control. Between 1991 and 2001, TB incidence rates in Russia increased from 34 to 88 per 100,000, and TB mortality climbed from 8.1 to 19.9 per 100,000. In the region of Orel, near Moscow, risk factors for mortality were unemployment and homelessness, highlighting the role of poverty in poor TB outcomes. A drastic rise in petty crimes created ideal conditions for generating a TB epidemic. Overcrowded prisons and pre-trial detention centres were crammed with individuals from the poorest sections of society, the alcoholic, homeless, and mentally ill. TB incidence rates in Russian prisons were as high as 7,000 per 100,000. In the 1990s, prisoners made up approximately 25 per cent of all newly diagnosed TB cases in Russia and approximately 30 per cent of newly diagnosed civilian cases had a history of prior imprisonment. Although the prison system may have functioned as an 'epidemiological pump', releasing tens of thousands of active TB cases into the civilian population, the same forces driving the prison epidemic were independently contributing to rising rates of TB in the civilian population (Keashavjee et al. 2008, Stuckler et al. 2008).

Tuberculosis remains a serious threat to public health in Russia and other former Soviet Union countries. Marx et al. (2009) examine this issue in terms of the characteristics of the traditional Russian TB control model inherited from the Soviet Union. They further note that in 2006, nearly 125,000 TB cases and 28,000 TB deaths were notified in the Russian Federation. The TB notification rate was 13 times higher than in Germany. Thus while there has been some improvement, economic marginalisation, high rates of imprisonment, and infrastructural and treatment problems have created a perfect storm for MDR-TB and potentially XDR-TB.

### Tuberculosis: A Local Picture

*TB and HIV in South Africa – Experiencing the Disease and the Loss of Civil Rights*

We now turn to South Africa and a national and localised picture in Africa that is 'facing the worst tuberculosis epidemic since the advent of the antibiotic era' (Chaisson and Martinson 2008, 1089). On this continent especially, the epidemic has been exacerbated by the presence of HIV infections which have also worsened life circumstances. This is particularly true for South Africa that remains the only high burden country (out of 22) where TB incidence is still increasing (WHO 2011). Local studies, such as that by Kritzinger et al. (2009) in Cape Town, indicate little progress in reducing the population burden of TB, with highest rates of increase found in the provinces KwaZulu-Natal and Eastern Cape.

The distribution of tuberculosis is associated with factors similar to those found in Russia. A low level of personal education, unemployment and a low level of household wealth were associated with increased odds of tuberculosis. Individuals living in areas of high inequality had an increased prevalence of tuberculosis disease, independent of their individual- and household-level risk factors. Alcohol abuse, cigarette smoking and low Body Mass Index (a proxy for poor or insufficient food intake) were each independently risk factors for tuberculosis in South Africa, even after adjusting for the SES of individuals. A recent meta-analysis found the relationship between smoking and tuberculosis to be statistically significant, and stronger in those studies which adjusted for SES than those that did not (Kritzinger et al. 2009; see also Lin et al. 2007; Harling et al. 2008). Furthermore, WHO (2012) estimated that there were 330,000 new HIV-positive TB cases in 2011 in South Africa, bringing the country's HIV prevalence in incident TB cases to 65 per cent, the highest level of co-infection globally. Furthermore, there seems to be a growing trend in levels of co-infection, with 2011 estimates being 5 per cent higher than those for the previous year (WHO 2011) and those identified by Corbett et al. (2003). On the positive side, multidrug resistancy still appears relatively low compared to other high-burden countries. MDR-TB was found in 1.8 per cent of new TB cases and 6.7 per cent of retreatment cases. Another recent national survey (see Weyer et al.2007) also commented at the relatively low rate of MDR-TB in South Africa, but they note that drug resistance is higher in retreatment patients as well, with them being 2.3 times more likely than new patients to have an increased risk of drug resistance. They also point to the relatively high rates of HIV-co-infection, with this varying from 28 (Western Cape) to 72 per cent (Free State) by province, with Mpumalanga and North West having over two-thirds of cases. They conclude (Weyer et al. 2007, 1127) that 'a history of sub-optimal TB control together with the rapidly progressing HIV epidemic has created a fertile environment for transmission of drug-resistant TB in South Africa'. This comment applies particularly to those living in rural and informal settlements (see also SA Dept

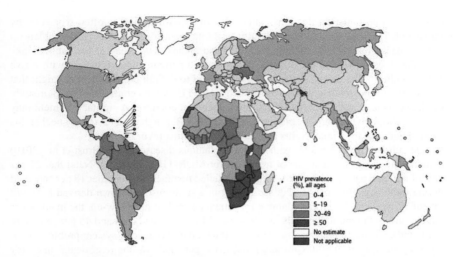

**Figure 14.2    Estimated HIV prevalence in new TB cases, 2011 (WHO 2012)**

of Health 2007). Hence, while MDR-TB rates are still relatively low, there is no room for complacency.

Overall, these factors have led to life expectancy declining by almost 20 years and infant and maternal mortality at their highest rates ever. Mean life expectancy is 48.4 years for men and 51.6 years for women today, implying that most adult South Africans are dying in the economically active period of their lives (Karim et al. 2009). While these issues are clearly a national problem, local effects can be identified. A community-based study in Johannesburg found a 2.5-fold increase in overall TB notification rates culminated in annual rates exceeding 1,400 cases per 100,000 persons. This is double the national rate, approximately nine-fold higher than the TB notification rate for sub-Saharan Africa and 280-fold greater than that for the United States. The epidemiology of TB in this community has changed profoundly over a short period of time. Historically, TB notification rates in this community have been highest among persons older than 60 years of age. However, in 2003–2004, the rates were highest among persons aged 30–49 years, indicating a major shift in the burden of disease to individuals in the economically productive age groups who also have the most dependents (Lawnet al. 2006).

XDR-TB and the socio-political challenges this brings are especially noticeable in South Africa. In this country, XDR-TB first emerged at a rural hospital in Tugela Ferry, KwaZulu-Natal. Of the 1,539 individuals tested for tuberculosis from January, 2005, to March, 2006, 542 had at least one culture that was positive for *M tuberculosis*. Of these 542 with confirmed tuberculosis, 53 had XDR tuberculosis. The median time of death from sputum collection was 16 days (range 2–210 days) for the 52 of 53 patients who died. Concern about hospital-acquired infection was triggered by the findings that 26 (55 per cent) of 47 patients with XDR tuberculosis had never been previously treated for tuberculosis and 28 (67 per cent) of 42 had reported a recent stay in hospital before their tuberculosis diagnosis (Jassal and Bishai 2009). As Singh et al. (2007) note, system characteristics are as important as patient-related ones, with poor institutional infection control procedures being indicted. Many hospital patients are often co-infected with HIV and other opportunistic infections. This issue of cross-infection is often worsened by those with TB being made to attend outpatient treatment for receipt of DOTS tablets on a daily basis in some jurisdictions. This demand means that spread of the bacillus may be assisted, especially where immune-compromised patients mix with those with active TB. In addition, the daily DOTS strategy may lead to default on treatment as might that of involuntary hospitalisation for those with XDR-TB. Atkins et al.(2010) in their study of Khayelitsha, Cape Town, call the former treatment coercive. A similar comment may be made about involuntary hospitalisation for XDR-TB. Singh et al. (2007) argue that this tension between individual rights and public health must favor the latter.

Default is a serious matter with such a contagious disease as TB. Brust et al. (2010) demonstrate from their analysis of treatment for MDR-TB in KwaZulu Natal that 21 per cent of initiated patients defaulted, 17 per cent failed treatment and another 18 per cent died during treatment. Botha et al. (2008a; 2008b) in a study of Cape Town derived a default rate of 17 per cent. When examining why patients were lost to follow-up, the main issues were found in finding individuals to interview (24 per cent had died and 45 per cent were not found). Of the 18 patients interviewed, 10 defaulted because of system problems (e.g. inconsistent test results, files missing) and 8 for personal reasons (e.g. denial that they interrupted treatment or started it late, considered TB not serious). A similar figure of 16 per cent defaulting was found in a recent study in the Western Cape (Jacobson et al. 2011).

Treatment success depends therefore on the system as well as the patient. Treatment of MDR-TB and XDR-TB requires a longer duration; is considerably more complicated, expensive, and toxic; and results in lower treatment success rates. HIV-infected individuals undergoing treatment for MDR-TB have lower rates of treatment success and higher mortality rates than do HIV-uninfected patients. One study of a case series of patients with MDR-TB in South Africa found that the treatment success rate for HIV-uninfected patients was 53 per cent, compared with 38 per cent for HIV-infected patients. These treatment success rates, even among HIV-uninfected individuals, are significantly lower than the international norms for a well-functioning MDR-TB program (Andrews et al. 2007). As indicated above, treatment success of both 'normal' and drug-resistant TB is not only relevant for the individual patient but for public health and the economy in general. Hence, understanding and addressing challenges impeding success at the health system level are important.

But the patients' broader social context cannot be ignored. In a review of patient perceptions, Munro et al. (2007) point out that for most, distance and access to available transport as well as their physical condition affect treatment uptake. Other issues concern long waiting times, queues, lack of privacy, inconvenient appointment times, and the poor upkeep of clinics' health care facility. TB also has consequences for employment and there is often a tension between adherence and work. Economic barriers are many. The influence of community members or peers on treatment-taking behaviour and the strong influence of stigma among family and friends may lead to TB patients hiding their diagnosis and feeling guilt and shame because of the disease with consequences for later productivity and the care of children.

## Experiencing TB and its Treatment at Urban and Rural Sites in South Africa

In order to contribute to the knowledge base needed to respond better to the TB epidemic, an analysis of patient experiences of TB and its co-infection with HIV was recently carried out in two urban and one rural area in South Africa. Part of a larger project on access to health care services, a patient-centred exploration of TB treatment and antiretroviral therapy (ART) was undertaken (see Chimbindi et al. 2012, Fried et al. 2012). Forty-five patients were interviewed in Bushbuckridge (Mpumalanga), Soweto (Johannesburg, Gauteng) and Mitchell Plain (Cape Town, Western Cape) on their life histories, with a special focus on their experiences with TB and access to related health care. Most of these patients were interviewed twice to further clarify and expand on their narratives. In addition to the patient interviews, 22 TB providers from the same health facility locations were also invited to share their experiences within TB health care provision and with TB patients. They were also specifically asked about the challenges patients are facing in accessing TB treatment. In the following analysis, all names mentioned are pseudonyms to protect the identity of our interviewees.

Some patients describe their many months of receiving treatment for TB. They emphasise the complexity of the treatment, especially in the context of poverty and the high rates of HIV co-infection, but also of the positive impact the availability of treatment has had on their lives. Treatment becomes the dominant dimension in life, impacting on social and economic life. For example, Nolwazi Mthembu, a 37-year-old, HIV-positive widow and mother of one surviving child in Bushbuckridge describes her experience after the HIV-related death of her husband and second-born child:

> Yes, they checked me for TB and HIV as well from the clinic. They referred me to the nearest clinic to receive the TB treatment for six months and I became well again after taking the treatment for six months. Thereafter, they referred me to (a nearby) Hospital that in January 2008 I should go there in regards with my HIV status.

Thulani Zondo, a 36-year-old Soweto resident, is on ART and TB treatment, but defaulted the former. He used to have a regular employment in the service industry, and suspects that he lost his job due to his illness. Now he earns money by being self-employed, selling ice cream. Describing the actual process of receiving DOTS, he says:

> When you get there, if you've just been infected, they give you a card and some pills to take or they give you pills to take in the clinic and you have to come to the clinic every time to take the pills. But if you know how to take the pills, they give you those pills until you recover. Then, after you have recovered well for them, they then give you more pills to take on your own. And then they count the number of days that you should come and collect another batch of treatment. For example, they can say next week Monday or Tuesday you should come collect another treatment. And then they change them after some time when they see that you are committed into taking your treatment.

A clinic nurse in Bushbuckridge aims to highlight the clinic's flexibility in enabling patients to fit the long-lasting treatment into patients' lives:

> If they are having a problem of not coming every two weeks, they do explain to us so that we increase the treatment. But we stress that usually we want to see the improvement when they come every two weeks. But sometimes they give reason "but I am working, I don't have a chance, please increase this treatment for me," so we increase.

Another man, 51-year-old Samuel Mhlongo, was diagnosed with HIV in 2007 and now receives ART as well as TB treatment. While both he and his wife are unemployed, he gets strength from his religion and from the support of his wife.

> I'm just living my life, doing what I can – trying to gain stamina, and drinking Mageu [a traditional non-alcoholic drink]. And when I was at the TB side, we were taught that when you are on treatment, you are not supposed to miss any dose. And you are also not supposed to drink any traditional muthi (medicine). That's what I always knew from when I was at the TB side when they educated us every day. (…) I was at home; they gave me appointment dates for follow up and to collect treatment. They would tell me that I was taking it properly. So I was taking it from home until they told me that I have finished.

Mvelo Moyo, also 51, a divorcee with one child who learnt of his HIV status in 2007 and had to quit his job because of deteriorating health, speaks of his treatment experiences that were also influenced by strong family support and a continued use of a traditional healer.

> I am feeling fine; I am feeling very much better. I am not really fine but I can work, even at home I am working on my own. (…) I was unable to drive, my only problem (are) my legs, because at some point, (they) are having numbness and it's continuing. It was also in the hand, but now it's not that much. It is only left in the legs but in terms of life, I am feeling very much better because of the HIV and the TB treatments. I am able to do everything at home, I even do washing my clothes, ploughing and also building houses (for the) chickens when it's necessary.

A 38-year-old Soweto mother of a 16-year-old son and 13-year-old daughter, Thabisa Zulu finished her schooling at standard nine. In the past, she used to have a regular job but is now self-employed. She describes her complicated diagnosis and successful treatment in the following story:

> I went for the TB test when I was losing weight. I had those signs, I was not eating and I was sweating. So I said, these are the symptoms of TB. Here they are, they are written at the clinic. I see them, I said alright let me go for a TB test. And then they give you a small plastic bottle to put sputum inside it and bring it back to the clinic. Then, when I went to get my results, my results were negative. But the signs are saying I am losing weight and all that. So, I asked why don't you get it. Then they said, let us take another sputum (sample). They took it three times. Going back to the clinic, the last TB test was taken by the doctor from the hospital. So he checked everything with the blood test and he discovered that I had TB of the blood. He told me that I will attend TB treatment. He asked me which is the nearest clinic? You must go there and get your treatment. He started me with multivitamin and gave me a referral letter to go and take TB treatment. That is how I got TB; I found that everything was O.K. I took my treatment, I went there every day to go and drink. (…) I think it was for two months, then they started to give me treatment for two weeks and every time after two weeks. And they would give me a green card to mark if have taken treatment and if haven't taken it. (…) It was for nine months and I finished it. They tested me and I was cured and I started my ARVs.

All the above stories speak of the promises of a successful TB therapy and the importance this has for the survival and ordinary lives of infected people. However, they also indicate some of the challenges related to treatment – the complexities in adjusting treatment to the daily life of people, the importance of traditional and religious beliefs as well as social support networks, the economic costs of treatment, difficult diagnosis and other health care provider challenges including the high level of HIV co-infection.

Fifty-three-year-old John Mayibuye, originally from Mozambique and working since the age of 10 in Johannesburg's mining industry, describes his approach to the double diagnosis. The married father of two children, despite being on TB treatment, also uses traditional medicine and considers himself a traditional healer and expresses his thoughts on the best treatment approach.

> As I am going to complete my TB course, I will go for check-up after this (for HIV). ( …) I don't want to mix the treatment because I am still taking six tablets for everyday and it will be too much to take another treatment, so I have to finish this one first. I know that when I get to mix the treatments, it would not come along. I have to go step by step.

There are many difficulties in accessing care. Some of these are also related to patients' knowledge and attitudes. One TB health care provider in Bushbuckridge considers stigma and inconvenience as some of the issues, leading to delay: 'You know, maybe they don't want to be seen when they are coming here, and sometimes they are just afraid of this long queue.'

However, it is not only health care providers who observe a delay in seeking treatment, often for competing interests such as work. John Mayibuye describes his own experience:

> I was suffering from this disease, TB and I didn't know in the beginning that I was suffering from TB. I felt tired when working, even when walking. And I didn't know what was what, so they took me to see a doctor. He examined me, he said that I have water in my stomach and I have to go for X- ray. But I didn't go for X-ray till the illness became worse and I got bedridden. My son called his mother at home to fetch and they took me to (the nearest) hospital.

Similarly, Mdiduzi Ndaba, a father of three children, had to stop working due to his illness, but took months to realise its seriousness:

> I was coughing, feeling hot when it's cold, and sweating and feeling cold when it's hot, and shivering. Until I came here to the clinic where I was diagnosed with TB. (…) It just took me over four months, if I am not mistaken. (…) I became ill for a long time while in Jo'burg. I was thinking that it was just a cough and (only when) I realised that it is becoming worse, then I came home (and went to the clinic).

This delay in seeking care does not only influence people's own well-being and the individual's chance to get healed, it also impacts on the treatment success rate. However, while attitudes can play a role in initiating contact with the health care system, there are also barriers once patients have started treatment. Treatment delays and barriers may come from lack of knowledge, transport issues and the debilitating nature of the illness. Concentrating on those affecting security and well-being, a TB co-ordinator talks of social and economic insecurity and the lack of financial resources:

> Because the issue of crime, I think it also contributes to the challenges that we are having. Because in our community, we have got the challenge of poverty where you find that at times people have got to take the treatment on an empty stomach. The food supplements that we are getting, it's only the (…) soft porridge type (…) Although it does help, but it's not enough.

Insufficient nutrition is especially problematic since it increases the chances of severe side effects and related treatment interruptions.

> Others just default, and then others, when we did the follow up treatment, you find that some are not taking treatment who are saying that we don't have something to eat, and this treatment (is) making us to be very hungry, so I can't take it because I don't have something to eat.

Similar issues are also identified by a DOTS treatment supporter in Mitchell's Plain:

> sometimes, they default because they say that they can't eat the tablets because they are hungry, they don't have food, that's why they default the treatment. The others, they said "No, we are working; we can't go to the clinic every time." We just explain to them, "we are here for you, that's why we are the community DOTS (supporters). To help those who are working, after work you just come to me and take your tablets and every day you must do that." (…) The other (patients), maybe they are far way, they are too far from the clinic, they don't have the money to come, they have to take the taxi. They can't walk each and every day, now it's raining. The others, even day before yesterday, it was raining miss, they didn't come. Yesterday, we just go to them to recall them, "Why didn't you come?" They said "It was raining, how can I go out, go the clinic, when it is raining?" We said, "But it is your health." (…) It was really raining hard, but they are supposed to make a plan. Don't know about a plan, but they are supposed to eat their treatment each and every day.

These insights by health care providers support the findings by Munro et al. (2007) about the ways in which poverty-related financial resource constraints can undermine physical access (e.g. transport) and treatment adherence (e.g. nutrition). These factors are seldom articulated by patients, except for their immediate physical condition. However, besides these difficulties there are also factors more directly linked to health facilities and the actual provision of services with staff shortages and overworked staff being often less than sympathetic. A resource-limited setting with patients having difficulty making ends meet can lead to communication difficulties, lack of trust and provider insensitivity, worsening the situation of suffering from TB.

For example, 38-year-old Lesedi Ledwaba from Johannesburg was diagnosed with an STI and HIV in 1996 and started a TB DOTS therapy. The mother of one son, she lives separated from her abusive husband and found strong support in her elderly neighbour, who treats her like her adopted daughter. Due to a lack of money for school fees, Lesedi Ledwaba had to leave school after standard four and now earns her living by doing laundry and ironing in other people's households. Being on TB DOTS and ART, she describes her experience of diagnosis, treatment side effects and subsequent complications within her clinic:

With TB, I don't know because I was sent there by the professional and they gave me two bottles for sputum. Then they tested my sputum and it all came back negative. Then the last test showed that I have TB. Then they started me on treatment for TB. Maybe I took them only three times because these big ones (tablets) where not fine for me. They used to make me sick because I used to vomit after taking them. Then I told my adopted mother that I am no longer going to the clinic to get the TB treatment because it is making me sick and I vomit all the time. Except for that this HIV treatment needs me to eat before I can take it, but now – because after eating I vomit because of these TB tablets – then I have to stop the treatment.

Perhaps due to a lack of trust, Lesedi Lewaba did not share her concerns with health care providers supervising her TB DOTS.

Then when I came back here the professional nurse shouted at me and told me that she will even stop my ARV treatment. (…) She said to me, "why are you infecting me with TB?" shouting at me as if I am a child. But because I am a quiet person I kept quiet, (while she was) banging her hand on the table at the same time. Then she took my file and we went to the TB side. (…) And when we got there we found another nurse lady and she told her that if I do not come for treatment that side then she will stop me from taking the ARVs also. And all that time I was quiet and I said nothing. (…) Then afterwards, when I left this place, on my way home I felt so numb, I couldn't feel myself walking. Even where I stay now, my adopted mother knows that you can be harsh on me, but not that harsh because I am not supposed to be stressed because of my health. What the professional nurse did to me, it was hurtful.

All these experiences also highlight the additional complications faced by a TB treatment programme in countries with very high-levels of HIV co-infections. In South Africa, where more than 60 per cent of all people with TB are HIV-positive, this is especially relevant and needs specific co-ordination efforts between the two, usually parallel implemented, health care provision areas in a resource-limited environment. One key ingredient in enabling continuing access to TB DOTS is the availability of sufficient resources, including necessary drugs and health care staff. Commenting on the former, a TB programme co-ordinator describes:

Yeah, I think TB drug supply is … it's adequate. Although we did have a little bit of a problem, but that was last year – we had a shortage of streptomycin – that is a TB injection for those that are on re-treatment – and we had a little bit of shortage of rifampicin as well, that is your rimactazid. But it was a specific rimactazid – 150 75. So we had a shortage of that, but that was for about four months, but it was four months too long, you know? (…) But we had a way of dealing with that because we were going from facility to facility to try and borrow from this facility and supply this facility and … It was a strain, but it did work, we didn't have a situation where people completely did not have treatment.

A nurse from Mitchell's Plain indirectly illustrates the resource limitation of staff shortages leading to increasing wait times, and thus perhaps reducing patients' willingness to regularly visit health facilities, especially at a later stage of treatment once their symptoms have improved.

It's never more than an hour, I would say, it's never more than an hour. (…) It's only, the only busy day that they will find themselves waiting is on Monday, when we've got a doctor and on Fridays where I am busy doing Mantoux's on children. So in between then, they will find themselves waiting especial the ones that are on Streptomycin or MDR, on Kanamycin. Those are the only ones that find themselves waiting. (…) Most of them are very impatient, but for some reason they manage to wait. Very few will say sister I can't wait I'll come back or very few would disappear for good. Some of them do wait, really (…).

Treating MDR-TB patients in hospital or community setting adds more problems, especially related to infection control.

And of course we have patients like our special patients, the MDR patients. In Bushbuckridge, we have 39 MDR patients that are actually in the community and we have three … two XDR patients and the one that is actually still on investigation but we are afraid … (it) looks like we're going to have three XDR patients. And all of those patients are in the community. So they have to be visited, and you know, re-adherence is strengthened on them and … re-educated on how to isolate these people, not in a way that they can actually feel like they are not wanted.

These experiences of TB and its treatment in the context of South Africa provide voice to those dealing with this epidemic, its impacts and context. South Africa is a middle-income country with great wealth disparities, exacerbated by its apartheid years. Resource limitations prevent good infection control, especially with MDR- and XDR-TB. Providers are stretched and while they recognise the economic pressures on patients, they can do little to mitigate them. Patients see their physical challenges and how complicated care is and how that, with possibly ART, be fitted into economically deprived but often socially resilient lives (Fried et al. 2012).

## Discussion and Conclusion

TB is back with a vengeance, although there have been some changes in locality and significant recent improvements as documented by WHO (2012). Treatment and infection control are central in managing this treatable disease. For this, a constant supply of quality-assured anti-TB drugs is fundamental. Directly Observed Treatment, Short-course (DOTS) is the systematic application of standardised and supervised drug therapy, along with diagnosis by sputum smears. DOTS has been practiced all over the world since 1999. But DOTS coverage is not the same as DOTS treatment and estimates of incidence are difficult to achieve (see Attaran 2005). As we have seen, DOTS does little with respect to drug-resistant TB and may provide a false sense of security or complacency. Questions have been raised over the efficacy of DOTS over other TB treatment approaches (see Davies 2003) or that direct observation enhances cure rates (see Volmink and Garner 2009). There are serious concerns as well over the accuracy of sputum tests. In a study in South Africa, Hassim et al. (2010) showed only one third of culture-positive patients were identified by smear. Depending on its implementation, DOTS also has implications for civil rights. The 'policing' of patients through direct observation and the uses of coercion and detention with MDR- and XDR-TB may delay treatment (see Coker 2003) and be difficult to enforce in resource-limited settings, while significant ethical issues remain (see London 2009). Such settings may also compromise infection control, making the impacts of the disease worse for its sufferers and their dependents. Infection control in countries undergoing rapid societal or political change or with large, poor and poorly housed populations is likely to be minimal. The experiences of our respondents in South Africa are likely to change slowly because of the inequitable development and distribution of resources. Low economic status, social stigma and the denial of opportunity will continue and reinforce the challenges in such societies and populations. The co-infections of TB and HIV result in opportunities, too, as there are similarities in their treatment regimes and thus potential for pooling resources (see Maher 2010). But as Horton (2009) noted, 'progress towards the Millennium Development Goals has been slow and uneven. Inequities in health are deep and intractable. Donor funding is unpredictable. International institutions suffer pervasive democratic deficits – the views of low-income and middle-income countries are too often marginalised or excluded'. Furthermore, 'evidence from past economic crises gives us reasonable precision about what is likely to happen … Government expenditures on health will be squeezed and likely fall, contributing to worse health outcomes. Household income to pay for health will drop. Insurance protection will decline. The cost of medicines will probably increase (because of currency devaluations). Patients will switch from the private to the public sector, putting an often unbearable burden on government-funded health services' while at the same time economic productivity is further compromised. Investing in public health needs to become a greater global priority since development of any kind is not possible without treating the diseases that sap the strength, hope and energy of individuals, communities and regions. TB is one of these.

## References

Andrews, J.R., Shah, N. Sarita et al. 2007. Multidrug-resistant and extensively drug-resistant tuberculosis: implications for the HIV epidemic and antiretroviral therapy rollout in South Africa. *Journal of Infectious Disease*, 196(Suppl 3), S482–490.

Atkins, S., Biles, D., Lewin, S. et al. 2010. Patients' experiences of an intervention to support tuberculosis treatment adherence in South Africa. *Journal of Health Services Research and Policy*, 15(3), 163–70.

Attaran, A. 2005. An immeasurable crisis? A criticism of the millennium development goals and why they cannot be measured. *PLoS Medicine*, 2(10): e318.

Barnes, D. 1995. *The Making of a Social Disease. Tuber culosis in Ninetheenth-Century France*. Berkeley: The University of California Press.

Benatar, S. and Upshur, R. 2010. Tuberculosis and poverty. *International Journal of Tuberculosis and Lung Disease*, 14, 1215–21.

Boseley, S. 2011. Drug-resistant TB rising in Europe. *The Guardian*, 18 March 2011 [online]. Available at: http://www.guardian.co.uk/society/sarah-boseley-global-health/2011/mar/18/tuberculosis-europe-news?CMP=twt_gu.

Botha, E., den Boon, S., Lawrence, K.A. et al. 2008a. From suspect to patient: tuberculosis diagnosis and treatment initiation in health facilities in South Africa. *International Journal of Tuberculosis and Lung Disease*, 12(8), 936–41.

Botha, E., den Boon, S., Verver et al. 2008b. Initial default from tuberculosis treatment: how often does it happen and what are the reasons? *International Journal of Tuberculosis and Lung Disease*, 12(7), 820–23.

Brust, J.C., Gandhi, N.R., Carrara, H. et al. 2010. High treatment failure and default rates for patients with multidrug-resistant tuberculosis in KwaZulu-Natal, South Africa, 2000–2003. *International Journal of Tuberculosis and Lung Disease*, 14(4), 413–19.

CDC. (2011). *Multi-drug resistant tuberculosis*. Atlanta: CDC.

Chaisson, R.E. and Martinson, N.A. 2008. Tuberculosis in Africa – Combating an HIV-driven crisis. *The New England Journal of Medicine*, 358(11), 1089–92.

Chimbindi, N., Bärninghausen, T. and Newell, M. 2012. Almost universal coverage: HIV testing among TB patients in a rural public programme. *International Journal of Tuberculosis and Lung Disease*, 16(4), 708.

Coker, R.J. 2003. Public health impact of detention of individuals with tuberculosis: systematic literature review. *Public Health*, 117(4), 281–7.

Corbett, E.L., Watt, C.J., Walker, N. et al. 2003. The growing burden of tuberculosis. *Archives of Internal Medicine* 163, 1009–21.

Davies, P.D. 2003. The role of DOTS in tuberculosis treatment and control. *American Journal of Respiratory Medicine*, 2(3), 203–9.

de Alencar Ximenes, R.A., de Fátima Pessoa Militão de Albuquerque, M., Souza, W.V. et al. 2009. Is it better to be rich in a poor area or poor in a rich area? A multilevel analysis of a case-control study of social determinants of tuberculosis. *International Journal of Epidemiology*, 38(5), 1285–96.

Delfino, D. and Simmons, P. 2005. Dynamics of tuberculosis and economic growth. *Environment and Development Economics*, 10(6), 719–43.

Dye, C. and Floyd, K. 2006. Tuberculosis, in *Disease Control Priorities in Developing Countries*, edited by D.T. Jamison, J.G. Breman and A.R. Measham. Washington, DC: World Bank.

Dye, C., Lönnroth, K., Jaramillo, E. et al. 2009. Trends in tuberculosis incidence and the determinants in 134 countries. *Bulletin of the WHO*, 87, 683–91.

Farmer, P. 2001. *Infections and Inequalities*. Berkeley: University Press of California

Fried, J., Harris, B. and Eyles, J. 2012. Hopes interrupted: accessing and experiences of antiretroviral therapy in South Africa. *BMJ Sexually Transmitted Infections*, 88(2), 147–51.

Gandhi, N.R., Shah, N.S., Andrews, J.R. et al. and on behalf of the Tugela Ferry Care and Research (TF CARES) Collaboration 2010. HIV coinfection in multidrug- and extensively drug-resistant tuberculosis results in high early mortality. *American Journal of Respiratory and Critical Care Medicine*, 181, 80–86.

Grimard, F. and Harling, G. (2004). The impact of tuberculosis on economic growth. Department of Economics, McGill University [online]. Available at: http://neumann. hec.ca/neudc2004/fp/grimard_franque_aout_27.pdf.

Harling, G., Ehrlich, R. and Myer, L. 2008. The social epidemiology of tuberculosis in South Africa. *Social Science and Medicine*, 66, 492–505.

Horton, R. 2009. The global financial crisis: an acute threat to health. *The Lancet*, 373(9661), 355–6.

Jacobson, K.R., Theron, D., Victor, T.C. et al. 2011. Treatment outcomes of isomazid-resistant tuberculosis patients, Western Cape Province, South Africa. *Clinical Infectious Diseases*, 53(4), 369–72.

Jassal, M. and Bishai, W.R. 2009. Extensively drug-resistant tuberculosis. *The Lancet Infectious Diseases*, 9(1), 19–30.

Karim, S.S., Churchyard, G.J., Karim, Q.A. and Lawn, S.D. 2009. HIV infection and tuberculosis in South Africa: an urgent need to escalate the public health response. *The Lancet*, 374, 921–33.

Keshavjee, S., Gelmanova, I., Pasechnikov, A. et al. 2008. Treating multi-drug resistant tuberculosis in Tomsk, Russia: Developing programs that address the linkage between poverty and disease. *Annals of the New York Academy of Science*, 1136, 1–11.

Kritzinger, F.E., Den Boon, S., Verver, S. et al. 2009. No decrease in annual risk of tuberculosis infection in endemic area in Cape Town, South Africa. *Tropical Medicine and International Health*, 14(2), 136–42.

Lawn, S.D., Bekker, L.G., Middelkoop, K. et al. 2006. Impact of HIV infection on the epidemiology of tuberculosis in a peri-urban community in South Africa: the need for age-specific interventions. *Clinical Infectious Diseases*, 42(7), 1040–47.

Lin, H.H., Ezzati, M. and Murray, M. 2007. Tobacco smoke, indoor air pollution and tuberculosis: A systematic review and meta-analysis. *PLoS Medicine*, 4(1), e20.

London, L. 2009. Confinement for extensively drug-resistant tuberculosis: balancing protection of health systems, individual rights and the public's health. *International Journal of Tuberculosis and Lung Disease*, 13(10), 1200–1209.

Lönnroth, K., Jaramillo, E., Williams, B. et al. 2010. Tuberculosis, in *Equity, Social Determinants and Public Health Programs*, edited by E. Blas and A.S. Kurup. Geneva: World Health Organization, 219–41.

Maher, D. 2010. Re-thinking global health sector efforts for HIV and tuberculosis epidemic control: promoting integration of programme activities within a strengthened health system. *BMC Public Health*, 10, 394.

Marx, F.M., Skachkova, E.I., Son, I.M. et al. 2009. Control of tuberculosis in Russia and other countries of the former Soviet Union. *Pneumologie*, 63(5), 253–60.

Meintjes, G., Schoeman, H., Morroni, C. et al. 2008. Patient and provider delay in tuberculosis suspects from communities with a high HIV prevalence in South Africa: A cross-sectional study. *BMC Infectious Diseases*, 8(72).

Munro, S.A., Lewin, S.A., Smith, H.J. et al. 2007. Patient adherence to tuberculosis treatment: A systematic review of qualitative research. *PLoS Medicine*, 4(7), e238.

Ott, K. 1996. *Fevered Lives*. Cambridge, MA: Harvard University Press.

Porter, J.D.H. and McAdam, K.P.W.J. 1994. The re-emergence of tuberculosis. *Annual Review of Public Health*, 15, 303–23.

Rasanathan, K., Sivansankara Kurup, A., Jaramillo, E. and Lönnroth, K. 2011. The social determinants of health: key to global tuberculosis control. *International Journal of Tuberculosis and Lung Disease*, 15(6), 530–36.

Schlipkoter, U. and. Flahault, A. 2010. Communicable diseases. *Public Health Reviews*, 32, 90–119.

Shilova, M.V. and Dye, C. 2001. The resurgence of tuberculosis in Russia. *Philisophical Transactions of the Royal Society of London Series B, Biological Sciences*, 356, 1069–75.

Singh, J.A., Upshur, R. and Padayatchi, N. 2007. XDR-TB in South Africa: No time for denial or complacency. *PLoS Medicine*, 4(1), e50.

South African Department of Health . 2007. *Tuberculosis Strategic Plan for South Africa, 2007–2011*. Johannesburg: DOH.

South African Medical Research Council. 2002. *National survey of tuberculosis drug resistance in South Africa: Second progress report*. Johannesburg: USAID.

Stuckler, D., Basu, S., McKee, M. and King, L. 2008. Mass incarceration can explain population increases in tuberculosis and multi-drug resistant tuberculosis in European and central Asian countries. *Proceedings of the National Academy of Sciences*, 105(36), 13280–85.

Tackling TB better. Weak human efforts are making a natural scourge worse. (2011, March 23). *The Financial Times*. Avaliable at: www.FT.com.

The Global Fund to Fight AIDS, tuberculosis and malaria (2012). [online]. Available at: http://www.theglobalfund.org/en/.

Udwadia, Z., Amale, R., Ajbani, K. and Rodrigues, C. 2012. Totally drug-resistant tuberculosis in India. *Clinical Infectious Diseases*, 54(4), 579–81, first published online December 21, 2011 doi:10.10933/cid/cir889.

Velayati, A., Masjedi, M., Farnia, P. et al. 2009. Emergence of new forms of totally drug-resistant tuberculosis bacilli: super extensively drug-resistant tuberculosis or totally drug-resistant strains in Iran. *CHEST*, 136(2), 420–25.

Weyer, J., Brand, J., Lancaster, J. et al. 2007. Determinants of multidrug-resistant tuberculosis in South Africa: results from a national survey. *South African Medical Journal*, 97(11), 1120–28.

WHO, 2005. *Addressing Poverty in TB Control*. Geneva: World Health Organization.

WHO, 2011. *The Global TB Control Report*. Geneva: World Health Organization.

WHO, 2012a. *Fact Sheet on Cuberculosis, No 104*, Geneva: World Health Organization.

WHO, 2012b. *The Global TB Control Report*. Geneva: World Health Organization.

Wright, A., Zignol, M., Van Deun, A. et al. 2009. Epidemiology of antituberculosis drug resistance 2002–07: an updated analysis of the Global Project Anti-Tuberculosis Drug Resistance Surveillance. *The Lancet*, 373(9678), 1861–73.

# Chapter 15

# Globalisation and the Misplacement of Health: An Emerging Agenda

Sarah Lovell and Mark M. Rosenberg

## Introduction

The history of globalisation is one of contradiction, politics, and protests. Alongside the benefits of globalisation that we unthinkingly take advantage of, from the opportunities for social networking to the growing range of products we consume, there are negative externalities (Barnett et al. 2008; Kelly 1999). In 2011, the implications of economic globalisation came to the fore as we witnessed the *Occupy* protesters in the West reject the economic system that allows wealth to be monopolised by an elite minority, we saw residents of Greece act out in rejection of the austerity measures deemed necessary to keep their economy afloat on a global stage, while worsening food security and dissatisfaction were a factor in the social media-facilitated *Arab Spring* that spread across the Middle East (Breisinger et al. 2011). The human cost of globalisation is increasingly occupying the public consciousness. In this chapter, we focus on health as one of the few *hard* indicators we have of the impacts of globalisation on the quality of life of individuals. We examine how global economic forces are shaping health and health care and the progress geographers have made in examining these relationships. We begin our discussion by delving into the contested nature of globalisation and its importance to debates on development.

## Globalisation and the (Mis)Use of Scale

Globalisation describes a process by which the *social*, the *political*, and the *economic* spread across space in new and faster ways creating interconnections that transcend national borders (Voisey and O'Riordan 2001, 26). The history of globalisation dates back to the 1400s but it is only in recent decades that we have experienced the profound economic and social shifts that have transformed the political and economic interdependence of the globe and our conceptualisations of it (Wallerstein 1974; Swynguedow 2000). The current era of globalisation has been dominated by discussion of two phenomena. First, the flow of information, at faster rates than ever before, has led to the *compression* of the social world and heightened our experience of global connectedness (Robertson 1992). Indeed, if we take the view of Yeung (2002), globalisation may be more active in our imaginings of space than in reality. Second, globalisation is deeply entwined with processes of economic liberalisation characterised by the loosening of government controls over the economy and increased exposure and integration with world markets. It is this second component of globalisation that is to be the focus of this chapter.

Above all, globalisation is a process. When we describe globalisation as a set of fixed material outputs, such as an integrated global economic system, we overlook the actions that transcend scale in order to constitute the global (Kelly 1999). For example, when the nation-state uses the World Trade Organisation (WTO) to oppose international trade sanctions, when workers' unions form international alliances in pursuit of labour rights, and when individual businesses use the internet to reach buyers around the world, all are participating in economic globalisation. None of these examples is scale neutral, rather, these examples draw on the strength of global connections to represent and reproduce relationships of power: 'scale does not provide a simple container for action, but rather a site for interaction between social forces operating across scales and a contested political construction of social processes' (Kelly 1999, 381). Engaging with globalisation thus becomes deeply political; even resistance to 'the totalising and globalising force of money and capital accumulation demands the forging of 'scalar' alliances that are sensitive to geographical differences and uniqueness' (Swyngedouw 2000, 74). Thus, elucidating the process of globalisation requires understanding how the messy, multi-scaled and geographically situated concept is leveraged as a tool for power.

Arguments in favor of globalisation have traditionally emphasised the economic benefits brought about by closer global connections; the economic benefits in turn translating into improved standards of living, including better health outcomes. Despite the systematic collection of population health indicators, such as infant mortality rates, the health impacts of globalisation are often overlooked in favour of monetary indicators of social wellbeing. Few studies have sought to quantify the health impacts of the broader concept of globalisation within low-income nations. Bergh and Nilsson (2010a) are one exception; using the KOF index of globalisation, they found that 'economic globalisation has a strong and robust positive effect on life expectancy' a trend that holds even when restricted to low-income countries (Bergh and Nilsson 2010b). Our understanding of the diverse ways in which globalisation is impacting on health has increased rapidly but there are several reasons why our current understanding of the health impacts of globalisation is incomplete. First, in most cases the health impacts of globalisation are indirect and very difficult to attribute quantitatively to globalisation. Secondly, the determinants of human health themselves are still being identified and are proving very difficult to pin down due to the sheer number of confounding factors. Our understanding of globalisation is contested, and our knowledge of the many ways in which it may be affecting human lives is still in its infancy and reliant on parallel developments in other disciplines. Thirdly, and finally, globalisation is a fairly new focus of research, and so the tools to measure its impacts are still being refined and in many cases we simply do not have the necessary historical data. The health effects of globalisation being explored here are predominantly an indirect result of neo-liberal policies that have prioritised the pursuit of economic growth.

This chapter seeks to highlight the impacts of economic globalisation on health and health care in developing nations. We begin by delving further into the contested nature of globalisation drawing on the work of key theorists from recent decades. Subsequently, our discussion focuses on three processes that are critical to the development and health agenda: first, we examine the nature of economic liberalisation policies in low-income countries to understand how globalisation has shaped the distribution of wealth. Second we explore how the liberalisation of health systems has impacted on health outcomes. Finally, we discuss the marginalisation of health relative to the international trade agenda. Throughout, we use the geographic literature on globalisation and health as a springboard for drawing the reader's attention to those themes which geographers have great potential to contribute to but have largely overlooked to date. Examples are used as illustrative devices, but should not be taken as the only research issues of importance or the limits of the research agenda we propose.

## Situating Globalisation and Development

Globalisation in its current capacity emerged out of the economic glut of the 1970s. Governments were led to reduce their role in the economy as the global flow of capital was seen as a means by which trade and financial profits could expand to a scale never experienced before (McMichael 2001; Taylor, Watts and Johnston 2001). Subsequently, economic globalisation has come to be understood as a philosophy to guide the restructuring of economies as Harvey (2005) explains:

> Neoliberalism is in the first instance a theory of political economic practices that proposes that human well-being can best be advanced by liberating individual entrepreneurial freedoms and skills within an institutional framework characterized by strong private property rights, free market and free trade. The role of the state is to create and preserve an institutional framework appropriate to such practices. (Harvey 2005, 2)

Neoliberal philosophy, and specifically the belief that economic growth would be stifled by excessive state intervention, came to shape the international development agenda of the 1980s and 1990s becoming entrenched through the introduction of structural adjustment programmes (SAPs). Founded on neoliberal ideals, SAP policies were grounded in the assumption that rapidly opening up a country's economy was key to economic development and would lead to newfound prosperity with trickle-down effects that would improve the well-being of a country's population (Stiglitz 2002). Structural Adjustment Programmes emerged out of the policies of global lending institutions such as the International Monetary Fund (IMF). The IMF is not a neutral observer and rapidly adopted the open market ideologies that infused economic policies in the 1980s including the lowering of taxes and interest rates in order to expand a nation's economy (Stiglitz 2002). The IMF was mandated to provide a steady hand at the global level by ensuring each country was adopting the macroeconomic policies deemed necessary to sustain growth and to provide stabilising loans in times of an economic downturn (Stiglitz 2002).

Termed SAPs, these loans were contingent upon the restructuring of internal economies to eliminate what were deemed to be the barriers to growth. Specifically, this involved the deregulating of employment markets, privatisation of services and assets, and a declining role for government. Critics of SAPs highlighted the growing income inequalities that resulted from less protection for the poor and vulnerable in the form of social security. Within the health sectors of affected countries, budgets were cut, reducing the resources and capital available for investment in programmes such as HIV prevention and treatment and more basic services such as sanitation with enormous negative implications for health (Baum 2001; Eyles 2002; Taylor, Watts and Johnston 2002; Lurie, Hintzen and Lowe 2004). In Africa, SAPs were implemented during a time of economic hardship serving to increase levels of risky sexual behaviour while minimising funding available for prevention and education (Lurie et al. 2004). The health sector changes conveniently took place during a period when the World Health Organisation (WHO) was particularly weak and 'WHO officials were unable or unwilling to respond to the new international political economy structured around neoliberal approaches to economics, trade, and politics' (Brown et al. 2006).

SAPs were introduced with the clear goal of increasing economic growth but, as we will illustrate with the following case study, the results were mixed. Following a period of economic decline in the 1970s East Asian countries such as Thailand and Indonesia, sought the assistance of the IMF and World Bank to stabilise their declining economies. The economic climate of these emerging economies improved in the 1980s as they became favoured by Japan as a destination for considerable foreign direct investment (Glassmand and Carmody 2001). Internationally, East Asia was known as the 'Asian Miracle' its development strongly influenced by economic and cultural links with Japan. Rejecting the SAPs that had come to accompany loans, the governments of these countries continued to secure investment from Japan and rejected liberalisation policies by retaining strong connections with business, and considerable control over local development and finance (Glassman and Carmody 2001; Beeson and Islam 2010). In 1997, a dramatic decline in the fortunes of these countries took place which neoliberals attributed to the 'crony capitalism' that had allegedly been implemented in East Asia (Beeson and Islam 2010). The Philippines was the exception. Having experienced years of political conflict, ready investment from Japan was not forthcoming and the country was forced to continue its reliance on IMF loans. The loans were contingent on meeting the terms of the World Bank's structural adjustment programmes. The Philippines undertook radical restructuring to reshape the protectionist policies that influenced its economy and began the rapid deregulation and privatisation of government assets, such as oil refineries and water supplies (Bello 1997). Today, the Philippines leads East Asia as a model of an open economy and has experienced some economic growth. The country, however, is still burdened by extreme debt, corruption, rising unemployment, and has become vulnerable to a cycle of recession and recovery (Bello 1997; Lim and Bautisa 2002; Urbano, 2011). The policies that have opened up the economy of the Philippines have led to wide scale emigration for labour and increased dependence on foreign investment and trade, as Lim and Bautisa (2002, 43) conclude: 'Overall, therefore, the combination of boom-bust or recession-recovery cycles with external liberalisation has not improved labour productivities, employment generation and factor income distribution in the last two decades.'

Where the IMF went wrong, Stiglitz (2002) argues, was in failing to acknowledge the important role governments play in mediating and protecting their industries and populations in order for markets to become competitive on the world stage. Strong welfare systems, the subsidisation of establishing industries, and placing tariffs on imported goods that threaten domestic industry all play a key role in ensuring a country develops a strong economy *prior* to liberalisation (Cornia 2001; Stiglitz 2002). To make matters worse, many low-income countries opened up their markets but the promise of investment and trade went un realised as they were left competing on a global stage with developed countries that retained measures aimed at protecting their own low-tech industries (Stiglitz 2002; Cornia 2003). As a result has been that the goal of SAPs, to increase economic growth, appears to have been largely ineffectual; observations of the performance of loan recipients over a five year period indicated that: 'greater IMF loan participation has a direct negative effect on economic growth' (Barro and Lee 2005, 1247). Furthermore, unequal access to such loans is implied by observations that the loans have been more common and more sizeable amongst larger countries with stronger political and economic connections to the US/Western Europe and with greater numbers of IMF staff (Barro and Lee 2005).

SAPs have led to decades of debt among many of the least developed countries (LDCs). Having opened up their borders to trade, a country is effectively backed into a corner as any attempts to recover protectionist ideologies face the threat of action by the WTO for restricting free trade. This phenomenon is now being addressed as political pressure from the accumulation of disease and poverty led G8 countries to recognise, grudgingly at least, some of the limitations of their policies with the decision to write off African debt at their 2005 meeting in Gleneagles, Scotland. More recent development initiatives in response to SAPs have increasingly emphasised national control over economic development; albeit in the case of Africa's New Partnership for Africa's Development (NEPAD) the growing importance of national economic determinism is constrained by neo-liberal philosophies. Owuso (2003) suggests this adherence to neo-liberal doctrines is a pragmatic acknowledgement of a route necessary to ensure continued international support. Described as a strategic approach to engaging with globalisation, NEPAD aims to both reduce poverty and produce sustainable economic growth. Its ability to succeed where past development programmes have failed will, however, be keenly watched (Owuso 2003).

## Growing Inequalities?

Widespread criticism of SAPs, and indeed neoliberal policies at large, have centred on the accusation that the economic boons of liberalised economies have benefited the minority and served to increase disparities between the rich and poor both within and between countries (Cornia 2003). Proponents of economic globalisation argue that participation in the global economy allows countries to specialise in producing the goods that are most competitive on a global stage creating a more efficient global economic system that enables individuals to consume more thus prompting economic growth (see Murray 2006). Yet, even the role of economic liberalisation in sustaining economic growth is questioned by Wesibrot, Baker and Rosnick (2005) who found rates of economic growth to be lower amongst low-middle income countries in the quarter century beginning in 1980 than was experienced by countries in this income range in the decades of the 1960s and 1970s.

Globalisation has long been anticipated to bring about geographical inequalities by theorists such as Gertler (1997), Harvey (1989), and Wallerstein (1974). Wallerstein's World-Systems Theory portrays a web of competition amongst those who emerge as the economically and politically core states and those subordinate and peripheral states (which include less developed countries and emerging economies respectively). Wallerstein (1974) saw the world system to be as strong as the sum of its parts, that is, the strength of individual nations and regions is important to the maintenance of the global economy. Wallerstein (1974, 348) argued: 'capitalism has been able to flourish precisely because the world-economy has had within its bounds not one but a multiplicity of political systems.' Equally, the potential for individual groups and nations to pursue their own interests is a vulnerability of the system. At a national scale, special interest groups have steadfastly lobbied their governments to retain the protectionist measures and subsidies that support their viability both nationally and within the global market (Stiglitz 2002). The extent to which we are a part of a global economic system and vulnerable to its fluctuations was highlighted in 2008 when the escalation of food and oil prices and a global banking crisis originating in the United States contributed to an international recession. Coordinated government efforts to stabilise the global economy warned of the potential harm of protectionist responses that could undermine the global system (see the Declaration of the Summit on Financial Markets and the World Economy 2008; NZ Herald 2008). While the nation-state is supported as a political entity in today's globalised world, its economic presence is less welcome.

> The rush to carve out ever new and ever weaker and less resourceful "politically independent" territorial entities does not go against the grain of the globalising economic tendencies; political fragmentation is not a "spoke in the wheel" of the emergent "world society", bonded by the free circulation of information. On the contrary – there seems to be an intimate kinship, mutual conditioning and reciprocal reinforcement between the globalisation of all aspects of the economy and the renewed emphasis on the "territorial principal". (Bauman 1998, 67)

Harvey's (1989) understanding of the outcomes of globalisation builds on Wallerstein's identification of the unevenness of the global economy by stressing the importance of the spatial to economic growth. Harvey (1989, 294) asserts that increased competition is serving to heighten the importance of space as we see locations competing against each other to attract industry: 'small differences in what the space contains in the way of labour supplies, resources, infrastructures, and the like become of increased significance.' Harvey argues that economic determinism encourages the individualising of places at all economic scales as a means of attracting capital (Harvey 1989). Within this ideology *place* is seen as a fundamental tool in determining competitiveness for attracting investment (Harvey 1989). If we are to take Harvey's (1989) conceptualisation of global competition more bleakly then we see what Gertler (1997) describes as a 'whipsaw' effect in which governments compete against each other to attract industries. Rather than focusing on the development of a distinct identity, countries instead focus on providing more tax cuts and other economic incentives for investment and trade. This is what has been termed a *race to the bottom* as impoverished countries attempt to attract industry, including multinational corporations, through tax breaks, limited labour regulations and a lack of environmental protection. Gertler (1997, 48) expands: '... the multinational basis of these firms' organisation allows them to shelter profits from taxation and continue to pursue socially or environmentally regressive practices in more permissive jurisdictions.' The implications for health are evident in the uneven distribution of waste and unmoderated labour practices that emerge as outputs of production. But this view is highly contested by Drezner (2000) who argues that multinationals are, in fact, driven primarily by their market and make locational decisions based upon the potential for market growth and largely adopt responsible environmental and labour practices to avoid alienating the local market.

This leads us to ask what are the health implications of the policies of economic liberalisation? Where economic growth reduces levels of poverty we see positive implications for the health and wellbeing of individuals (Stiglitz 2002; Marmot 2005). With few exceptions (e.g., Feachem 2001), reviews of the health outcomes of economic liberalisation indicate that the health benefits associated with development are tied to increases in a country's wealth. Recent work by Clark (2011), for example, concluded that while increases in life expectancy across poor countries between 1995 and 2005 could be attributed to economic development. Yet, social and political context remains important, as Chowdury and Islam (2011) remind us, policies of economic liberalisation often fail to produce sufficient growth to improve the outcomes of a population. Indeed, macroeconomic policies appear to have undermined the Millennium Development Goals by failing to generate enough economic growth to significantly reduce poverty (Chowdury and Islam, 2011). The sustained increases to life expectancy anticipated amongst low-middle income countries as they experienced economic growth between 1980 and 2005 were not realised, instead, increases to life expectancy halted in part due to the rise of HIV/AIDS, itself exacerbated by processes of globalisation (Weisbrot, Baker and Rosnick 2005). A great deal more attention has been awarded to documenting changing levels of inequality within developed countries. These trends are attributed to policies of economic liberalisation as countries experiencing high levels of income inequality are more likely to encounter worse social and health outcomes (see Wilkinson and Pickett 2010). Indeed, in *A Brief History of Neoliberalism* (2005) Harvey draws on the work of Dumenil and Levy (2004) to suggest that the pursuit of neoliberalism has been a conscious undertaking to re-secure class privileges.

The analysis provided by such authors as Stiglitz (2002) and Weisbrot, Baker and Rosnick (2005, 24) does brings into question the benefits of economic liberalisation policies and recommends a more measured consideration to the adoption of such policies. This is in contrast to the unquestioned and widespread adoption of such measures in the 1980s. Particularly within developed countries, it is the dramatic increases in income inequality that has been pinpointed as a side effect of liberalisation and a major cause of heightening health disparities between the rich and poor. The relationship between income inequality and health is documented extensively elsewhere and is believed to be influenced by such factors as status and social capital that are also shaped by income (see Kaplan et al. 1996; Wilkinson, 1996; Kawachi and Kennedy 1997). A weakness of this literature, however, is its limited ability to make direct connections with the specific economic policies shaping health outcomes (Wilkinson 2000).

## The Liberalising of Health Systems

The liberalisation of health systems is one of a set of policies that falls under the broad umbrella of neoliberalism, a contentious term that, so far as health care is concerned, includes deregulation, privatisation, downloading of services to the voluntary sector, and a discourse centring on competition and efficiency (Beeson and Firth 1998). The process of health care liberalisation was instituted in many low-income countries as a necessary component of IMF loans and was adopted voluntarily in developed countries beginning in the 1980s under the rubric of *restructuring*. The 1980s and early 1990s was a period where many governments were facing growing external debt and increased urbanisation while health care budgets were ballooning due to accelerations in the availability of new drugs and health care technology, the response to these problems was, overwhelmingly, the liberalisation of health care systems (Kleinke 2001; Okanade and Murthy 2001).

Work by health geographers has examined the implementation and effects of neoliberal shifts in health policy, primarily within developed countries, and highlights the spatiality of health care rationalisation (Atkinson 1995; Hanlon and Rosenberg 1998; Cloutier-Fisher and Skinner 2006). Amongst the liberalisation strategies geographers have documented is the imposition of competition into the health care environment, for example, via the separation of the purchaser and provider of health services (Cloutier-Fisher and Joseph 2000; Moon and Brown 2000; Barnett and Barnett 2004), the introduction of user fees and the growing role of private health care providers in the health care landscape (Kearns and Joseph 1997; Barnett and Brown 2004; Cloutier-Fisher and Skinner 2006). Informal health services operating on a user pays basis dominate the health care landscape for the poor in many low-income countries (Mackintosh 2006, 396). Consistent with the conditions of SAPs, primary health care in many sub-Saharan African countries was privatised at a time of economic vulnerability, as Mackintosh (2006, 396) explains: '... the poorer the country, the more dominant out-of-pocket spending on health care is likely to be.' Health insurance is rare and the burden of disease, and thus cost, is felt most heavily by the poor (Mackintosh 2006). In low-income countries the privatisation of primary care and imposition of user charges has had direct implications for health service use. Lurie et al. (2004) report that a charge of US$2.15 for an STD clinic in Kenya led to a 35 to 60 per cent decline in use.

The liberalisation of health care may have created a legacy of undermining national health systems. International trade agreements, enforceable by the WTO, mean that opening up a health care system to commercial competition would likely lead to lofty fines should a nation choose to retreat from privatisation at a later date (Commission on the Future of Health Care in Canada 2002; Smith 2004). Fear that privatisation could lead to escalating health care costs and a two-tiered health care system – with the potential to undermine access to health services – prompted the former Liberal government of Canada to ensure the integrity of the public health system by directing the country's provinces to cease the establishment of private clinics (Commission on the Future of Health Care in Canada 2002). Spurring on this trend are the health care and pharmaceutical industries which are using free trade agreements and the media to challenge their right to a market share in countries where competition in health care is frowned upon.

There is abundant evidence of the positive population health impacts of the distribution of modern contraceptives, refrigeration techniques, and antibiotics (Yach and Bettcher 1998); yet the failure to provide equitable access to drugs to prevent malaria or antiretroviral medication for HIV/AIDS are some of society's most easily addressed public health failures. The pharmaceutical industry initially used the signing of the Agreement on Trade-Related Aspects of Intellectual Property Rights (TRIPS) as a tool to protect their market share and promote their products as global solutions (Findlay and Hoy 2000, 211). The TRIPS agreement ensures pharmaceutical companies gain 20 years of intellectual property rights over their product allowing them free reign over pricing decisions (Pollock and Price 2003). The agreement counters the practice adopted by many low-income countries of excluding drugs from patent protection in order to develop their domestic drug industries and to meet the needs of their populations (Barton 2004; Cohen-Kohler 2007). The arguments of the pharmaceutical industry that producing drugs on patent is necessary to fund further investment in drug research and development falls flat when we look at the data indicating that only a minimal amount of money invested – less than five per cent of global expenditure – addresses diseases most common in low-income countries (Pollock and Price 2003). The Doha round of the WTO negotiations secured the legal right for drugs created under patent to be distributed to low-income countries under strict licensing rules (Messerlin 2005); yet, even under these allowances the distribution of drugs has been delayed by years due to complicated approval processes (International Centre for Trade and Sustainable Development 2008).

**The Trade Agenda – Its Triumph and Failure?**

A new level of global trade interdependence was formalised in 1995 with the development of the World Trade Organisation (WTO), which became responsible for facilitating and policing international trade agreements. The WTO capitalises on the interdependence of relationships, captured by Wallerstein's World-Systems Theory (1974), in which he argues that most scales of society, such as the nation-state, fail to comprise a whole system because of their interdependence with the global economy (see also Cooke 2005). This argument was taken up by politicians and chief executives on the world stage who portrayed globalisation as an evolutionary process – and even a moral imperative – through arguments that 'there is no alternative' (Koechlin 2006; Sparke 2006). As a result, the WTO has the potential to enforce or override a government's policies to protect a country's population where such policies may influence the availability or consumption of goods.

The promise of trade liberalisation to create a global economy more efficient than the sum of its parts – with the potential to resolve world hunger – has faced a series of blows. In the name of efficiency, the production of food has become a transnational affair (Lang et al. 2001, 540) and certainly a case study in cultural diffusion. Of increasing pertinence to public health is the impact of food exports on domestic economies (Patel 2007). Many countries have experienced increases in the availability of imported foods (often processed and thus higher in fats and sugars) at lower costs than the healthier, locally produced alternative (Athukorala and Jayasuriya 2003; Patel 2007). Forming an effective public health response to the widespread availability of unhealthy foods is complicated by the enforcement of WTO rules. Governments have relative freedom to limit the availability and accessibility of alcohol and tobacco but resisting rules of free trade is difficult where the product is not deemed a drug. Western food, typically high in fat and refined sugar, is a prime contributing factor in increased rates of obesity and related diseases within low-income countries and amongst indigenous populations in developed countries, yet it is virtually impossible to prove under WTO rules that banning such products would positively impact the health of the population (Spiegel et al. 2004).

Rates of diabetes in the Pacific are amongst the highest in the world; the prevalence rate in Western Samoa is reported by the WHO as 23.1 per cent, with obesity affecting 57 per cent of the population (WHO, 2008). Samoa has long sought to gain membership into the WTO having first applied in 1998. In 2011, Samoa had its 'accession cleared' by the WTO contingent upon a series of policy changes including lifting a ban on the sale of turkey tails and related turkey tail products. The Pacific region represents a significant market – valued at US$30 million back in 2003 – for turkey tails and other low-grade meat exported from Western countries where the fatty products are rarely eaten (FAO 2003). The WTO press release states that a 24 month transition will see 'a domestic ban on the sale of turkey tails and turkey tail products would be in place and an import duty of 300% would apply to the imports' (WHO 2008, 2). This delay is to allow the country to develop and implement a national health promotion programme and, subsequently, domestic sales would be permitted and import duty reduced to 100% (WHO, 2008: 2). While this sounds reasonable Evans et al. (2001) found that dietary educational programmes in Tonga have had little effect on the population as the foods of poor nutritional value are available at lower prices than their healthier alternatives.

Were Samoa to argue that turkey tails represent a threat to their country's public health in a WTO forum the onus would be on the country to provide the evidence and shoulder the financial burden of arguing their case. The rulings of the WTO on health and environmental safety disputes have, to date, established a high benchmark for scientific evidence, as illustrated by France's ban on Asbestos being one of a few successfully upheld, suggesting the strategy may be beyond the means of a small, low-income nation (Kelly 2003, 139). By joining the WTO, the Samoan example illustrates the reduced capacity of developing nations to implement healthy public policy to reduce the impacts of non-communicable disease.

This chapter engages specifically with the literature on economic globalisation as a first step to destabilising the discourse of inevitability and helplessness that surrounds discussions of health and health care in a global economic system. Liberal economic ideology espouses distance between politics and the economy in much the same way as positivism sought to eliminate the researcher's presence in science. It is clear that health has systematically been positioned as subordinate to economic needs through global political will. Rather than being a matter of *no alternative*, the WTO has the power to facilitate or block access to cheap drugs (Findlay and Hoy 2000, 211), to protect government funded health care or allow multinational investment in national health systems (Barnett and Brown 2004), and to enforce public health legislation, or the rights of multinational corporations to sell products that play a role in harming the health of populations (Commission on the Future of Health Care in Canada 2002). While the impact of economic globalisation has not all been negative, and indeed has been positive in many cases, it is the positioning of economic activities at the expense of health that is cause for global health concern.

Arguably, the most obvious manifestation of the concern for global health and indirectly, the failure of the global economic system to address the growing gap in health inequalities between the 'North' and the 'south' in the 1990s came in 2000 when the United Nations adopted the Millennium Development Goals (MDGs). Of the eight MDGs: Goal 4 – Reduce Child Mortality; Goal 5 – Improve Maternal Health; and Goal 6 – Combat HIV/AIDS, Malaria and Other Diseases; speak directly to the ongoing need to improve global health. Indirectly, Goal 1 – Eradicate Extreme Poverty and Hunger might also be included in this list. Unfortunately, as the target date, 2015 quickly approaches, the likelihood of meeting these four goals and the targets which define them will only be partially met (http://www.un.org/millenniumgoals/index.shtml).

**Summary**

Neoliberal policies espoused by institutions such as the IMF have become ingrained in the global health and health care landscapes. At their most extreme, these policies were implemented as SAPs, which are now widely acknowledged for their negative impact on the health of populations (Lurie, Hintzen and Lowe 2004). SAPs have led to decades of debt amongst many low-income countries. Having opened up their borders they face the threat of action by the WTO for restricting free trade should they attempt to reinstate protectionist policies. More recent development initiatives emerging in response to SAPs have emphasised national control over economic development (see for example, Africa's New Partnership for Africa's Development), however, adherence to neoliberal philosophies appear to be well entrenched. Owuso (2003) suggests this adherence to neoliberal doctrines is a pragmatic acknowledgement of a route necessary to ensure continued international support.

In restricting the scope of this chapter to the impact of economic globalisation on health we omit a sizeable body of work addressing the social and cultural dimensions of health in an era of globalisation. Amongst this large body of work research is being carried out into such diverse themes as the implications of the rapid diffusion of medical knowledge and resources across the globe (Brown and Bell 2008), and urbanisation and health (Affonso, Andrews and Jeffs 2004). We have also not discussed the health and health care implications of the movement of people that are, so often, tied to global migration trends that see low-income countries consistently dispossessed of their most skilled workers, including health care professionals. While clearly connected to processes of globalisation (including the increased commercialisation of health care), we believe this issue is deserving of its own research agenda having been overlooked by all but a few geographers and gains attention in this volume (see Massey 2007).

For decades, lack of financial and political will on the part of nation states has been a barrier to addressing the basic public health needs of low-middle income countries. This era of economic globalisation is significant for exacerbating health inequalities (Wilkinson 1996), undermining health sector resources and shifting attitudes toward individual responsibility (Peacock, Bissell, and Owen 2014). The neoliberal call for the state to untangle itself from economic activities has been broadened by neoliberal interests into a widely accepted assertion that governmental influence over individual behaviour impinges on a fundamental right to economic choice (Labonte and Laverack 2008). Ultimately, health is bigger than the WTO. It is shaped by ideology, politics, the environment, and society as well as by economics. As Smith (2000, 3) says in his editorial: 'There absolutely have to be decent social, environmental, and work standards in the global economy, but only a fool would trust an organisation devoted to trade and managed by the profit-taking beneficiaries of that trade to implement them.' Inroads have been made within the WTO to address health-related trade, particularly in terms of the TRIPS agreements, but ultimately the role of the organisation is to support trade not to promote health.

We have witnessed resistance and criticism of public health initiatives aimed at reducing smoking, drinking, improving diet etc. associated with what is sometimes labelled a 'nanny state' (Johnston 2007; Macey 2009). Often unacknowledged are the WHOs normative powers to: 'propose conventions, agreements and regulations, and make recommendations with respect to international health matters and perform such duties as may be assigned thereby to the Organisations and are consistent with its objective' (Minelli 2008). Yet, the Framework Convention on Tobacco Control of the WHO has been the only effort to exercise these powers. The WHO instead largely constrains its authoritative powers to the development of technical guidelines and has been eclipsed by the World Bank as the largest funder of health activities (Beyer et al. 2000; Minelli 2008). Like the environmental movement, public health appears paralysed by the neoliberal ideologies that render any legislation that may constrain the pursuit of profits as a threat.

With 'The Collapse of Globalism', John Ralston Saul (2005) suggested that the end to globalisation is in sight. Saul (2004, 3) sees the fundamental weakness of the global model as resting on economic agreements in which human welfare: 'is treated as a secondary outcome of trade and competition and self-interest.' This is the principle on which the WTO has grown as its jurisdiction extends to treat anything involving commercial interest as being *'fundamentally* commercial' (Saul 2004, 12). We, however, are more cynical and draw attention to the ongoing globalisation of health care where we see the privatisation of health systems taking new forms, consumers finding new ways to transcend national borders in their pursuit of health care, and growing inequalities heightening disparities in health outcomes (Messerlin 2005; Connell 2006; Maarse 2006).

## References

[No Author]. 2008. *Declaration of the Summit on Financial Markets and the World Economy*. The White House, G20 Summit on the Financial Markets and World Economy. [Online]. Available at: http://www.whitehouse.gov/news/releases/2008/11/20081115–1.html [accessed: 18 November 2008].

Affonso, D.D., Andrews, G.J. and Jeffs, L. 2004. The Urban Geography of SARS: Paradoxes and dilemmas in Toronto's Health Care. *Nursing and Health Care Management and Policy*, 45(6), 56–78.

Athukorala, P. and Jayasuriya, S. 2003. Food Safety Issues, Trade and the WTO: A developing country perspective. *The World Economy*, 26(9), 1395–416.

Atkinson, S. 1995. Restructuring Health Care: Tracking the decentralization debate. *Progress in Human Geography*, 19, 486–503.

Barnett, J.R. and Barnett, P. 2004. Primary health care in New Zealand: Problems and policy approaches. *Social Policy Journal of New Zealand*, 21, 49–66.

Barnett, R. and Brown, L. 2008. 'Getting into Hospitals in a Big Way': The corporate transformation of hospital care in Australia. *Environment and Planning D: Society and Space*, 24, 283–10.

Barro, R.J. and Lee, J. 2005. IMF Programmes: Who is chosen and what are the effects? *Journal of Monetary Economics*, 52, 1245–69.

Barton, J.H. 2004. TRIPS and the Global Pharmaceutical Market. *Health Affairs*, 23(3), 146–54.

Baum, F. 2001. Health, Equity, Justice and Globalisation: Some lessons from the People's Health Assembly. *Journal of Epidemiology and Community Health*, 55, 613–16.

Bauman, Z. 1998. *Globalisation: The Human Consequences*. Cambridge: Polity Press.

Beeson, M. and Firth, A. 1998. Neoliberalism as a Political Rationality: Australian public policy since the 1980s. *Journal of Sociology*, 34, 215–31.

Beeson, M. and Islam, L. 2010. Neo-Liberalism and East Asia: Resisting the Washington Consensus. *Journal of Development Studies*, 41(2), 197–219.

Bello, W. 1997. *Unfinished Business: The Bretton Woods Twins and Southeast Asia*. [Online]. Available at: http://www.focusweb.org/publications/1997/Unfinished%20Business.htm [accessed: 21/1/2012].

Bergh, A. and Nilsson, T. 2010a. Do Liberalisation and Globalisation Increase Income Inequality? *European Journal of Political Economy*, 26(4), 488–505.

Bergh, A. and Nilsson, T. 2010b. Good for Living? On the relationship between globalisation and life expectancy. *World Development*, 38(9), 1191–203.

Berk, M. and Monheit, A. 2001. The Concentration of Health Care Expenditures, Revisited. *Health Affairs*, 20(2), 9–18.

Beyer, J., Preker, A. and Feachem, R. 2000. The Role of the World Bank in International Health: Renewed commitment and partnership. *Social Science & Medicine*, 50, 169–76.

Breisinger, C., Ecker, O. and Al-Riffai, P. 2011. Economics of the Arab Awakening: From revolution to transformation and food security. *IFPRI Policy Brief 18*. May 2011. [Online]. Available at: http://www.ifpri.org/sites/default/files/publications/bp018.pdf [accessed: 27 January 2011].

Brown, T. and Bell, M. 2008 Imperial or Postcolonial Governance? Dissecting the genealogy of a global public health strategy. *Social Science & Medicine*, 67, 1571–9.

Brown, T., Cuento, M. and Fee, E. 2006. The World Health Organization and the Transition from 'International' to 'Global' Public Health. *American Journal of Public Health*, 96(1), 62–75.

Chowdhury, A., Islam, I. 2011. Attaining the Millenium Development Goals: The role of macroeconomic policies. *International Journal of Social Economics*, 38(12), 930–52.

Clark, R. 2011. World Health Inequality: Convergence, divergence, and development. *Social Science & Medicine*, 72, 617–24.

Cloutier-Fisher, D. and Skinner, M. 2006. Levelling the playing field? Exploring the implications of managed competition for voluntary sector providers of long-term care in small town Ontario. *Health & Place*, 12(1), 97–109.

Cloutier-Fisher, D. and Joseph, A.E. 2000. Long-term care restructuring in rural Ontario: retrieving community service user and provider narratives. *Social Science and Medicine*, 50, 1037–45.

Cohen-Kohler, J. 2007. The Morally Uncomfortable Global Drug Gap. *Clinical Pharmacology and Therapeutics*. 82(5), 610–14

Commission on the Future of Health Care in Canada. 2002. *Issue/Survey Paper: Globalisation and Canada's Healthcare System*. Commission on the Future of Health Care in Canada: Ottawa, July 2002.

Connell, J. 2006. Medical Tourism: Sea, sun, sand, and … surgery. *Tourism Management*, 27, 1093–1100.

Cornia, G. 2001, Globalisation and Health: Results and options. *Bulletin of the World Health Organization*, 79(9), 834–41.

Cornia, G. 2003. The Impact of Liberalisation and Globalisation on Within-country Income Inequality. *CESifo Economic Studies*, 49(4), 581–616.

Cooke, P. 2005. Regionally Asymmetric Knowledge Capabilities and Open Innovation. Exploring 'Globalisation 2' – A new model of industry organisation. *Research Policy*, 34, 1128–49.

Drezner, D. 2000. Bottom Feeders. *Foreign Policy*. November/December, 64–70.

Evans, M., Sinclair, R.C., Fusimalohi, C. and Liava'a, V. 2001. Globalisation, Diet and Health: An example from Tonga. *Bulletin of the World Health Organization*, 79(9), 856–62.

Eyles, J. 2002. Global change and patterns of death and disease, in *Geographies of Global Change*, edited by R.J. Johnston. Oxford: Blackwell, 216–35.

Feachem, R. 2001. Globalisation is Good for your Health, Mostly. *BMJ*, 323, 504–6.

Findlay, A.M. and Hoy, C. 2000. Global Population Issues: Towards a geographical research agenda. *Applied Geography*, 20, 207–19.

Food and Agriculture Organization of the United Nations. 2007. *WTO Agreement on Agriculture: The Implementation Experience – Developing Country Case Studies*. Fiji. [Online]. Available at: http://www.fao.org/DOCREP/005/Y4632E/y4632e)d.htm#bm13.2 [accessed: 23 January 2011].

Gertler, M.S. 1997. Between the Global and the Local: The spatial limits to productive capital, in *Spaces of Globalisation: Reasserting the Power of the Local*, edited by K. Cox. New York: The Guilford Press, 45–63.

Glassman, J. and Carmody, P. 2001. Structural Adjustment in East and Southeast Asia: Lessons from Latin America. Geoforum, 32, 77–90.

Hanlon, N. and Rosenberg, M. 1998. Not-so-new public management and the denial of geography: Ontario health care reform in the 1990s. *Environment and Planning C: Government and Policy*, 16(5), 559–72.

Harvey, D. 1989. *The Condition of Postmodernity: An Enquiry into the Origins of Cultural Change*. Oxford: Blackwell.

Harvey, D. 2005. *A Brief History of Neoliberalism*. New York: Oxford.

International Centre for Trade and Sustainable Development. 2008. First Generic Drugs En Route to Africa under 5-Year-Old WTO Deal. *ICTSD*. [Online]. Available at: http://ictsd.net/i/news/bridgesweekly/29778/ [accessed: 19 January 2009].

Johnston, M. 2007. Principles Lash Out at 'Food Police' Diet. *NZ Herald*. [Online]. Available at: http://www.nzherald.co.nz/nz/news/article.cfm?c_id=1&objectid=10445049 [accessed: 28 July 2009].

Kaplan, G.A., Pamuk, E.R., Lynch, J.W. et al. 1996. Inequality in income and mortality in the United States: analysis of mortality and potential pathways. *British Medical Journal*, 312, 999–1003.

Kawachi, I. and Kennedy, B.P. 1997. The relationship of income inequality to mortality: does the choice of indicator matter? *Social Science and Medicine*, 45(7), 1121–7.

Kearns, R.A. and Joseph, A.E. 1997. Restructuring Health and Rural communities in New Zealand. *Progress in Human Geography*, 21(1), 18–32.

Kelly, P. 1999. The Geographies and Politics of Globalisation. *Progress in Human Geography*, 23(3), 379–400.

Kelly, T. 2003. The WTO, the Environment, and Health and Safety Standards. *The World Economy*, 26(2), 131–51.

Kleinke, J. 2001. The Price of Progress: Prescription costs in the health care market. *Health Affairs*, 20(5), 43–60.

Koechlin, T. 2006. Stiglitz and his Discontents. *Review of Political Economy*, 18(2), 253–64.

Labonte, R. and Laverack, G. 2008. *Health Promotion in Action: From Local to Global Empowerment*. Houndmills: Palgrave Macmillan.

Lang, T., Barling, D. and Caraher, M. 2001. Food, Social Policy and the Environment: Toward a New Model. *Social Policy & Administration*, 35(5), 538–58.

Lim, J. and Bautista, C. 2002. *External Liberalisation, Growth and Distribution in the Philippines*. External Liberalisation, Growth, Development and Social Policy Conference. Hanoi, Vietnam. 18–20 January 2002. [Online]. Available at: http://www.upd.edu.ph/~cba/bautista/docs/cepa-phil-0102.pdf [accessed: 29 January 2011].

Lurie, P., Hintzen, P. and Lowe, R.A. 2004. Socioeconomic Obstacles to HIV Prevention and Treatment in Developing Countries: The Roles of the International Mondetary Fund and the World Bank, in *HIV & AIDS in Africa: Beyond Epidemiology*, edited by E. Kalipeni, S. Craddock, J.R. Oppong and J. Ghosh. Malden, MA: Blackwell Publishing Ltd, 204–12.

Maarse, H. 2006. The Privatisation of Health Care in Europe: An eight-country analysis. *Journal of Health Politics, Policy and Law*, 31(5), 981–1014.

Macey, J. 2009. Abott Slams 'Trivial' Smoking Ban. *ABC*. [Online]. Available at: http://www.abc.net.au/news/stories/2009/07/02/2614334.htm [accessed: 28 July 2009].

Mackintosh, M. 2006. Commercialisation, Inequality and the Limits to Transition in Health Care: A polyanyian framework for policy analysis. *Journal of International Development*, 18, 393–406.

Marmot, M. 2005. Social Determinants of Health Inequalities. *The Lancet*, 365(9464), 1099–104.

Massey, D. 2007. *World City*. Oxford: Polity Press.

McMichael, T. 2001. *Human Frontiers, Environments and Disease: Past Patterns, Uncertain Futures*. Edinburgh: Cambridge University Press.

Messerlin, P., 2005. Trade, Drugs and Health Care. *The Lancet*, 365(9465), 1198–200.

Minelli, E. 2008. *World Health Organization: The mandate of a specialized agency of the United Nations.* Geneva Foundation for Medical Education and Research. [Online]. Available at: http://www.gfmer.ch/TMCAM/WHO_Minelli/Index.htm [accessed: 14 July 2009].

Moon, G. and Brown, T. 2000: Governmentality and the spatialized discourse of policy: the consolidation of the post-1989 NHS reforms'. *Transactions Of The Institute of British Geographers*, 25(1), 65–76.

Murray, W. 2006. *Geographies of Globalisation.* New York: Routledge.

NZ Herald. 2008. World's Leaders Waiting for Obama. *New Zealand Herald.* [Online] Available at: http://www.nzherald.co.nz/world/news/article.cfm?c_id=2&objectid=10544685 [accessed: 24 November 2008].

Okanade, A. and Muthy, V. 2001. Technology as a 'Major Driver' of Health Care Costs: A cointegration analysis of the Newhouse conjecture. *Journal of Health Economics*, 21(1), 147–59.

Owusu, F. 2003: Pragmatism and the Gradual Shift from Dependency to Neoliberalism: The World Bank, African Leaders, and Development Policy in Africa. *World Development*, 31(10), 1655–72.

Patel, R. 2007. *Stuffed and Starved: Markets, Power and the Hidden Battle for the World Food System.* Melbourne: Black Inc.

Peacock, M., Bissell, P. and Owen J. (2014). Dependency Denied: Health inequalities in the neo-liberal era. *Social Science & Medicine*, 118, 173–80.

Pollock, A.M. and Price, D. 2003. The Public health Implications of World Trade Negotiations on the General Agreement on Trade in Services and Public Services. *The Lancet*, 362, 1072–5.

Robertson, R. 1992. *Globalisation: Social Theory and Global Culture.* London: Sage.

Saul, J.R. 2004. The End of Globalism. *Australian Financial Review.* [Online]. Available at: http://afr.com/articles/2004/02/19/1077072774981.html [accessed: 14 August 2005].

Saul, J.R. 2005. *The Collapse of Globalism: And the Reinvention of the World.* Toronto: Viking Canada.

Smith, N. 2000. Guest Editorials: Global Seattle. *Environment and Planning D: Society and Space*, 18, 1–13.

Smith, R. 2004. Foreign Direct Investment and Trade in Health Services: A review of the literature. *Social Science & Medicine*, 59, 2313–23.

Sparke, M. 2006. Political Geography: Political geographies of globalisation (2) – governance. *Progress in Human Geography*, 30(3), 357–72.

Spiegel, J.M., Labonte, R. and Ostry, A.S. 2004. Understanding 'Globalisation' as a Determinant of Health Determinants: A Critical Perspective. *International Journal of Occupational and Environmental Health*, 10, 360–67.

Stiglitz, J. 2002. *Globalisation and its Discontents.* London: Penguin.

Swyngedouw, E. 1997. Neither Global nor Local: 'Glocalization' and the politics of scale, in *Spaces of Globalisation: Reasserting the power of the local*, edited by K.R. Cox. New York: The Guilford Press, 137–66.

Swyngedouw, E. 2000. Authoritarian Governance, Power, and the Politics of Rescaling, in *Environment and Planning D: Society and Space*, 18, 63–76.

Taylor, P.J., Watts, M.J. and Johnston, R.J. 2002. Geography/Globalisation, in *Geographies of Global Change: Remapping the World – Second Edition*, edited by R.J. Johnston, P.J. Taylor and M.J. Watts. Malden, MA: Blackwell Publishing, 1–18.

United Nations. 2012. *Millenium Development Goals.* [Online]. Available at: http://www. un.org/millenniumgoals/index.shtml [accessed: 10 March 2012].

Urbano, R. 2011. Global Justice and the Plight of Filipino Domestic Migrant Workers. *Journal of Asian and African Studies*, 47, 605–19.

Voisey, H. and O'Riordan, T. 2001. Globalization and localization, in *Globalism, Localism and Identity*, edited by T. O'Riordan. London: Earthscan, 25–42.

Wallerstein, I.M. 1974. *The Modern World-System: Capitalist Agriculture and the Origins of the European World-Economy in the Sixteenth Century.* New York: Academic Press.

Weisbrot, M., Baker, D. and Rosnick, D. 2005. *The Scorecard on Development: 25 Years of Diminished Progress.* Washington, DC: Centre for Economic and Policy Research, 1–24. [Online]. Available at: http://www.cepr.net/documents/publications/ development_2005_09.pdf [accessed 11 December 2008].

Wilkinson, R.G. 1996. *Unhealthy Societies. The Afflictions of Inequality.* London: Routledge.

Wilkinson, R.G. 2000. 'Deeper than Neoliberalism: A reply to David Coburn'. *Social Science & Medicine*, 51, 997–1000.

Wilkinson, R. and Pickett, K. 2010. *The Spirit Level: Why Equality Is Better For Everyone.* London: Penguin.

World Health Organization Regional Office for the Western Pacific. 2008. *'Health Situation and Trend'.* [Online]. Available at: http://www.wpro.who.int/countries/2008/sma/ health_situation.htm [accessed: 23 January 2012].

Yach, D. and Bettcher, D. 1998. The Globalisation of Public Health I: Threats and opportunities. *American Journal of Public Health*, 88(5), 735–8.

Yeung, H. 2002. The Limits to Globalisation Theory: A geographic perspective on global economic change. *Economic Geography*, 78(3), 285–305.

# Chapter 16
# Global Reach, Local Depth, and New Cartographies of Metropolitan Health

Ted Schrecker

## Introduction

*Global Reach* (Barnet and Müller 1974) was one of the first popular books on the growing significance of transnational corporations as global economic actors. Since it was published, production, consumption and finance have all been reorganised across national borders (Dicken 2007) to an extent that was difficult to imagine in the 1970s. One of the most familiar manifestations is the deindustrialisation of much of the high-income world, as manufacturing reconcentrated in jurisdictions where wages are low, employment relations are 'flexible', and working conditions are reminiscent of those that drove trade union organising and fuelled public outrage in high-income countries a century ago. Another manifestation is the emergence of global financial markets, which have shifted power from national governments to investors whose priorities constitute the collective wisdom of 'the markets' (see Schrecker 2009). In the aftermath of the financial crisis that swept across the world in 2008, it should no longer be controversial to assert that new forms of predatory capitalism can devastate the lives of people half a world away, as well as those living in the shadow of bank towers who had no role in the origins of the crisis and no control over its resolution.

This chapter is organised around three propositions. The first is that contemporary geographies of health and development must incorporate new understandings of how globalisation – 'transnational economic integration animated by the ideal of creating self-regulating global markets for goods, services, capital, technology, and skills' (Eyoh and Sandbrook 2003, 252) – has redrawn literal and metaphorical maps based on the terms on which individuals, households and communities are connected to or excluded from macro-scale economic and social processes. Nothing is new about dramatic juxtapositions of wealth and privation. However, as globalisation magnifies and transforms these juxtapositions, processes that operate on a global scale have penetrated deeply into the intra-national organisation of economies and societies: hence, local depth. William Robinson (2002b), a leader in the emerging transdiscipline of critical globalisation studies (Appelbaum and Robinson 2005), therefore argues that studies of development must transition 'from a territorial to a social cartography' and indeed that as a consequence of globalisation so that 'a sociology of *national* development is simply no longer a tenable undertaking' (Robinson 2002b, 1061). With specific reference to the urban or metropolitan context, urbanist and sociologist Saskia Sassen (2012a, 323–9) refers to the need for a new geography of centres and margins. Whatever the chosen terminology, development can no longer be understood as a process that occurs within and is tied to territorial boundaries; rather, it must be understood with reference to the map of 'new globalised circuits' of production and capital accumulation (Robinson 2002b, 1060).

The second, superficially paradoxical proposition is that globalisation has generated distributions of resources and driven the emergence of politics that are in some respects more territorial than ever, while reflecting new fault lines and axes of conflict that do not correspond to national borders, but rather exist within and often cross them. Thus, the chapter's focus is on processes of reterritorialisation that link the global and the local. A corollary of these first two propositions, taken together, is that Tobler's 'first law of geography: everything is related to everything else, but near things are more related than distant things' (Tobler 1970, 236), is simply wrong with respect to many manifestations of contemporary globalisation. This point is exemplified, and underscored, by anthropologist James Ferguson's (2005) description of the contemporary political economy of the oil industry in sub-Saharan Africa. He points out that capital, as invested by transnational oil companies, does not 'flow' but rather 'hops' from financial centres to extractive industry enclaves, 'neatly skipping over most of what lies in between' while interacting minimally with local economies, perhaps apart from offering the prospect of local employment in the privatised security forces that are becoming commonplace (Soares de Oliveira 2007, 114, 283).

The relevance of this analysis to health depends on a third proposition: disparities in health status reflect not only inequalities in access to health care, which is critically important and often increasingly problematic under conditions of globalisation (Lister and Labonté 2009), but also social determinants of health: the conditions of life and work that make it relatively easy for some individuals to lead long and healthy lives, and all but impossible for literally billions of others. The lives of those others are dominated by the quotidian constraints of poverty and inequality (Paluzzi and Farmer 2005), leading to widespread death and disability from causes that are routinely avoided or successfully treated elsewhere on the planet, sometimes elsewhere in the same neighbourhood for those who can pay the price of admission. Thus, an understanding of the 'causes of the causes' of disparities in health – a phrase that originated with Geoffrey Rose, but was popularised by Michael Marmot (2005) – must be sought 'upstream' (Marmot 2000) from what happens to and with people on a daily basis, based on the choices and processes that affect those experiences and exposures.

These insights are far from new, although underscored by recent demonstrations of the omnipresence of socioeconomic gradients in health within and across societies (Murray et al. 2006; Gwatkin et al. 2007; James et al. 2007). Rather, they represent a return to earlier, less biomedicalised understandings of population health exemplified by the work of the nineteenth century public health pioneer Rudolf Virchow. More recently, researchers like Link and Phelan (1995) have revisited the role of social conditions as fundamental causes of disease, as did the World Health Organisation's landmark Commission on Social Determinants of Health (2008), chaired by Marmot. Although the point cannot be explored further here, focusing on social determinants of health as a priority for research and policy must be understood as constituting both an epistemological and a political challenge to the 'biomedical individualism' (Baum et al. 2009, 1968–9) that dominates health research and practice.

## Focus on Metropolitan Areas: Selected Pathways of Influence

Anthropologist James Holston (1998, 37) eloquently observes: 'Cities are plugged into the globe of history like capacitors; they condense and conduct the currents of social time.'

Urbanisation is an almost universal demographic trend, with some of the poorest regions of the world urbanising the fastest (World Health Organisation and United Nations Human Settlements Programme 2010); it has been estimated that the number of people living in slums will rise from more than 850 million *circa* 2003 to 1.4 billion in 2020, in the absence of decisive policy intervention (Garau, Sclar, and Carolini 2005). 'Slum' is an admittedly problematic category, but on almost any definition living within a settlement defined as a slum does not offer abundant opportunities for healthy living. The future of population health worldwide will therefore increasingly be determined by what happens within metropolitan areas (a term I prefer to cities because it captures the connections among cities and their surrounding suburbs, exurbs and edge cities) and to their inhabitants. The metropolitan frame of reference provides striking concrete illustrations of how globalisation generates new social cartographies that territorialise differences in exposure and vulnerability – mid-level categories borrowed from Diderichsen, Evans and Whitehead (2001) – and new challenges to the political possibilities for eliminating those disparities.

Urban health as a subfield of research and practice now supports at least one major journal and an international scientific society, and in 2009–2010 was the topic of an international research network funded by the Rockefeller Foundation, but researchers who identify themselves with this subfield generally neglect such connections. In the discussion that follows, I present a relatively mechanistic view of how globalisation has transformed metropolitan areas and opportunities to lead healthy lives within them. While aware of the case-specific complexity that may be overlooked by this approach, critically including the extent to which global influences are mediated by national political institutions, I have adopted it in the interests of analytical clarity, and because focusing on the commonalities among social processes occurring in disparate contexts is essential to understanding macro-micro linkages for explanatory purposes, despite the unavoidable loss of contextual detail (for a contrary view, see Ong 2011). Much of the evidence to which I refer to is drawn from the high-income world. This is because health geography, and studies in population health more generally, must acknowledge that development (and the reversal of development) are processes that unfold not only at a safe territorial distance from bourgeois academia, but also within what older bodies of development studies research would characterise as the core or the imperial centre.

*Deindustrialisation and 'Labour Arbitrage'*

As noted at the start of the chapter, perhaps the most familiar manifestation of globalisation is the reorganisation of manufacturing, and an expanding range of service industries, across multiple national boundaries. This process was already under way by the late 1970s (Fröbel, Heinrichs and Kreye 1980) and has since accelerated with the emergence of China as the workshop of the world (Fallows 2007; Duhigg and Barboza 2012; Duhigg and Bradsher 2012) and the integration of not only China but also India and the economies of the former Soviet bloc into the global labour market (Freeman 2007). A fundamental dynamic here was described in a trade journal in 2002 as labour arbitrage: 'the ability to pay one labour pool less than another labour pool for accomplishing the same work, typically by substituting labour in one geography for labour in a different locale' (Ong 2006, 161). The locales in question may be elsewhere in the same country (Gringeri 1994), or half a world away. Thus, the incomes of the working class in a particular location may have more to do with the price of labour in (say) China or India than closer to home, with even the threat to relocate production leading to substantial pressure for the 'recommodification' of labour

(Standing 2007; see also Choi 2002) – one illustration, among many, of the limitations of Tobler's approach.

In high-income countries such as the United States and more recently Canada, deindustrialisation involved catastrophic job losses in older industrial cities such as Chicago, Philadelphia, Detroit, Gary (Indiana) and Hamilton (Ontario) (Abu-Lughod 1999, 323–44; Hodos 2002, 365; Savitch 2003, 592; DeLuca, Buist and Johnston 2012). By the end of the century and despite downtown 'revivals', deindustrialisation had transformed many metropolitan landscapes: 30,000 housing units were vacant or abandoned in Philadelphia (Jacobs 2000) and 40,000 housing units in Baltimore (Levine 2000, 138), with 15,000 recently demolished or slated for demolition (Rozhon 1999). Wilgoren (2002) observed that 28,000 abandoned housing units had been demolished over the previous decade in Detroit, the former Motor City. Furthermore, between 1950 and 2000 'the city of Detroit lost nearly 1 million residents, 165,000 industrial jobs, and 147,000 housing units. The city is now left with an average annual income that is half that of its surrounding counties, 37,000 vacant housing units, and well over 66,000 vacant lots' (Hall 2010, 7; see also McGreal 2010; Seelye 2011).

Drastic losses of relatively well-paid manufacturing jobs accessible to those with limited formal credentials occurred in most high-income countries (Nickell and Bell 1995; Wood 1998), but urban deindustrialisation and informalisation have often followed the integration of low- and middle-income countries (LMICs) into the global economy. For example in Ghana, a decade after the start of a structural adjustment programme in 1983, impressive economic growth rates had been accompanied by a decline in overall formal sector employment of more than 50 per cent (Songsore 2008); in Accra, '[p]overty and marginality within the city [had] become structural with a growing number of youth who have nothing to offer to the globalising and liberalised economy' (Songsore and McGranahan 2007, 136). Unemployment in Mumbai 'more than doubled' between 1981 and 1996 (Patel 2004, 335), while informal employment and self-employment increased substantially. In São Paulo and Rio de Janeiro, hundreds of thousands of Brazilian manufacturing jobs disappeared between 1985 and 2003, as import-substitution industrialisation was abandoned in favor of opening to international markets, which resulted in casual or precarious labour became the norm (Perlman 2005, 21; Buechler 2006). As South Africa's newly democratised government effectively abandoned employment creation as a policy objective while accelerating neoliberalisation, informal employment increased as a percentage of total employment in Johannesburg from 9.6 per cent to 16 per cent in just three years (1996–1999); in 2001 the city's official unemployment rate was 37 per cent (Mabin 2007). Nationally, the official unemployment rate in 2010 was 24 per cent, and 42 per cent among people under 30 (National Treasury Department 2011). Not surprisingly, of 109 cities selected for inclusion in a UN Habitat study, eight South African cities were found to have the highest Gini coefficients (United Nations 2008, 72–3).

Sassen's early work (Sassen 1991, Sassen 2001) described such polarised labour markets and income distributions in so-called world cities, such as New York, London and Tokyo, that host the command and control centres of the world economy. In these cities the concentration of highly paid individuals working in so-called producer services generates a parallel demand for legions of low-wage service workers who clean the buildings, drive the taxis, cook and deliver the restaurant meals, and often provide child care (see e.g. Abu-Lughod 1999, 285–320, Herod and Aguilar 2006, Moody 2007, 245–54, 286–90, Sassen 2012a, 241–72); exploiting these workers offers new opportunities to accumulate fortunes

(Winerip 1998). The importance of the new geography of centres and margins referred to by Sassen is underscored by research findings like those from Judith Hellman's interview-based study of undocumented immigrants living in New York City which described a 'basement shared by eighteen single men, an unheated garage that is home to two Mexican families, an abandoned tractor trailer ... and an abandoned tugboat and barge, both vessels half in and half out of the water, and each providing housing to another two or three men' (Hellman 2008, 159) – within sight of the glittering towers of a world financial centre.

An important contextual element is the fact that segments of the United States economy as diverse as landscaping and garment manufacturing in southern California, meatpacking in the Midwest, and poultry processing in the southeast rely on the work of several million undocumented immigrants (Delgado Wise and Covarrubias 2008; Shavers 2009) whose marginal legal status renders them a highly exploitable reserve army of labour, with few or no legal protections (Compa 2005; Fussell 2011; Quesada, Hart and Bourgois 2011; Sarabia 2011). In the United States as elsewhere, such precarious and hazardous work often represents the end point of global 'survival circuits' (Sassen 2002) that begin in LMICs where livelihoods have been destroyed – for example, in Mexico by liberalisation of agricultural trade with the United States and in Central America by the devastating US-supported proxy wars at the end of the Cold War era. Crucially, the new geographies (Sassen, 2002) or new cartographies (Robinson, 2002a) are not restricted to the high-income world (Robinson 2002a; Gugler 2004; Lemanski 2007), *or* to cities at or near the top of conventional hierarchies of global or world cities. Indeed, some of the most dramatic negative effects of global reorganisation of labour markets affect smaller metropolitan areas or districts within them that are closely connected to global flows without in any way controlling them.

## Gentrification and Real Estate Capitalism

In contrast to the North American instances of deindustrialisation and abandonment cited earlier in the chapter, which have their counterparts in some LMIC settings like the cities of South Africa, globalisation often raises the stakes, and the price, in economic contests for urban space; downtowns, at least some parts of them, may be or become highly desirable locations. Gentrification has become familiar to metropolitan residents in much of the high-income world, along with conflicts on the ground that often result as the working class is displaced from affordable housing and established communities (see for example, Hartman and Carnochan 2002; Hackworth 2007, 77–149). The term was originally coined to describe the 'rehabilitation' of residential areas by middle-class consumers, with limited attention to the macro-scale economic and political context, but by 1991 Sassen (in the first edition of *The Global City*) had formulated a more expansive and analytically sophisticated understanding:

> [B]y the early 1980s, it was becoming evident that residential rehabilitation was only one facet of a far broader process linked to the profound transformation in advanced capitalism: the shift to services and the associated transformation of the class structure and the shift toward the privatisation of consumption and service provision. Gentrification emerged as a visible spatial component of the transformation. It was evident in the redevelopment of waterfronts, the rise of hotel and convention complexes in central cities, large-scale luxury office and residential developments, and fashionable, high-priced shopping districts. (Sassen 1991, 255, see also Slater 2011)

Gentrification also reflects a decline in the importance of cities as sites for production (at least, manufacturing production) and an expansion in their role as sites for consumption (Sassen and Roost 1999), with urban environments, or at least tourism-oriented enclaves, themselves becoming marketed commodities (Fainstein and Judd 1999; Eisinger 2000; Murray 2002; Silk 2007). In addition to obvious issues of affordability, aspects of the built environment may reflect and contribute to the exclusionary aspects of this urban redesign, notably by replacing public spaces with enclosed ones to which access can be controlled by owners and managers (Davis 1990, 221–63; Boddy 1992; Newman 2002; Kohn 2004).

Gentrification, in the broad sense defined by Sassen, has now emerged in a number of LMIC cities, to the point where the largest-scale variants are referred to by one author as 'megagentrification' (Lees 2012). Harris (2008) has pointed out both the parallels between gentrification in London and Mumbai and its more brutal dimensions in the latter city, where it has been described in terms of 'class cleansing' (Whitehead and More 2007; see also Appadurai 2000) – an issue revisited in the next section of the chapter. This superficial introduction suffices as background to the question: What connects contests over urban space with globalisation? At least two distinct, although interdependent, pathways can be identified.

First, as production and finance are reorganised across national borders, economic inequality within those borders – in particular the concentration of wealth – tends to increase. Although there are exceptions to this rule, a remarkable 2003 study of *The Challenge of Slums*, incorporating findings from 29 city case studies, describes the spatial consequences succinctly: '[T]he prime resources of the city are increasingly appropriated by the affluent. And globalisation is inflationary as the new rich are able to pay more for a range of key goods, especially land' (United Nations 2003, 52). For example, after economic liberalisation and a dramatic increase in foreign direct investment, in the mid-1990s portions of Mumbai's central business district temporarily became 'the most expensive in the world'; residential real estate prices, and therefore opportunities for profit, likewise increased (Grant and Nijman 2004; see also Nijman 2000) – in a city where it was estimated contemporaneously that '[m]ore than half' of the population live 'in slums and on pavements or under bridges and near railway tracks' (Patel 2007, 76). In Accra, Grant (2009) describes a pattern in which, even as unemployment was growing, new residential developments proliferated that were unaffordable for the overwhelming majority of the city's residents but affordable for some entrepreneurial Ghanaians living abroad, and for domestic elites seeking rental income and capital appreciation. A new middle class whose fortunes are closely tied to South Africa's integration into the global marketplace has also driven the gentrification of portions of central Cape Town (Visser and Kotze 2008).

This might be called the demand-driven link between gentrification (broadly defined, as by Sassen) and globalisation. The second, supply-driven link is the emergence of real estate investment and provision of associated infrastructure and financing as a major theatre of capital accumulation for both domestic and transnational investors outside the high-income world, where it had earlier become well established (see e.g. Moody 2007 on New York City). In cities as diverse as Accra, Beirut, Santiago, Johannesburg and Bangalore, to name just a few, the prospect of real estate profits has attracted capital to residential and commercial projects oriented toward corporate clients and rich individuals (Makdisi 1997; Murray 2008, 191–209; Grant and Yang 2009, 18–89; López-Morales 2010; Goldman 2011). Although these may involve new construction at relatively distant suburban sites, as in the case of Johannesburg's Sandton district, often substantial displacement (by various means) of existing populations is required (see Murray 2008, 202–24, on Johannesburg). The Bangalore case is especially interesting: although Bangalore is widely identified as the center of India's information technology (IT) industry, Goldman (2011) shows that high-end real estate developments and construction of the requisite subsidised airports and highways have become more profitable, for major foreign investors and for IT firms. Major entertainment and sporting mega-events such as the Olympic games and Grand Prix auto races are also highly profitable (Lefebvre and Roult 2011; Scherer 2011), and – along with certain kinds of infrastructure and amenities associated with such events or generically oriented to the needs of the rich – are viewed, at least for public consumption and to justify public subsidy, as economically valuable because they brand a city as a world-class location suitable for foreign investment as well as directly attracting wealthy visitors.

This said, gentrification must be understood 'not solely as a 'top-down' project driven by globalisation's domestic winners and key players in the globalised property market, but also as a 'bottom-up' project resulting from the needs of local capitalists to find a new way of realising profits after the collapse of the urban economy based on traditional industrial production' (Rousseau 2012, 50). The critical point is that gentrification reterritorialises class conflict locally (Slater 2011) by excluding those who lack the price of admission, within a cost structure now defined at least partly by global distributions of resources and investment strategies: 'speculative urbanism', Bangalore-style (Goldman 2011) has little or nothing to offer the working class. Half a world away, a similar point can be made about the so-called revitalisation of deindustrialised cities like Baltimore (Levine 2000) and Detroit (McCarthy 1997; McCarthy 2002), where as long ago as 1981 it was observed that 'the family of the unemployed auto worker is not saved by employing one daughter as a file clerk at the Renaissance Center or one son as a security guard at Riverfront West', two early and heavily subsidised instances of Detroit's efforts to reinvent itself as a site of consumption (Luria and Russell 1981, 5).

## The Role of the State

The state has been a key protagonist in the developments I have described. Governments have responded to external pressures for policy convergence on a model that has been described as the competition state, prioritising 'promotion of economic activities, whether at home or abroad, which will make firms and sectors located within the territory of the state competitive in international markets' (Cerny 2000, 136). Competition state policies involve not only the retreat from certain kinds of state functions, for instance through privatisation and retrenchment of social provision, but also expansion of state intervention in other areas, such as the 'discipline of labour' that Amsden (1990, 18) identified as a necessary condition for late industrialisation and a variety of more or less coercive workfare policies in high-income countries (Wacquant 2009, 76–109). Governments at various levels ranging from local to national have also initiated and aggressively pursued policies that accelerate and entrench global influences on intra-national social *and* territorial cartographies in other ways, for instance through support of gentrification. Economic (class) interests are still implicated, and many such policies reflect complex alliances between state elites and economic actors both domestic and international. At the same time, these alliances provide only a partial explanation of public policies that have affected social determinants of health in the metropolis. Some are best characterised as 'tectonic policies' (Young 1991) designed to reconfigure the political terrain in ways both metaphorical and literal, as part of a larger, transnational class project (Harvey 2006). This discussion demonstrates the value of Peck and Tickell's (2002)'s distinct yet interdependent categories of 'roll-out' and 'roll-back neoliberalism' (see also Ward and England 2007); only a few illustrations can be offered here.

In the high-income world, some of the most striking illustrations come from the United States. Starting in the mid-1970s with the fiscal crisis of New York City, the federal government began to retreat from its earlier support for cities (Moody 2007). The retreat gathered speed under the right-wing administrations of Presidents Reagan and Bush I (Caraley 1992; Caraley 1996; Judd 1999), magnified the effects of deindustrialisation, and intensified the competition among jurisdictions for investment and local tax revenue that is intrinsic to how US urban government and services are financed (Weir 1994; Savitch 2003, 594). Equally important were long standing 'stealth urban policies' (Dreier, Mollenkopf and Swanstrom 2005, 114–23) including federal subsidies for interstate highway construction that facilitated commuting from the suburbs and often bisected established urban neighbourhoods, the deductibility of mortgage interest for income tax purposes, and federal mortgage subsidy programmes that favoured the suburbs. Such policies both initiated and reinforced a shift of political gravity to the suburbs, creating a powerful positive feedback loop. Reagan-era patterns of defence procurement decisively shifted industrial activity toward the south and west and away from the traditional industrial heartland (Markusen, Hall, Campbell and Deitrick 1991; see also Kirby 1992), creating 'new cities, life-styles, and real-estate markets that [were] highly praised by their partisans' (Markusen et al. 1991, 245). The inter-regional shift of economic activity, including major foreign direct investments, to the US south was facilitated by the strongly anti-union stance of many state and local governments in the region (Maunula 2005), and by the subsidies and tax holidays they offered in order to attract investment (Guthrie-Shimizu 2005). It can also be argued that welfare 'reforms' signed into law by President Clinton in 1996 (Wacquant 2009, 76–109) were likewise a stealth urban policy, given their disproportionate impact on inner cities and inner suburbs with high proportions of poor residents (Wolch 1998; Accordino 1998; Peck and Tickell 2002).

Poor neighbourhoods in New York City suffered large-scale housing destruction and population displacement as a consequence of overt local government policies of 'benign neglect and planned shrinkage' in municipal service provision, the initiation of which in the 1970s predated the fiscal crisis (Wallace and Wallace 1998, 21–77). Even when local opposition was strong, many cities in the United States and Canada promoted gentrification (packaged using rubrics like revitalisation) as an economic development strategy, often with public subsidies that were justified by invoking increased local employment and an expanded property tax base (McCarthy 1997; Judd 1999; Levine 2000; Eisinger 2000). Whether or not these benefits materialised, the development strategies tended to be highly profitable for property developers and financial institutions, while changing the character and class composition of affected neighbourhoods (see e.g. Hartman and Carnochan 2002 on San Francisco). British examples show a similar pattern of state initiative. In addition to selling off council houses, creating 'new stakeholders in private property' (Young 1991, 138), the Thatcher government created the London Docklands Development Corporation (LDDC) to bypass a local council whose 'priorities were to preserve traditional land uses and activities employing the existing working-class population; LDDC, however, saw the future in terms of an international economy and was determined to attract jobs in activities serving this and to build homes for the predominantly middle-class people who would work in it' (Buck, Gordon, Hall, Harloe and Kleinman 2002, 64; see also Smith 1989). LDDC spent £3.9 billion, at 1998 currency values, in the process (Deas and Ward 1999, 122); many 'middle-class people' as well as property developers and their financiers no doubt made fortunes in ensuing property booms.

More dramatic instances of both roll-back and roll-out neoliberalism are observable in many LMIC metropolitan areas, and the canvass provided here is especially selective and incomplete. The *Challenge of Slums* study, for which 23 of the case studies were from LMICs, concluded that '[t]he main single cause of increases in poverty and inequality during the 1980s and 1990s was the retreat of the state' from a variety of redistributive policies (United Nations 2003, 43). That retreat can often be traced to the debt crises and subsequent structural adjustment programmes of the same period (United Nations 2003, 45–6; Davis 2006, 152–68), thus illustrating with special clarity the long-distance connections between global and local processes as well as showing the need to consider the spatial dimensions of policies that at first glance are spatially neutral in their incidence and impact.

Such policies are often adopted proactively, rather than reactively. For example, in South Africa post-1994, both local and national governments embraced strategies of neoliberalisation (Ward and England 2007), bolstered by the legitimacy associated with institutions of democracy, that systematically marketwise metropolitan and national economies, with indisputably destructive consequences (see Bond 2006, Mabin 2007, McDonald 2008, among many other sources). In explaining such policies, the fact that they enabled political elites with strong connections to the governing African National Congress to accumulate world-scale fortunes cannot be ignored (Smith 2012). In India, another formally democratic country undergoing internal transformations as a result of rapid state-initiated integration into the global economy, various governments have been clearing out urban shantytowns in favour of higher-value residences, commercial space and technoparks (Appadurai 2000; Banerjee-Guha 2009; Bhan 2009), with an official of one state government quoted as saying that: 'With the slum demolitions [in Mumbai], we showed political courage for the first time and sent a strong signal that you cannot expect free space in this city anymore' (Lakshmi 2005). Hosting of mega-events like the FIFA World Cup (South Africa, 2010, Brazil 2014); the Commonwealth Games (Delhi 2010), and of course the Olympic games (Beijing 2008, Rio de Janeiro 2016) has routinely been associated with large-scale forced evictions (Centre on Housing Rights and Evictions 2007; Fowler 2008; Burke 2010; Broudehoux 2013); whether or not they involve mega-events, such evictions in the service of 'development' are sufficiently widespread that they have been recognised as a significant human rights problem by United Nations observers (Kothari 2007). A related issue of particular spatial significance involves infrastructure investment priorities that favour car-owning minorities or wealthy business travelers, tourists and commuters, literally casting certain kinds of social exclusion and segregation in concrete (Leaf 1996; Alcantara de Vasconcellos 2005; Pucher, Korattyswaropam, Mittal and Ittyerah 2005; Bond 2006, 116; Rodgers 2007; Goldman 2011, 570). Globalisation drives those priorities directly through new accumulations of wealth, as in the case of contests over urban land, and indirectly through the perceived need to provide infrastructure appropriate for transnational business and tourism.

## Making Connections: Globalisation, Post-Crisis Cartographies, and Health

The 2008 financial crisis revealed new dimensions of globalisation's 'disequalising' potential (Birdsall 2006). Spreading from the United States, the crisis quickly compounded the effects on people in low-income countries of a spike in food prices (Hossain and McGregor 2011; Samuels et al. 2011) that was driven in part by the financialisation of transnational agricommodity markets (United Nations 2009, 53–79). At the epicentre an estimated 14 million US households, a substantial proportion consisting of tenants living in mortgaged properties, faced dispossession by foreclosure (Sassen 2011).

The crisis must be recognised as a consequence, perhaps an inevitable one, of the combination of domestic financial deregulation (especially in the US); a global financial marketplace that enabled and rewarded the packaging (securitisation) and selling on of high-risk mortgages as just one more addition to the dizzying array of financial instruments already on offer; and the ability of that global marketplace to transmit shocks around the world, revealing what the Bank of England (2008, 9) described with masterful understatement as 'underappreciated, but potent, interconnections between firms in the global financial system'. Once transmitted, those shocks fed back into local and national economies through multiple channels including the contraction of lending; the cost of bailouts and stimulus measures needed to avoid an even more serious crisis; subsequent public sector austerity measures that were defended with reference to the need for deficit reduction; and drastic increases in unemployment. The high-risk mortgage racket itself has been characterised as 'an efficient mechanism for getting at the savings of households ... that moves faster than extracting profit from lowering wages' (Sassen 2009, 412), suggesting an important homology between this form of exploitation and established patterns of labour arbitrage and offshoring.

The spatial consequences may also turn out to be comparable. Sassen (2012b, 78) compares the neighbourhood-scale impacts of foreclosures with what happened in the city of Detroit as a result of deindustrialisation but so far, and inevitably given the time frame, only limited evidence exists (in particular from outside the US) on the intra-metropolitan impacts of the crisis and its aftermath. In the US, relatively low-income and minority households and neighbourhoods were a major target market for such mortgages, and were disproportionately likely to face foreclosure in the recession that followed the crisis (Wyly et al. 2009; Darden and Wyly 2010). In at least one case, the San Francisco-Oakland metropolitan area, the effect was to increase already dramatic intra-metropolitan differences in property values, and therefore household wealth (Schafran 2012). Yet while some neighbourhoods were being eviscerated by foreclosures and recession-driven budget cuts to local services, in 2010 there were *more* 'high net worth individuals' with financial assets of more than $1 million in nine out of the 10 largest US metropolitan areas than in 2007; the exception was Detroit, which saw only a slight decline (Capgemini 2011). As per Sassen's comparison, it is certainly not implausible to anticipate deepening intra-metropolitan inequality and segregation, compounded by the effects of post-crisis austerity measures worldwide, including in many LMICs (Ortiz, Chai and Cummins 2011).

Multidisciplinary narratives that connect global processes, intra-metropolitan social cartographies and health disparities remain scarce. This is partly because of the difficulty in tracing the relevant pathways to health outcomes over time, in a way that meets epidemiological standards of proof. As Pfeiffer and Chapman (2010) have suggested in reviewing the evidence on structural adjustment programmes and health, the problem in such cases has to do with the choice of a standard of proof that is inappropriately difficult to meet, rather than with the overall strength of evidence. A more basic problem is conceptual, and involves a misguided assumption about the spatial proximity of causes and exposures (broadly defined). Thus, Schulz and Northridge (2004) argue that 'within areas of greater concentrations of wealth live individuals and groups with the social and economic resources to influence political decisions; this is less likely to be the case in areas of greater concentrations of poverty' (457).

No doubt this is true, and such insights are important to understanding power relations as they operate on a local or metropolitan level. At the same time, they radically understate the range of pathways that link macro-scale processes with local differences in exposure and vulnerability. Diderichsen, Evans and Whitehead (2001) correctly insisted on the need for policy analysis to connect such differences with 'those central engines in society that generate and distribute power, wealth and risks' (Diderichsen, Evans and Whitehead 2001, 16). Those engines may in fact be driven by choices made or dynamics set in motion half a world away, or in situations where spatial proximity is irrelevant. Closings of manufacturing plants and changes in the location of outsourced contract production are routinely driven by the priorities of far-away investors and the corporate managers who must meet their demands for returns on investment; foreclosures have a lot to do with where the target households live, but nothing at all to do with where the financial racketeers live or where they sold their 'toxic' asset-backed securities.

A far more productive approach to research on connections among globalisation, new cartographies and health outcomes is suggested, perhaps unintentionally, by an article on health and urban planning in which the authors noted that '[r]ich and poor people live in very different epidemiological worlds, even within the same city' (Rydin et al. 2012, 2079). The authors did not further theorise the concept of an epidemiological world at the core of this statement, yet the concept offers a valuable starting point for examining the full range of influences on health in metropolitan areas – and, indeed, everywhere. Explanations of how and why epidemiological worlds differ are, in fact, best advanced on the basis of research in multiple disciplines in addition to epidemiology, as suggested (for example) by the work of Pfeiffer and Chapman. In order to be comprehensive they must, in contrast to the framework described by Schulz and Northridge, explicitly consider influences that originate in locations far from where their consequences are manifested. Multidisciplinary research organised around the epidemiological world concept will inevitably foreground the fact that some people have *far less control* than others over their epidemiological worlds, and direct attention to why that is the case. The effect will be to create opportunities for explicit recognition of how health is affected by 'the inequitable distribution of power, money, and resources' that was the focus of one of the three policy directions recommended by the Commission on Social Determinants of Health; to trace the origins of such inequities back to the 'central engines' referred to by Diderichsen and colleagues; and ultimately to transform research on place and health into an enterprise more relevant to the moral imperative of reducing health inequities.

## Acknowledgements

Research was partially supported by Canadian Institutes of Health Research grant no. 80070. Portions of the argument were presented to a pre-conference workshop on global health justice at the annual meeting of the International Studies Association, Montréal, March 2011. Very special thanks to Theresa Grant for an intellectual jump-start at a crucial point in completion of the chapter, and to K.S. Mohindra for ongoing exchanges.

## References

Abu-Lughod, J. 1999. *New York, Chicago, Los Angeles: America's Global Cities.* Minneapolis: University of Minnesota Press.

Accordino, J. 1998. The Consequences of Welfare Reform for Central City Economies. *Journal of the American Planning Association*, 64, 11–15.

Alcantara de Vasconcellos, E. 2005. Urban change, mobility and transport in São Paulo: three decades, three cities. *Transport Policy*, 12, 91–104.

Amsden, A. 1990. Third World Industrialization: 'Global Fordism' or a New Model. *New Left Review*, no. 182, 5–31.

Appadurai, A. 2000. Spectral Housing and Urban Cleansing: Notes on Millennial Mumbai. *Public Culture*, 12, 627–51.

Appelbaum, R.P. and Robinson, W.I., eds 2005. *Critical Globalisation Studies.* London: Routledge.

Banerjee-Guha, S. 2009. Neoliberalising the 'Urban': New Geographies of Power and Injustice in Indian Cities. *Economic and Political Weekly*, 44(22), 95–107.

Bank of England 2008. *Financial Stability Report* No. 24. London: Bank of England. [Online]. Available at: http://www.bankofengland.co.uk/publications/fsr/2008/fsrfull0810.pdf.

Barnet, R.J. and Müller, R.E. 1974. *Global Reach: The Power of the Multinational Corporations.* New York: Touchstone.

Baum, F.E., Bégin, M., Houweling, T.A.J., and Taylor, S. 2009. Changes Not for the Fainthearted: Reorienting Health Care Systems Toward Health Equity Through Action on the Social Determinants of Health. *American Journal of Public Health*, 99, 1967–74.

Bhan, G. 2009. 'This is no longer the city I once knew'. Evictions, the urban poor and the right to the city in millennial Delhi. *Environment and Urbanization*, 21, 127–42.

Birdsall, N. 2006. *The World is Not Flat: Inequality and Injustice in our Global Economy*, WIDER Annual Lecture. Helsinki: World Institute for Development Economics Research. [Online]. Available at: http://www.wider.unu.edu/publications/annual-lectures/en_GB/AL9/_files/78121127186268214/default/annual-lecture-2005.pdf.

Boddy, T. 1992. Underground and Overhead: Building the Analogous City, in *Variations on a Theme Park*, edited by M. Sorkin. New York: Hill & Wang, 123–53.

Bond, P. 2006. Johannesburg: Of Gold and Gangsters, in *Evil Paradises*, edited by M. Davis. New York: New Press, 114–26.

Broudehoux, A-M. 2013. Neo-liberal exceptionalism in Rio de Janeiro's Olympic port regeneration, in *Routledge Companion to Urban Regeneration*, edited by M. Leary and J. McCarthy. London: Routledge, 558–68.

Buck, N., Gordon, I., Hall, P. et al. 2002. *Working Capital: Life and Labour in Contemporary London.* London: Routledge.

Buechler, S. 2006. São Paulo: Outsourcing and Downgrading of Labour in a Globalizing City, in *The Global Cities Reader*, edited by N. Brenner and R. Keil. London: Routledge, 238–45.

Burke, J. 2010. 'Shining India' makes its poor pay price of hosting Commonwealth Games. *The Guardian*, 11 July.

Capgemini. 2011. *US Metro Wealth Index 2011 Findings.* New York: Capgemini. [Online]. Available at: http://www.capgemini.com/m/en/doc/2011_US_Metro_City_Wealth_Index_small.pdf.

Caraley, D. 1992. Washington Abandons the Cities. *Political Science Quarterly*, 107, 1–30.

Caraley, D. 1996. Dismantling the Federal Safety Net: Fictions versus Realities. *Political Science Quarterly*, 111, 225–58.

Centre on Housing Rights and Evictions. 2007. *Fair Play for Housing Rights: Mega-Events, Olympic Games and Housing Rights*. Geneva: Centre on Housing Rights and Evictions. [Online]. Available at: http://iocc.ca/documents/FairPlayForHousingRights-COHRE.pdf.

Cerny, P.G. 2000. Restructuring the Political Arena: Globalisation and the Paradoxes of the Competition State, in *Globalisation and its Critics: Perspectives from Political Economy*, edited by R.D. Germain. Houndmills: Macmillan, 117–38.

Choi, M. (2002). *Essays on the threat effects of foreign direct investment on labour markets.* PhD dissertation, University of Massachusetts Amherst.

Commission on Social Determinants of Health. 2008. *Closing the Gap in a Generation: Health equity through action on the social determinants of health (final report)*. Geneva: World Health Organization. [Online]. Available at: http://whqlibdoc.who.int/publications/2008/9789241563703_eng.pdf.

Compa, L. 2005. *Blood, Sweat and Fear: Workers' Rights in U.S. Meat and Poultry Plants*. New York: Human Rights Watch. [Online]. Available at: http://www.hrw.org/sites/default/files/reports/usa0105.pdf.

Darden, J. and Wyly, E. 2010. Cartographic Editorial: Mapping the Racial/Ethnic Topography of Subprime Inequality in Urban America. *Urban Geography*, 31, 425–33.

Davis, M. 1990. *City of Quartz: Excavating the Future in Los Angeles*. London: Verso.

Davis, M. 2006. *Planet of Slums*. London: Verso.

Deas, I. and Ward, K.G. 1999. The song has ended but the melody lingers. *Local Economy*, 14, 114–32.

Delgado Wise, R. and Covarrubias, H.M. 2008. Capitalist Restructuring, Development and Labour Migration: the Mexico-US case. *Third World Quarterly*, 29, 1359–74.

DeLuca, P., Buist, S. and Johnston, N. 2012. The Code Red Project: Engaging Communities in Health System Change in Hamilton, Canada. *Social Indicators Research*, 108, 317–27.

Dicken, P. 2007. *Global Shift: Reshaping the Global Economic Map in the 21st Century*. 5th edition. New York: Guilford Press.

Diderichsen, F., Evans, T. and Whitehead, M. 2001. The Social Basis of Disparities in Health, in *Challenging Inequities in Health: From Ethics to Action*, edited by M. Whitehead, T. Evans, F. Diderichsen et al. New York: Oxford University Press, 13–23.

Dreier, P., Mollenkopf, J. and Swanstrom, T. 2005. *Place Matters: Metropolitics for the Twenty-first Century*. 2nd edition. Lawrence: University Press of Kansas.

Duhigg, C. and Barboza, D. 2012. In China, Human Costs Are Built Into an iPad. *New York Times*, 26 January.

Duhigg, C. and Bradsher, K. 2012. How U.S. Lost Out on iPhone Work. *New York Times*, 22 January.

Eisinger, P. 2000. The Politics of Bread and Circuses: Building the City for the Visitor Class. *Urban Affairs Review*, 35, 316–33.

Eyoh, D. and Sandbrook, R. 2003. Pragmatic neo-liberalism and just development in Africa, in *States, Markets, and Just Growth: Development in the Twenty-first Century*, edited by A. Kohli, C. Moon, and G. Sørensen. Tokyo: United Nations University Press, 227–57.

Fainstein, S. and Judd, D. 1999. *The Tourist City.* New Haven, CT: Yale University Press.

Fallows, J. 2007. China Makes, The World Takes. *Atlantic*, 300, July/August, 48–72.

Ferguson, J. 2005. Seeing Like an Oil Company: Space, Security, and Global Capital in Neoliberal Africa. *American Anthropologist*, 107, 377–82.

Fowler, D. 2008. *One World, Whose Dream? Housing Rights Violations and the Beijing Olympic Games*. Geneva: Centre on Housing Rights and Evictions. [Online]. Available at: http://sheltercentre.org/sites/default/files/COHRE_OneWorldWhoseDreamHousing RightsViolationsAndTheBeijingOlympicGames.pdf.

Freeman, R.B. 2007. The Challenge of the Growing Globalisation of Labour Markets to Economic and Social Policy, in *Global Capitalism Unbound: Winners and Losers from Offshore Outsourcing*, edited by E. Paus. Houndmills: Palgrave Macmillan, 23–40.

Fröbel, F., Heinrichs, J. and Kreye, O. 1980 [orig. German publication 1977]. *The New International Division of Labour*. Cambridge: Cambridge University Press.

Fussell, E. 2011. The Deportation Threat Dynamic and Victimization of Latino Migrants: Wage Theft and Robbery. *The Sociological Quarterly*, 52, 593–615.

Garau, P., Sclar, E.D. and Carolini, G.Y. 2005. *A Home in the City: UN Millennium Project Task Force on Improving the Lives of Slum Dwellers*. London: Earthscan. [Online]. Available at: http://www.millenniumproject.org.

Goldman, M. 2011. Speculative Urbanism and the Making of the Next World City. *International Journal of Urban and Regional Research*, 35, 555–81.

Grant, R. 2009. *Globalizing City: The Urban and Economic Transformation of Accra, Ghana*. New York: Syracuse University Press.

Grant, R. and Nijman, J. 2004. Globalisation and the Hyperdifferentiation of Space in the Less Developed World, in *Globalisation and Its Outcomes*, edited by J. O'Loughlin and E. Greenberg. New York: Guilford Press, 45–66.

Grant, T. and Yang, J. 2009. Immigrants take brunt of recession, recover less quickly. *The* [Toronto] *Globe and Mail*, 25 July.

Gringeri, C.E. 1994. Assembling 'genuine GM parts': rural homeworkers and economic development. *Economic Development Quarterly*, 8, 147–57.

Gugler, J. 2004. *World Cities Beyond the West: Globalisation, Development and Inequality.* Cambridge: Cambridge University Press.

Guthrie-Shimizu, S. 2005. From Southeast Asia to the American Southeast: Japanese Business Meets the Sun Belt South, in *Globalisation and the American South*, edited by J.C. Cobb and W. Stueck. Athens: University of Georgia Press, 134–65.

Gwatkin, D.R., Rutstein, S., Johnson, K. et al. 2007. *Socio-Economic Differences in Health, Nutrition and Population Within Developing Countries: An Overview*. Washington, DC: World Bank. [Online]. Available at: http://go.worldbank.org/XJK7WKSE40.

Hackworth, J. 2007. *The Neoliberal City: Governance, Ideology, and Development in American Urbanism*. Ithaca: Cornell University Press.

Hall, P.A. 2010. *The Regeneration of Urban Empty Space/Detroit.* MCP thesis, University of Cincinnati, Cincinnati. [Online]. Available at: http://rave.ohiolink.edu/etdc/ view?acc_num=ucin1282170030.

Harris, A. 2008. From London to Mumbai and Back Again: Gentrification and Public Policy in Comparative Perspective. *Urban Studies*, 45, 2407–28.

Hartman, C. and Carnochan, S. 2002. *City for Sale: The Transformation of San Francisco* (revised and updated edition). Berkeley: University of California Press.

Harvey, D. 2006. Neo-liberalism and the restoration of class power, in *Spaces of Global Capitalism*. London: Verso, 9–68.

Hellman, J.A. 2008. *The World of Mexican Migrants: The Rock and the Hard Place*. New York: The New Press.

Herod, A. and Aguilar, L. 2006. The Dirty Work of Neoliberalism: Cleaners in the Global Economy [journal issue]. *Antipode*, 38, 3.

Hodos, J. 2002. Globalisation, Regionalism, and Urban Restructuring: The Case of Philadelphia. *Urban Affairs Review*, 37, 358–79.

Holston, J. 1998. Spaces of Insurgent Citzenship, in *Making the Invisible Visible: A Multicultural Planning History*, edited by L. Sandercock. Berkeley: University of California Press, 37–56.

Hossain, N. and McGregor, J.A. 2011. A 'Lost Generation'? Impacts of Complex Compound Crises on Children and Young People. *Development Policy Review*, 29, 565–84.

Jacobs, A. 2000. A City Revived, but With Buildings Falling Right and Left. *New York Times*, 31 August.

James, P.D., Wilkins, R., Detsky, A.S. et al. 2007. Avoidable mortality by neighbourhood income in Canada: 25 years after the establishment of universal health insurance. *Journal of Epidemiology and Community Health*, 61, 287–96.

Judd, D. 1999. Constructing the Tourist Bubble, in *The Tourist City*, edited by D. Judd and S. Fainstein. New Haven, CT: Yale University Press, 35–55.

Kirby, A. 1992. The Pentagon *versus* the Cities?, in *The Pentagon and the Cities: Urban Affairs Annual Reviews 40*, edited by A. Kirby. Newbury Park, CA: Sage, 1–22.

Kohn, M. 2004. *Brave New Neighborhoods: The Privatization of Public Space*. New York: Routledge.

Kothari, M. 2007. *Report of the Special Rapporteur on adequate housing as a component of the right to an adequate standard of living, Miloon Kothari*, A/HRC/4/18. New York: United Nations. [Online]. Available at: http://daccessdds.un.org/doc/UNDOC/GEN/ G07/106/28/PDF/G0710628.pdf?OpenElement.

Lakshmi, R. 2005. Bombay Moves to Push Out the Poor: Slums Are Razed as Plans Envisage Reinvented City. *Washington Post*, 5 August.

Leaf, M. 1996. Building the road for the BMW: Culture, vision, and the extended metropolitan region of Jakarta. *Environment and Planning A*, 28, 1617–35.

Lees, L. 2012. The geography of gentrification. *Progress in Human Geography*, 36, 155–71.

Lefebvre, S. and Roult, R. 2011. Formula One's new urban economies. *Cities*, 28, 330–39.

Lemanski, C. 2007. Global Cities in the South: Deepening social and spatial polarisation in Cape Town. *Cities*, 24, 448–61.

Levine, M.V. 2000. 'A Third-World City in the First World': Social Exclusion, Racial Inequality, and Sustainable Development in Baltimore, Maryland, in *The Social Sustainability of Cities: Diversity and the Management of Change*, edited by M. Polèse and R. Stren. Toronto: University of Toronto Press, 123–56.

Link, B.G. and Phelan, J. 1995. Social Conditions As Fundamental Causes of Disease. *Journal of Health and Social Behavior*, 35, 80–94.

Lister, J. and Labonté, R. 2009. Globalisation and Health Systems Change, in *Globalisation and Health: Pathways, Evidence and Policy*, edited by R. Labonté, T. Schrecker, C. Packer and V. Runnels. New York: Routledge, 181–212.

López-Morales, E.J. 2010. Real Estate market, state-entrepreneurialism and urban policy in the 'gentrification by ground rent dispossession' of Santiago de Chile. *Journal of Latin American Geography*, 9, 145–73.

Luria, D. and Russell, J. 1981. *Rational Reindustrialization: An Economic Development Agenda for Detroit*. Detroit: Widgetripper Press.

Mabin, A. 2007. Johannesburg: (South) Africa's Aspirant Global City, in *The Making of Global City Regions: Johannesburg, Mumbai/Bombay, Sao Paulo, and Shanghai*, edited by K. Segbers. Baltimore: Johns Hopkins University Press, 32–63.

Makdisi, S. 1997. Laying Claim to Beirut: Urban Narrative and Spatial Identity in the Age of Solidere. *Critical Inquiry*, 23, 660–705.

Markusen, A., Hall, P., Campbell, S. and Deitrick, S. 1991. *The Rise of the Gunbelt: The Military Remapping of Industrial America*. New York: Oxford University Press.

Marmot, M. 2000. Inequalities in health: causes and policy implications, in *The Society and Population Health Reader, vol. 2: A State and Community Perspective*, edited by A. Tarlov and R. St. Peter. New York: New Press, 293–309.

Marmot, M. 2005. Social determinants of health inequalities. *The Lancet*, 365, 1099–104.

Maunula, M. 2005. Another Southern Paradox: The Arrival of Foreign Corporations – Change and Continuity in Spartanburg, South Carolina, in *Globalisation and the American South*, edited by J.C. Cobb and W. Stueck. Athens: University of Georgia Press, 164–84

McCarthy, J. 1997. Revitalization of the core city: the case of Detroit. *Cities*, 14, 1–11.

McCarthy, J. 2002. Entertainment-led Regeneration: the Case of Detroit. *Cities*, 19, 105–11.

McDonald, D.A. 2008. *World City Syndrome: Neoliberalism and Inequality in Cape Town*. New York: Routledge.

McGreal, C. 2010. Detroit mayor plans to shrink city by cutting services to some areas. *The Guardian*, 17 December.

Moody, K. 2007. *From Welfare State to Real Estate: Regime Change in New York City, 1974 to the Present*. New York: New Press.

Murray, C.J.L., Kulkarni, S.C., Michaud, C. et al. 2006. Eight Americas: Investigating Mortality Disparities across Races, Counties, and Race-Counties in the United States. *PLoS Medicine*, 3(260).

Murray, M. 2002. City Profile: Denver. *Cities*, 19, 283–94.

Murray, M.J. 2008. *Taming the Disorderly City: The Spatial Landscape of Johannesburg after Apartheid*. Ithaca: Cornell University Press.

National Treasury Department. 2011. *Confronting youth unemployment: policy options for South Africa*, Discussion Paper. Pretoria: Government of South Africa. [Online]. Available at: http://www.treasury.gov.za/documents/national%20budget/2011/Confronting%20youth%20unemployment%20-%20Policy%20options.pdf.

Newman, H.K. 2002. Race and the Tourist Bubble in Downtown Atlanta. *Urban Affairs Review*, 37, 301–21.

Nickell, S. and Bell, B. 1995. The collapse in demand for the unskilled and unemployment across the OECD. *Oxford Review of Economic Policy*, 11, 40–62.

Nijman, J. 2000. Mumbai's Real Estate Market in 1990s: De-Regulation, Global Money and Casino Capitalism. *Economic and Political Weekly*, 35, 575–82.

Ong, A. 2006. *Neoliberalism as Exception: Mutations in Citizenship and Sovereignty*. Durham, NC: Duke University Press.

Ong, A. 2011. Introduction: Worlding Cities, or the Art of being Global, in *Worlding Cities* edited by A. Roy and A. Ong. New York: Wiley-Blackwell, 1–26.

Ortiz, I., Chai, J. and Cummins, M. 2011. *Austerity Measures Threaten Children and Poor Households: Recent Evidence in Public Expenditures from 128 Developing Countries*, Social and Economic Policy Working Paper. New York: UNICEF. [Online]. Available at: http://www.unicef.org/socialpolicy/files/Austerity_Measures_Threaten_Children.pdf.

Paluzzi, J.E. and Farmer, P.E. 2005. The Wrong Question. *Development*, 48(1), 12–18.

Patel, S. 2004. Bombay/Mumbai: Globalisation, inequalities, and politics, in *World Cities Beyond the West: Globalisation, Development and Inequality*, edited by J. Gugler. Cambridge: Cambridge University Press, 328–47.

Patel, S. 2007. Mumbai: The Mega-City of a Poor Country, in *The Making of Global City Regions: Johannesburg, Mumbai/Bombay, Sao Paulo, and Shanghai*, edited by K. Segbers. Baltimore: Johns Hopkins University Press, 64–84.

Peck, J. and Tickell, A. 2002. Neoliberalizing Space. *Antipode*, 34, 380–404.

Perlman, J.E. 2005. The Myth of Marginality Revisited: The Case of Favelas in Rio de Janeiro, 1969–2003, in *Becoming Global and the New Poverty of Cities*, edited by L.M. Hanley, B.A. Ruble and J.S. Tulchin. Washington, DC: Comparative Urban Studies Project, Woodrow Wilson International Center for Scholars, 9–54.

Pfeiffer, J. and Chapman, R. 2010. Anthropological Perspectives on Structural Adjustment and Public Health. *Annual Review of Anthropology*, 39, 149–65.

Pucher, J., Korattyswaropam, N., Mittal, N. and Ittyerah, N. 2005. Urban transport crisis in India. *Transport Policy*, 12, 185–98.

Quesada, J., Hart, L.K. and Bourgois, P. 2011. Structural Vulnerability and Health: Latino Migrant Labourers in the United States. *Medical Anthropology*, 30, 339–62.

Robinson, J. 2002a. Global and world cities: A view from off the map. *International Journal of Urban and Regional Research*, 26, 531–54.

Robinson, W.I. 2002b. Remapping development in light of globalisation: from a territorial to a social cartography. *Third World Quarterly*, 23, 1047–71.

Rodgers, D. 2007. 'Nueva Managua': The Disembedded City, in *Evil Paradises: Dreamworlds of Neoliberalism*, edited by M. Davis and B. Monk. New York: New Press, 127–93.

Rousseau, M. 2012. Post-Fordist Urbanism in France's Poorest City: Gentrification as Local Capitalist Strategy. *Critical Sociology*, 38, 49–69.

Rozhon, T. 1999. Old Baltimore Row Houses Fall Before Wrecking Ball. *New York Times*, 13 June.

Rydin, R., Bleahu, A., Davies, M. et al. 2012. Shaping cities for health: complexity and the planning of urban environments in the 21st century. *The Lancet*, 379, 2079–108.

Samuels, F., Gavrilovic, M., Harper, C. and Niño-Zarazúa 2011. *Food, finance and fuel: the impacts of the triple F crisis in Nigeria, with a particular focus on women and children*, Background Note. London: Overseas Development Institute. [Online]. Available at: http://www.odi.org.uk/resources/docs/7359.pdf.

Sarabia, H. 2011. Perpetual Illegality: Results of Border Enforcement and Policies for Mexican Undocumented Migrants in the United States. *Analyses of Social Issues and Public Policy*. Available at: http://dx.doi.org/10.1111/j.1530–2415.2011.01256.x.

Sassen, S. 1991. *The Global City: New York, London, Tokyo*. Princeton: Princeton University Press.

Sassen, S. 2001. *The Global City: New York, London, Tokyo*. 2nd edition. Princeton: Princeton University Press.

Sassen, S. 2002. Global Cities and Survival Circuits, in *Global Woman: Nannies, Maids, and Sex Workers in the Economy*, edited by B. Ehrenreich and A. Hochschild. New York: Metropolitan Books, 254–74.

Sassen, S. 2009. When Local Housing Becomes an Electronic Instrument: The Global Circulation of Mortgages – A Research Note. *International Journal of Urban and Regional Research*, 33, 411–26.

Sassen, S. 2011. Beyond Social Exclusion: New Logics of Expulsion. Presented at 6th Annual Research Conference on Homelessness in Europe: Homelessness, Migration and Demographic Change in Europe, Pisa, Italy. [Online video]. Available at: http://www.dailymotion.com/video/xl7upb_saskia-sassen-logics-of-expulsion-a-savage-sorting-of-winners-and-losers_news.

Sassen, S. 2012a. *Cities in a World Economy*. 4th edition. Thousand Oaks, CA: Pine Forge Press.

Sassen, S. 2012b. Expanding the Terrain for Global Capital: When Local Housing Becomes an Electronic Instrument, in *Subprime Cities: The Political Economy of Mortgage Markets*, edited by M.B. Aalbers. Oxford: Blackwell, 74–96.

Sassen, S. and Roost, F. 1999. The City: Strategic Site for the Global Entertainment Industry, in *The Tourist City*, edited by S. Fainstein and D. Judd. New Haven, CT: Yale University Press, 143–54.

Savitch, H. 2003. How Suburban Sprawl Shapes Human Well-Being. *Journal of Urban Health*, 80, 590–607.

Schafran, A. 2012. Origins of an Urban Crisis: The Restructuring of the San Francisco Bay Area and the Geography of Foreclosure. *International Journal of Urban and Regional Research*. Available at: http://dx.doi.org/10.1111/j.1468–2427.2012.01150.x.

Scherer, J. 2011. Olympic Villages and Large-scale Urban Development: Crises of Capitalism, Deficits of Democracy? *Sociology*, 45, 782–97.

Schrecker, T. 2009. The Power of Money: Global Financial Markets, National Politics, and Social Determinants of Health, in *The Crisis of Global Health Governance: Political Economy, Ideas and Institutions*, edited by O. Williams and A. Kay. Houndmills: Palgrave Macmillan, 160–81.

Schulz, A. and Northridge, M. 2004. Social Determinants of Health: Implications for Environmental Health Promotion. *Health Education & Behavior*, 31, 455–71.

Seelye, K.Q. 2011. Detroit Census Confirms a Desertion Like No Other. *New York Times*, 22 March.

Shavers, A.W. 2009. Welcome to the Jungle: New Immigrants in the Meatpacking and Poultry Processing Industry. *Journal of Law Economics & Policy*, 5, 31–86.

Silk, M.L. 2007. Come Downtown & Play. *Leisure Studies*, 26, 253–77.

Slater, T. 2011. Gentrification of the City, in *The New Blackwell Companion to the City*, edited by G. Bridge and S. Watson. Oxford: Blackwell, 571–85.

Smith, A. 1989. Gentrification and the Spatial Constitution of the State: The Restructuring of London's Docklands. *Antipode*, 21, 232–60.

Smith, P. 2012. How state capitalism helps the super-rich. *Africa Report*, 38, 4.

Soares de Oliveira, R. 2007. *Oil and Politics in the Gulf of Guinea*. New York: Columbia University Press.

Songsore, J. 2008. *The Urban Transition in Ghana: Urbanization, National Development and Poverty Reduction*. London: International Institute for Environment and Development. [Online]. Available at: http://pubs.iied.org/pdfs/G02540.pdf.

Songsore, J. and McGranahan, G. 2007. Poverty and the Environmental Health Agenda in a Low-income City: The Case of the Greater Accra Metropolitan Area (GAMA), Ghana, in *Scaling Urban Environmental Challenges: From Local to Global and Back*, edited by P.J. Marcotullio and G. McGranahan. London: Earthscan, 132–55.

Standing, G. 2007. Offshoring and Labor Recommodification in the Global Transformation, in *Global Capitalism Unbound: Winners and Losers from Offshore Outsourcing*, edited by E. Paus. Houndmills: Palgrave Macmillan, 41–60.

Tobler, W.R. 1970. A Computer Movie Simulating Urban Growth in the Detroit Region. *Economic Geography*, 46, 234–40.

United Nations Human Settlements Programme. 2003. *The Challenge of Slums*. London: Earthscan. [Online]. Available at: http://www.unhabitat.org/pmss/getPage. asp?page=bookView&book=1156.

United Nations Human Settlements Programme. 2008. *State of the World's Cities 2010/2011 – Cities for All: Bridging the Urban Divide*. London: Earthscan. [Online]. Available at: http://www.unhabitat.org/pmss/getElectronicVersion.aspx?nr=2917&alt=1.

United Nations Conference on Trade and Development. 2009. *Trade and Development Report, 2009: Responding to the global crisis; climate change mitigation and development*. New York: United Nations. [Online]. Available at: http://www.unctad. org/en/docs/tdr2009_en.pdf.

Visser, G. and Kotze, N. 2008. The State and New-build Gentrification in Central Cape Town, South Africa. *Urban Studies*, 45, 2565–93.

Wacquant, L. 2009. *Punishing the Poor: The Neoliberal Government of Social Insecurity*. Durham, NC: Duke University Press.

Wallace, R. and Wallace, D. 1998. *A Plague on Your Houses: How New York was Burned Down and National Public Health Crumbled*. London: Verso.

Ward, K. and England, K. 2007. Introduction: Reading Neoliberalization, in *Neoliberalization: States, Networks, People*, edited by K. England and K. Ward. Oxford: Blackwell, 1–22.

Weir, M. 1994. Urban Poverty and Defensive Localism. *Dissent*, Summer, 337–42.

Whitehead, J. and More, N. 2007. Revanchism in Mumbai? Political Economy of Rent Gaps and Urban Restructuring in a Global City. *Economic and Political Weekly*, 42, 2428–34.

Wilgoren, J. 2002. Detroit Urban Renewal Without the Renewal. *New York Times*, 8 July.

Winerip, M. 1998. The Blue-Collar Millionaire. *New York Times Magazine*, 7 June, 72–6.

Wolch, J.R. 1998. America's New Urban Policy: Welfare Reform and the Fate of American Cities. *Journal of the American Planning Association*, 64, 8–11.

Wood, A. 1998. Globalisation and the Rise in Labour Market Inequalities. *The Economic Journal*, 108, 1463–82.

World Health Organization and United Nations Human Settlements Programme. 2010. *Hidden cities: unmasking and overcoming health inequities in urban settings*. Nairobi: UN-HABITAT and WHO. [Online]. Available at: http://www.hiddencities.org/ downloads/WHO_UN-HABITAT_Hidden_Cities_Web.pdf.

Wyly, E., Moos, M., Hammel, D. and Kabahizi, E. 2009. Cartographies of Race and Class: Mapping the Class-Monopoly Rents of American Subprime Mortgage Capital. *International Journal of Urban and Regional Research*, 33, 332–54.

Young, R.A. 1991. Tectonic Policies and Political Competition, in *The Competitive State*, edited by A. Breton, B. Galeotti, P. Salmon and R. Wintrobe. Dordrecht: Kluwer, 129–45.

# Chapter 17
# Medical Migration From Zimbabwe:
# Towards New Solutions?

Abel Chikanda and Belinda Dodson

## Introduction

Health worker migration presents a daunting challenge to health systems in many sub-Saharan African countries (Anyangwe and Mtonga 2007; Conway et al. 2007; Crush and Pendleton 2011). In fact, the World Health Organisation (WHO) has identified the migration of health workers as probably the most critical problem facing health systems in Africa today (Hussey 2007). Global health indicators show that Africa bears one quarter of the burden of disease around the world when only 3 per cent of all health professionals are found on the continent (WHO 2006). The shortage of health professionals in Africa has been further worsened by the HIV and AIDS pandemic, which has severely overburdened health systems across the continent. Not surprisingly, the migration of health workers presents a major obstacle to the continent's quest to attain the Millennium Development Goals (MDGs).

Consequently, the migration of health professionals from Africa has attracted the attention of both academics and policy makers (Awases et al. 2004; Liese and Dussault 2004). Recent research has highlighted the magnitude, causes and impacts of the migration of health professionals from the continent. Some of the studies have focused on specific professionals such as nurses (Chikanda 2005; Kingma 2006) and medical doctors (Chikanda 2011; Mills et al. 2011). Medical doctors, in particular, seem to be drawing the largest attention because their rate of attrition has increased considerably over the past two decades. As Clemens and Pettersson (2006) have shown, about 11 per cent (or 53,298) of the African-born nurses and 28 per cent (or 36,653) of the African-born medical doctors were working in nine major immigrant receiving countries in 2000. Furthermore, the Global Commission on International Migration (GCIM) estimates that there are currently more Malawian doctors practising in the northern English city of Manchester than in the whole of Malawi (GCIM 2005). Some more developed countries in Africa such as South Africa have lost a significant number of doctors to developed countries such as Australia, Canada, the United Kingdom and the United States, but have also attracted medical doctors from other southern African countries such as Zimbabwe, Zambia and Namibia. These movements have been described as a 'global conveyor belt' of health personnel, 'global health chain', or 'medical carousel', which channels skilled professionals from poor to rich countries (Schrecker and Labonte 2004; Eastwood et al. 2005).

It is not surprising that the notion of 'brain drain' has become the primary mode of understanding the migration of medical doctors (Raghuram 2009). Developing countries such as those on the African continent labour to produce medical doctors at heavily subsidised rates only to have them move to more developed countries in search of greener pastures. Therefore, the loss of medical doctors from the continent is argued to represent a loss of both skills and capital. Calls have been made by some scholars for countries which benefit from the medical doctors to offer financial compensation to the countries which bore the costs of educating the professionals (Bhagwati 1976; Mensah et al. 2005). This seems unlikely to happen any time in the future because the medical doctors move voluntarily to destinations where they achieve economic, social and professional advancement. Nonetheless, this has not stopped some researchers from attempting to put a dollar value on the professionals who are lost through migration. In Kenya, for example, Kirigia et al. (2006) have calculated the cost of training a medical doctor from primary school to university to be US$65,997. More recently, Mills et al. (2011) estimated that the subsidised cost of educating a doctor to be US$58,698 in South Africa and US$38,620 in Zimbabwe. Considering the number of doctors who have moved to Australia, Canada, the United Kingdom and United States, this translates into US$1.41 billion in lost investment for South Africa and US$40 million for Zimbabwe (Mills et al. 2011). Not surprisingly, as Connell (2008) observes pejoratives such as 'poaching', 'looting', 'stealing' and the 'new slave trade' have entered the discourse on medical migration from Africa.

This chapter considers the migration of medical doctors in the light of emerging views on the role of migrants (or diaspora) in the development of their countries of origin. It uses evidence from Zimbabwe, which provides a good case of an African country which has lost a substantial number of its medical doctors through migration. It is important to examine the losses that Zimbabwe has experienced in view of the potential gains the country is likely to experience through remittances, return migration and other diaspora engagement initiatives. This 'new' literature questions the concept of a 'brain drain' by highlighting the positive impacts of migration to the sending region. The chapter argues that the feedback returns which Zimbabwe can derive from its emigrant medical doctors are limited and there is utility in describing the flow of medical doctors from the country as a 'brain drain'. As will be shown later in the chapter, the concept of a 'brain drain' is still relevant when analysing the migration of medical doctors, especially in view of the impacts of the movements on service delivery on the African continent.

## Medical Migration from Zimbabwe

Zimbabwe exemplifies a country whose health system has been negatively affected by the emigration of a large number of its medical doctors. The number of medical doctors who have left the country is not known since the country does not keep a record of the departing professionals. However, destination country data can be used to shed light on the volume of medical migration from Zimbabwe. Using data compiled by Clemens and Pettersson (2006) as well as that by Dumont and Zurn (2007), it is possible to generate a global distribution of Zimbabwean doctors in 2000 (Table 17.1). By that time, Zimbabwe had at least 1,662 doctors working in nine major immigrant receiving countries, with the majority based in South Africa, the United Kingdom and the United States. This is in stark contrast to the 1,530 medical doctors registered to practice in Zimbabwe at that time (Clemens and Pettersson 2006). The number of emigrant medical doctors is likely to have increased significantly over the past decade as a result of the intensification in emigration pressures in the country since 2000.

Using data from a World Bank study by Docquier and Bhargava (2006) which documented the size of the domestic medical labour force of several countries, Chikanda (2011) showed that the number of medical doctors practicing in Zimbabwe fell from 1,425

**Table 17.1    Location of Zimbabwean Medical Doctors Worldwide, 2000**

| Country | No. of doctors | Percentage (%) of emigrant Zimbabwean doctors |
|---|---|---|
| South Africa | 643 | 38.7 |
| UK | 553 | 33.3 |
| USA | 235 | 14.1 |
| Australia | 97 | 5.8 |
| New Zealand | 60 | 3.6 |
| Canada | 55 | 3.3 |
| Portugal | 12 | 0.7 |
| Belgium | 6 | 0.4 |
| Spain | 1 | 0.1 |
| Total abroad | 1,662 | 100.0 |

*Source:* Chikanda (2011) based on Clemens and Pettersson (2006); Dumont and Zurn (2007).

in 1991 to only 751 in 2004 (Figure 17.1). This supports observations by other scholars which show that the rate of attrition of medical doctors from Zimbabwe quickened in the 1990s. For instance, Liese and Dussault (2004) have noted that only 360 of the 1,200 medical doctors trained in Zimbabwe during the 1990s were still practising in the country in 2000. In fact, as shown in Figure 17.1, adding the number of new medical doctors trained and controlling for deaths and retirement, it can be demonstrated that Zimbabwe lost nearly 1,800 medical doctors through emigration during the period 1990–2004.

Medical migration from Zimbabwe has been promoted by a wide range of factors. In the 1980s, the political environment was cited as the leading cause of migration (Chikanda, 2011). The colonial policies favored whites over blacks, hence the medical workforce was dominated by white doctors. The country gained its independence in 1980 and a black dominated government was established. The exodus of medical doctors in the 1980s was connected to the 'white flight' (Zinyama 1990), which occurred as a result of security concerns among the white professionals in a black dominated government that had stated its commitment to the establishment of a socialist state. In the late 1980s and early 1990s, newly trained black Zimbabwean medical doctors also moved to South Africa, which was recruiting doctors to work in the rural areas which were shunned by its own citizens (Grant 2006). This also came at a time when the rate of production of doctors at Zimbabwe's only medical school failed to keep pace with the demand for specialist training. Hence, a large number of medical doctors left Zimbabwe in the early 1990s to pursue specialist training in South Africa (Chikanda 2011). The adoption of the World Bank/International Monetary Fund-driven structural adjustment programme in the early 1990s resulted in runaway inflation levels that eroded the real wages of professionals. Migration to South Africa and other destinations such as the United Kingdom, United States and Australia became a viable alternative for the medical doctors. By migrating, the doctors essentially 'voted with their feet' (Gaidzanwa 1999) and made a statement of their dissatisfaction with the economic and political climate prevailing in the country. A further deterioration of the political and economic conditions, which started with the chaotic land reform and the violence that marred the 2000's, and subsequent elections, have been the leading causes of medical migration from Zimbabwe over the past decade. The destruction of the country's

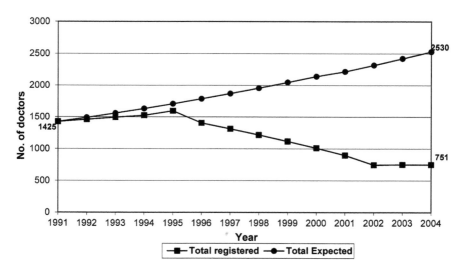

**Figure 17.1    Number of Doctors in Zimbabwe, 1991–2004**

*Source:* Chikanda (2011) based on Docquier and Bhargava, 2006.

agro-based economy led to the soaring of inflation, which officially peaked at 231 million per cent in 2008, although independent estimates suggest that the inflation levels at that time were as high as 89.7 sextillion (1021) per cent (Hanke 2008).

Medical migration from Zimbabwe has adversely affected the quality of care offered in health institutions. Chikanda (2008) has identified several effects of medical migration. First, medical migration has increased the workload of staff who choose not to migrate. Since the shortage of medical doctors was most acute in rural and remote locations, doctors posted in these locations bore the heaviest workload. Mutizwa-Mangiza (1999) attribute the 'uncaring and abusive' attitudes toward patients of some health staff as a direct result of low morale caused by excessive workload associated with dealing with so many patients. Second, some patients who were turned away from the busy public health institutions were forced to access care in the more expensive private clinics. This has an obvious effect on equity of access to health care for the poorest. In fact, some patients have been forced to visit traditional and faith healers as a direct result of shortage of qualified health personnel in the country's health institutions. Finally, medical training schools have also been affected by migration as they have lost experienced teaching staff. The workload for the remaining lecturers has increased and this is likely to affect the quality of training which the medical students receive.

**Debating Medical Migration**

Even though the Zimbabwean case demonstrates the negative impacts of medical migration on the quality of care in Africa, there is still considerable debate on whether such movements can be described as a 'brain drain'. There are arguments that the 'brain drain' is deceptive, outmoded or even dead (Teferra 2005; Skeldon 2008). Clemens

(2009, 34), for example, suggests that 'it is time to bury the unpleasant and judgmental term 'brain drain' in favour of a 'brief, accurate and neutral' term such as 'skill flow'.

Criticism of the brain drain phenomenon has been informed by recent advances in migration theory. By definition, the phrase 'brain drain' implies a one-way loss of skilled professionals who are lost to another country. Transnationalism theory, which describes the connections forged by migrants between host and home countries, has demonstrated the role of migrants in the development of their home countries. In other words, skilled professionals do not need to be located in their home country in order to contribute to its development. As Mohan (2002) notes, the activities of migrants are increasingly challenging development studies' conventional and analytical attachment to territories such as states and regions. In the case of medical doctors, Raghuram (2009, 31) notes that 'a more transnational approach towards addressing brain drain recognises the benefits and opportunities of medical worker mobility and aims to maximise and disperse the benefits of such mobility across origin and destination countries'. The migration and development literature shows that migrants can be engaged for the development of their sending states in at least three different ways.

Firstly, some studies suggest that migrant remittances can offset the 'brain drain' suffered by developing countries when their skilled professionals migrate to overseas destinations. Staubhaar and Vadean (2005), for instance, argue that remittances can compensate for the human capital loss suffered by developing countries through migration. World Bank data show a phenomenal rise in remittances to developing countries, which rose from US$81.3 billion in 2000 to US$325.5 in 2010 (World Bank 2011). Thus, remittances are argued to constitute an important source of development finance for developing countries and are capable of turning the drain of professionals into a gain. The second argument is that contemporary migration is dominated by cyclical migration, with migrants eventually returning home after working abroad for a certain number of years. It is argued that brain circulation has replaced the brain drain (Castles and Miller 2009). Return migration, or 'brain circulation' is expected to benefit the sending country through the provision of skills, knowledge and capital transfer. The third argument is that migrant sending states can tap into the professional expertise of their citizens abroad through a number of diaspora engagement programmes. This includes temporary returns on short term contracts, virtual participation through various information and communication technologies, and capacity building in home country (Bhargava and Sharma 2008; Raghuram 2009).

Therefore, the migration of skilled professionals becomes a zero-sum as the losses which sending countries experience are offset to varying degrees by the activities of the diaspora. This chapter examines these arguments using primary data collected in a study of emigrant Zimbabwean medical doctors in 2008–2009. The study comprised of an online survey with emigrant Zimbabwean medical doctors and in-depth qualitative interviews with a purposively selected group of Zimbabwean medical doctors working in South Africa.

## Medical Remittances

The issue of remittances has been addressed indirectly in the medical 'brain drain' debate. This is illustrated by the two conflicting viewpoints in the literature on the impacts of medical migration to the sending countries. Proponents of the 'brain drain' have sought to show the size of the brain drain by quantifying in dollar terms the losses experienced by the sending countries when skilled professionals leave for developed countries. It is argued that their movements constitute a loss of investment because most African countries subsidise the cost of training. It is obvious that there are significant differences among scholars on how to quantify the cost of the brain drain. In the case of South Africa, for example, the subsidised portion of training medical doctors varies from US$58,698 (Mills et al. 2011) to US$97,000 (Alkire and Chen 2004). Remittances feature prominently in the 'revisionist approach' to the medical brain drain debate. It is argued that the losses, which the sending country suffers, are offset to some extent by the remittances which it receives (Skeldon 2008; Clemens 2010). Individual African doctors in the United States and Canada are said to send at least US$6,500 per annum to family, friends and charitable organisations on the continent, which translates into an average cumulative amount of US$130,000 for those staying long term outside their countries of birth (Clemens 2010).

These conflicting viewpoints were put to the test in a study of emigrant Zimbabwean medical doctors. A comprehensive understanding of the remitting behaviour of migrants is needed before conclusions can be drawn on the extent to which the remittances they send can offset their training costs. Perhaps the most revealing aspect of the Zimbabwean study was that not all migrants send remittances and those sending money do so at varying levels. In the case of the Zimbabwean medical doctors, the proportion of remitters varies according to race with only 33 per cent of the white doctors sending remittances to Zimbabwe compared with 94 per cent of the black doctors. Race therefore plays a crucial mediating role in the remitting practices of Zimbabwean medical doctors. Context is therefore important in examining the remitting behaviour of migrants. White Zimbabwean medical doctors might lack family ties that bind them to the country because a significant number of white farmers have left since the start of the land reform programme in the country in 1999. Zimbabwe is not alone in this predicament: South Africa too has lost a significant number of its white citizens since the fall of apartheid in 1994 (Crush and Pendleton 2011). Therefore, it is unrealistic to expect the emigrant white medical doctors to send money to their countries of birth when they clearly lack family ties in those countries.

In terms of the volume of remittances, the Zimbabwean study showed that the emigrant doctors send on average US$2,000 annually to the country, an amount which includes remittances sent in the form of cash or goods. This amount is less than a third of the US$6,500 which African doctors in the United States and Canada are said to send to their countries of birth annually (Clemens 2010). More than a third (36.5 per cent) of the emigrant medical doctors who took part in the Zimbabwean survey are based in South Africa where salaries are lower than in Canada or the United States. Migrants based in developed countries are likely to earn higher salaries, and therefore have a greater potential for developing their home countries than those working in developing countries. These comparisons shed light into the importance of south-south migration in developing countries, a phenomenon which is usually neglected in most migration studies (Crush and Frayne 2007). Discussions on migrant remittances should not neglect migrants based in other developing countries. Ignoring this reality in contemporary migration trends would ultimately lead to erroneous policy decisions.

Evaluating the net potential contribution of migrants is not a simple linear relationship. In the case of African doctors in the United States and Canada, we cannot simply compute their potential contribution through remittances using a formula such as obtaining the average remittances sent by an individual annually (US$6,500, in the case of Clemens 2010 study) and multiplying this by the total number of years they will be based abroad (20 years) to arrive at an attractive sum of US$130,000 per migrant. The process of remitting is a complex one in itself and there are several factors which affect the remitting patterns of migrants. Factors in the home country such as the state of the economy, the financial standing of the family, and presence of close family members may play a crucial role in determining whether migrants send money to the home country and how much they send. In the host country, factors such as job security and integration of migrants may play a crucial role in influencing the remittance behaviour of migrants. In fact, insights from the integration literature show that migrants' remitting frequency and volume are affected by their level of integration in the host country (Marcelli and Lowell 2005). A linear model that estimates the cumulative volume of remittances which migrants send in their lifetime suffers the problem of overestimation as remittances are likely to fall due to a combination of factors operating either in the migrants' host or home countries.

Perhaps at this point it is crucial to evaluate the importance of remittances in the development process of countries which lose medical doctors through migration. Could the remittances which they send to their home countries lead to a zero-sum? It is a fact that remittances constitute an important facet in the development process as they provide the necessary financial resources that are needed to drive economic development in the regions lacking in capital resources. However, an important point that is not addressed by scholars who view remittances as the 'new development mantra' (Kapur 2005) is that they ignore the value of human capital in the development process. In the case of medical doctors, they contribute to the development process by ensuring the presence of a healthy population and thus contribute directly to the formation and maintenance of a country's human capital. Even though there is value in touting remittances as a source of development finance, it is questionable that they can compensate for the loss of skills a country suffers when doctors migrate. In other words, the remittances which a medical doctor sends to the home country cannot compensate for the loss of skills which are experienced by the users of the health system. As Mills et al. (2011) have demonstrated in the case of Zimbabwe, the country has suffered a cumulative loss of US$700 million as a result of medical migration from the country. A case can be made for 'medical exceptionalism' (Alkire and Chen 2004) because no amount of migrant remittances can compensate for the doctors who are leaving for developed countries. At present there is still value in describing the flow of professionals such as medical doctors from countries such as Zimbabwe as a brain drain and it cannot be described merely as a 'skill flow' (Clemens 2010).

**Return Migration**

Return migration has been projected to be an important feature of contemporary migration trends (Padarath et al. 2003; Tanner 2005; Faist 2008). The return option presents interesting opportunities for countries that have lost a substantial proportion of their skilled professionals as this would effectively help transform the brain drain into a brain gain (Skeldon 2008). Agencies such as the United Nations (2006) believe that return migration is more common than is normally believed. However, available evidence seems to contradict this claim. There have been reports of 'brain waste' in some regions where the return of professionals has occurred (Connell et al. 2007). Ray et al. (2006) cite studies in the South Pacific which have shown that between 10–20 per cent of migrant health workers return to their countries of origin, but only a few returned to the health sector. The rest are absorbed into non-medical fields. Studies in India have shown that some of the returnees who rejoin the medical field are absorbed in the medical tourism industry which serves the foreign instead of the local population (Khadria 2004).

Research evidence suggests that return migration to Zimbabwe among emigrant medical doctors is likely to be limited. Recognising the impact of the present economic and political challenges facing Zimbabwe on return intentions, the survey asked the medical doctors to look beyond the present circumstances facing the country and provide their own opinion on whether they would consider returning in the future. The survey results indicate that only 28.7 per cent of the respondents are likely to return permanently to Zimbabwe anytime in the future. Nearly half of the respondents (47.8 per cent) categorically stated that they do not see themselves returning to Zimbabwe to either live or work there. Clearly, the benefits of return of professionals are not likely to be experienced in Zimbabwe in the foreseeable future. The survey results showed that the intention to return varied according to race and age of migrants. Thus, 53.1 per cent of black medical doctors are likely to return to Zimbabwe compared to only 11.5 per cent of the white doctors. The possibility to return was higher amongst the young doctors and lower in the older doctors. Thus, 78.3 per cent of those in the 31–40 age group are likely to return to Zimbabwe, while 23.5 per cent in the 41–50 age group, 9.7 per cent in the 51–60 age group and none of those aged above 60 years are likely to return to Zimbabwe in the future. It can be inferred that increased integration in host countries explains the low likelihood to return expressed by the older medical doctors. Other studies have shown that return of older migrants may be hindered by problems associated with the payment of pension benefits (Klinthäll 2006; Yahirun 2009).

Again, the foregoing demonstrates that literature on return migration does not pay attention to the role integration into the host country played in influencing the decision to return. The interviews showed that the emigrant medical doctors have become entrenched into the societies in which they are living. Migrants as active agents are able to turn their host country into a new 'home' where they have emotional, social and economic attachments. As indicated by the research participants, most of them have made long term commitments in South Africa. These include loans acquired from banks to acquire property such as houses and motor vehicles as well as other business commitments. So even if things were to change dramatically in Zimbabwe, it would be difficult for them to leave as they would need to meet their obligations first. As indicated by Dr John Mandaza (not his real name, pseudonyms are used in this chapter) in the interviews:

> There are a lot of things that would make it difficult for me to simply uproot and go. Coming here is not like a visit. You come here and you have to settle as much as possible. And if you are settled you cannot just leave, it's not that easy. I mean, the banks will be interested in knowing where I am going – we have got car loans, houses on mortgages, bank overdrafts, contracts that are running and so forth. So even if things were to be okay today and I really want to go back home it would take me a bit of time to clear up all my obligations.

The transition from South Africa to Zimbabwe would not be a seamless one in professional terms. As noted by Dr Simon Chiremba in the interviews, the returning doctors are bound to face open hostility from their colleagues who will view them as 'traitors' who left at the height of a major crisis in Zimbabwe and return when stability has been reached:

> Some guys tried to go back but they found the environment so hostile in several ways. Any professional returning to Zimbabwe is bound to face open hostility from fellow

professional colleagues who will look at you and say "You are a traitor, why don't you stay at your overseas bases."

Dr Chiremba noted that this would be worsened by the fact that the returning professionals would possess superior qualifications and they would be viewed as a threat by the professionals who did not migrate. Such a hostile environment would make it difficult for the returning medical doctors to operate effectively. Again, this finding may not be limited to the case of Zimbabwe and may be a limiting factor to the professionals elsewhere returning to their countries of origin. Williams and Balaz (2008) documented similar results in their study of Slovak medical doctors who experienced power struggles at clinics on their return to Slovakia.

Zimbabwe, like many other African countries, lags behind developed regions in terms of the adoption of medical technology. This was identified in the interviews as a limiting factor in re-attracting doctors back to Zimbabwe. The majority of emigrant doctors have become specialists and use specialised equipment which is currently not available in Zimbabwe. These differences in levels of technology need to be addressed first before any meaningful attempts can be made to lure the professionals back to Zimbabwe. Such factors, coupled with policies that do not recognise the realities of contemporary migration patterns by denying migrants the right to dual citizenship, are likely to limit the rate of return migration.

It is therefore unlikely that migrant sending countries such as Zimbabwe will experience a substantial return of some of their professionals from abroad anytime in the future. Hence, the notion of return migration is not an attractive one when discussing the movement of skilled professionals such as medical doctors from developing countries, especially those on the African continent. That does not mean to say that no return movement is likely to occur between sending and receiving countries. The main argument is that the rate of permanent return migration among skilled professionals is low and has been overstated in the literature.

## Towards New Solutions: Diaspora Engagement Initiatives

Diaspora engagement has been advanced as a possible solution to the skills problems facing developing countries (Kuznetsov 2006). Agencies such as the International Organisation for Migration (IOM) acknowledge that tapping into the diaspora presents a more realistic way of utilising the skills of emigrant professionals compared to initiatives that seek the permanent return of professionals (IOM 2006). It is important at this stage to investigate the importance of diaspora engagement initiatives, particularly the role which they can play in resolving the human resource crisis in the health system.

The current literature on diaspora engagement show at least four different ways in which the diaspora can contribute to their country of origin's development. First, diasporas can play a critical role in the transfer of technology to their home country. The Indian diaspora features prominently in this regard especially in the role which they played in the growth of the IT industry in India (Aikins et al. 2009). Second, through temporary returns, the diaspora can provide a stop-gap measure of addressing skills shortages in their home countries. The Ghanaian Health Project, part of the Migration for Development in Africa (MIDA) programme which is run by the IOM, is an example of such a programme which facilitates the temporary return of the medical doctors to hospitals and medical training institutions in Ghana (Ndiaye et al. 2011). Third, through contributions to philanthropic activities, diasporas can play a significant role in the development of their country of origin. A useful example in this regard is the American Association of Physicians of Indian Origin (AAPIO) which mobilises resources for the health sector in India and funds clinics, equipment supplies and provides fellowship and support in Mumbai (Aikins et al. 2009). Finally, diasporas can contribute through virtual (cyberspace) return (Brinkerhoff 2008), which may take the form of e-learning in higher institutions and may bridge the skills gap resulting from migration (Ndiaye et al. 2011).

These new ideas of engaging the diaspora were applied to the Zimbabwean case in order to establish the exact nature of the potential diaspora's contribution to the country's health delivery system. Interviews with Zimbabwean medical doctors in South Africa revealed a number of ways in which the medical diaspora can be engaged to address the challenges facing the health system. Temporary returns were mentioned by the respondents as one crucial area where the diaspora could make a difference in Zimbabwe's health delivery system. The temporary returns could target the medical school and hospitals. The medical school in particular has been severely affected by the exodus of professors. Press reports in February 2010 indicated that three departments at the medical school namely Anaesthetics, Anatomy and Haematology had two lecturers each instead of the required 16, 11 and 10 respectively (*The Herald* 16 February 2010). Most of the medical doctors in South Africa who were interviewed have managed to specialise and were willing to become part of the solution to the problem of the shortage of lecturers at the medical school. In 2009, efforts were underway by the IOM to bring back medical doctors based in the United Kingdom to come and teach at the medical school for short periods of time. Similar programmes have been implemented by IOM such as the MIDA's Great Lakes Program covering Burundi, the Democratic Republic of Congo and Rwanda which enables university lecturers based abroad to teach courses in these countries (Ndiaye et al. 2011). Temporary returns could also be in the form of short-term hospital visits which allows the medical diaspora to be directly involved in alleviating the shortage of doctors in the country's hospitals. As noted by Dr Chiremba in the interviews: 'Most of us would be happy to go, say when I am on leave, to help for a week or two with difficult cases or even easy ones, just to clear up some of the operations that need to be done.'

While temporary returns by the doctors aimed at capacity building at the medical school or provision of critical skills in Zimbabwean hospitals yield undeniable results, the long term sustainability of such programmes are questionable. Short term returns can at best yield only short-term benefits and do not address the problem of the long term supply of medical doctors in the country. These criticisms raise questions on the feasibility of the diaspora option as a long term measure of strengthening health systems of countries affected by emigration.

Diaspora philanthropic activities could also make a significant impact on Zimbabwe's healthcare system. The medical diaspora can play a role in raising funds for hospitals as well as sourcing drugs and equipment. A good example of philanthropic activities by the medical diaspora is provided by the case of the Ethiopian medical diaspora living in the United States who recently donated equipment worth nearly US$2 million and trained the local staff on how to use the technology (Ndiaye et al. 2011). The Zimbabwean medical diaspora mentioned some of the ways in which they could be involved in philanthropic activities that might benefit the country's health system. For instance, they could help in sourcing and donating books to the medical school. Others would prefer to source drugs and medical equipment for the local hospitals. Many of the emigrant Zimbabwean doctors are working in developed countries where technology is constantly changing, thereby making redundant some equipment that might still be in good and usable state. The hospitals in such countries are willing to give away such equipment if it is going to be put to good use. As noted by Dr Henry Porter: 'The doctors can also help by sourcing equipment from their hospitals which is not being used. Most of the equipment is still usable but is lying idle in some hospitals. These could be utilised in the hospitals in Zimbabwe.'

Finally, the medical diaspora could make a difference in Zimbabwe through telemedicine. Even though telecommunications systems are not well developed in Africa, the adoption of telemedicine seems to be on the rise. Ghanaian-born doctors working in the Netherlands, for example, have provided patient diagnosis to hospitals in Accra, while Ethiopian-born doctors in the diaspora have assisted in health policy training in Ethiopia through videoconferencing (Brinkerhoff 2012). As noted by one interview participant, Dr Ron Johnson, telemedicine can potentially be the solution to Zimbabwe's brain drain problem:

> ... you can explore some new ways of using the skills of medical doctors who are based overseas; I mean ways that do not require them to be physically present in Zimbabwe. I think telemedicine offers an exciting option as it allows the doctors who are in Zimbabwe to connect with the overseas based specialists. I think it is quite an interesting option.

Telemedicine is highly dependent on access to reliable telecommunication systems which makes its adoption questionable in African countries. Ironically, rural areas in Africa which have the greatest need for telemedicine also have the worst telecommunication infrastructure. Therefore, telemedicine cannot provide a viable solution for the provision of expertise in areas that are underdeveloped.

## The Brain Drain of Medical Doctors: An Exceptional Case?

This chapter has analysed the 'brain drain' and 'drain gain' debate using field evidence from Zimbabwe. At this point, it is necessary to address some of the major points which the 'revisionists' offer on the brain drain debate. It has been argued that the migration of skilled professionals such as medical doctors can lead to a brain gain as it leads to increased demand for education among the population with the hope of migrating (Skeldon 2008). This might be true in the case of countries such as the Philippines which have adopted a deliberate 'brain export' policy of nurses. However, in the case of medical doctors in Africa, the capacity of medical schools to increase their medical student intake is hampered by institutional capacity constraints as well as the lack of lecturers at universities. This is true in the case of Zimbabwe where the medical school has been affected by the exodus of lecturers from the medical school who have not yet been replaced. In addition, Zimbabwe has only one medical school at the University of Zimbabwe and it does not make sense to expand the number of medical schools in the country when the present one is struggling for survival.

Could the brain drain be 'more perceived than real' as Skeldon (2008, 10) argues? The migration of health professionals has clear demonstrable impacts as the Zimbabwean case has shown. The users of the health system, particularly the poor, are usually the worst affected as they rely on healthcare service offered in public institutions and cannot afford to pay for the fees charged in the better staffed private health centres. It is probably this point which makes the case of medical doctors exceptional as their migration leads to some negative outcomes on the quality of health care in the sending country. In this case, it can be argued that the loss of doctors results in real and not perceived negative impacts to countries in the global south.

The debate on the impacts of medical migration on sending countries continues to have a polarising effect. At the heart of the debate is whether sending countries experience a brain drain when their skilled professionals such as medical doctors depart for more developed destinations. In its original formulation, the brain drain notion denotes a one-way flow of skilled human resources and does not pay attention to the potential contribution of diasporas to the home country's development. The brain drain notion is effective though in showing the net losses that occur to the sending state as a result of the departure of its skilled citizens. Contrary to the observations elsewhere (see Raghuram 2009), this makes the state a suitable unit of analysis as the effects of migration are felt at the national level. At the transnational level, it can be pointed out that sending states can potentially derive numerous benefits from their citizens in the diaspora through various diaspora engagement initiatives. This chapter acknowledges the unique contributions which diasporas make but argues that positioning diasporas as agents of development fails to acknowledge the human resource crisis which sending countries face as a direct result of migration. The right to health of citizens of developing countries needs to be acknowledged but that should not result in curtailing the right of medical doctors to migrate. In fact, medical doctors like other professionals have a right to seek employment wherever they might wish to do so. It is the responsibility of sending countries to ensure that they meet the right to health of their population by introducing policies that make it attractive for medical doctors to stay in the country.

The medical brain drain is therefore not dead as claimed by Skeldon (2008). It is a reality that is faced by many countries in the developing world. The impacts of the brain drain are experienced daily by the citizens of developing countries. Even though remittances which emigrant doctors send to their countries can offset some of the training costs and may stimulate development (Clemens 2010), it needs to be highlighted that these are private flows and they have limited impacts on the health care system, let alone on the supply of medical doctors. Remittances may not be the panacea for health systems in Africa. Engaging the diaspora may at best be described as a short term solution to Africa's medical human resource crisis. A long term solution lies in the introduction of policies that reduce the attrition of medical doctors from the continent from the current unsustainably high brain drain levels.

## References

Aikins, K., Sands, A. and White, N. 2009. *The Global Irish Making A Difference Together*. Dublin: The Ireland Funds.

Alkire, S. and Chen, L. 2004. Medical exceptionalism in international migration: Should doctors and nurses be treated differently?, in *Globalising Migration Regimes: New Challenges to Transnational Cooperation*, edited by K. Tamas and J. Palme . Aldershot: Ashgate, 100–117.

Anyangwe, S.C.E. and Mtonga, C. 2007. Inequities in the Global Health Workforce: The Greatest Impediment to Health in Sub-Saharan Africa. *International Journal of Environmental Research and Public Health*, 4(2), 93–100.

Awases, M., Gbary, A., Nyoni, J. and Chatora, R. 2004. *Migration of Health Professionals in Six Countries: A Synthesis Report*. Brazzaville: WHO Regional Office for Africa.

Bhagwati, J. 1976. The brain drain. *International Social Science Journal*, 28, 691–729.

Bhargava, K. and Sharma, J. 2008. *Building Bridges: A Case Study on the Role of the Indian Diaspora in Canada*. Kingston: Centre for the Study of Democracy.

Brinkerhoff, J.M. 2008. 'The potential of diasporas and development', in *Diasporas and Development: Exploring the Potential*, edited by J.M. Brinkerhoff. London: Lynne Reiner Publishers, 1–15.

Brinkerhoff, J.M. 2012. Creating an enabling environment for diasporas' participation in homeland development. *International Migration*, 50(1), 75–95.

Castles, S. and Miller, M.J. 2009. *The Age of Migration: International Population Movements in the Modern World*. New York and London: The Guilford Press.

Chikanda, A. 2005. Nurse migration from Zimbabwe: Analysis of recent trends and impacts. *Nursing Inquiry*, 12(3), 162–74.

Chikanda, A. 2008. The migration of health professionals from Zimbabwe, in *The International Migration of Health Workers*, edited by J. Connell. New York and London: Routledge, 110–28.

Chikanda, A. 2011. The changing patterns of physician migration from Zimbabwe since 1990. *International Journal of Migration, Health and Social Care*, 7(2), 77–92.

Clemens, M.A. 2009. 'Skill Flow: A Fundamental Reconsideration of Skilled Worker Mobility and Development'. *Human Development Research Paper 2009/08*. New York, United Nations Development Programme.

Clemens, M.A. 2010. The Financial Consequences of High-Skill Emigration: Lessons from African Doctors Abroad, in *Diaspora for Development in Africa*, edited by S. Plaza and D. Ratha. Washington, DC: World Bank, 165–82.

Clemens M.A. and Pettersson, G. 2006. *A New Database for Health Professional Emigration from Africa*. Washington, DC: Centre for Global Development.

Connell, J. (2008) Toward a global health care system?, in *The International Migration of Health Workers*, edited by J. Connell. New York: Routledge, 1–29.

Connell, J., Zurn, P., Stilwell, B. et al. 2007. Sub-Saharan Africa: Beyond the health worker migration crisis? *Social Science & Medicine*, 64, 1876–91.

Conway, M.D., Gupta, S. and Khajavi, K. 2007. Addressing Africa's Health Workforce. *The McKinsley Quarterly*, 1–11.

Crush, J. and Frayne, B. 2007. The migration and development nexus in Southern Africa: An introduction. *Development Southern Africa*, 24(1), 1–23.

Crush, J., and Pendleton, W. 2011. Brain flight: the exodus of health professionals from South Africa. *International Journal of Migration, Health and Social Care*, 6(3), 3–18.

Docquier, F. and Bhargava, A. 2006. *The Medical Brain Drain: A New Panel Data Set on Physician's Emigration Rates (1991–2004)*. Washington, DC: World Bank.

Dumont, J.C. and Zurn, P. 2007. Immigrant health workers in OECD countries in the broader context of highly-skilled migration. *International Migration Outlook* (pp. 162–228), Part III. Paris: OECD.

Eastwood, J., Conroy, R., Naicker, S. et al. 2005. Loss of health professionals from sub-Saharan Africa: The pivotal role of the UK. *The Lancet*, 365, 1893–900.

Faist, T. 2008. Migrants as transnational development agents: an inquiry into the newest round of the migration-development nexus. *Population, Space and Place*, 14(2), 21–42.

Gaidzanwa, R. 1999. *Voting with their Feet: Migrant Zimbabwean Nurses and Doctors in the Era of Structural Adjustment*. Uppsala: Nordiska Afrikainstitutet.

Global Commission on International Migration. 2005. *Migration in an Interconnected World: New Directions for Action*. Geneva: Global Commission on International Migration.

Grant, H. 2006. From the Transvaal to the Prairies: The migration of South African physicians to Canada. *Journal of Ethnic and Migration Studies*, 32, 681–96.

Hanke, S.H. 2008. *New Hyperinflation Index (HHIZ) Puts Zimbabwe Inflation at 89.7 Sextillion Percent*. Washington, DC: Cato Institute.

Hussey, P.S. 2007. International migration patterns of physicians to the United States: A cross-national panel analysis. *Health Policy*, 84, 298–307.

Kirigia, J.M., Gbary, A.R., Nyoni, J. et al. 2006. The cost of health related brain drain to the WHO African Region. *African Journal of Health Sciences*, 13(3–4), 1–12.

IOM. 2006. *A Global Strategy of Migration for Development Beyond the MIDA Approach to Mobilizing and Sharing of Human and Financial Resources of the Overseas African Community 2006 – 2010*. Geneva: IOM.

Kapur, D. 2005. Remittances: The new development mantra?, in *Remittances: Development Impact and Future Prospects*, edited by S.M. Maimbo and D. Ratha. Washington, DC: The World Bank, 331–60.

Khadria, B. 2004. *Perspectives on Migration of Health Workers from India to Overseas Markets: Brain Drain or Export?* IOM's International Dialogue on Migration. Seminar on Health and Migration. [Online]. Available at: http://www.iom.int [accessed: 5 June 2006].

Kingma, M. 2006. *Nurses on the Move: Migration and the Global Health Care Economy*. Ithaca, NY: Cornell University Press.

Klinthäll, M. 2006. Retirement return migration from Sweden. *International Migration*, 44(2), 153–180.

Kuznetsov, Y. 2006. 'Leveraging diasporas of talent: Toward a new policy agenda.', in *Diaspora Networks and the International Migration of Skills: How Countries Can Draw on Their Talent Abroad*, edited by Y. Kuznetsov. Washington, DC: The World Bank, 221–37.

Liese, B. and Dussault, G. 2004. *The State of the Health Workforce in Sub-Saharan Africa: Evidence of Crisis and Analysis of Contributing Factors*. Washington, DC: World Bank.

Marcelli, E.A. and Lowell, B.L. 2005. Transnational twist: Pecuniary remittances and the socioeconomic integration of authorized and unauthorized Mexican immigrants in Los Angeles County. *International Migration Review*, 39(1), 69–102.

Mensah, K. Mackintosh, M. and Henry, L. 2005. *The Skills Drain of Health Professionals from the Developing World: A Framework for Policy Formulation*. London: Medact.

Mills, E.J., Kanters, S., Hagopian, A. et al. 2011. The financial cost of doctors emigrating from sub-Saharan Africa: human capital analysis. *British Medical Journal*, 343. doi: 10.1136/bmj.d7031.

Mohan G. 2002. Diaspora and Development, in *Displacement and Development*, edited by J Robinson. Oxford: Oxford University Press, 77–139.

Mutizwa-Mangiza, D. 1999. *Doctors and the State: The Struggle for Professional Control in Zimbabwe*. Aldershot: Ashgate.

Ndiaye, N., Melde, S. and Ndiaye-Coic, R. 2011. 'The Migration for Development in Africa experience and beyond', in *Diasporas for Development in Africa*, edited by S. Plaza and D. Ratha. Washington, DC: World Bank, 231–59.

Padarath, A., Chamberlain, C., McCoy, D. et al. 2003. *Health Personnel in Southern Africa: Confronting Maldistribution and Brain Drain*. Equinet Discussion Paper No. 3. Harare: Regional Network for Equity in Health in Southern Africa (EQUINET).

Raghuram, P. 2009. Caring about the 'brain drain' in a postcolonial world. *Geoforum*, 40, 25–33.

Ray, K.M., Lowell, B.L. and Spencer, S. 2006. International health worker mobility: causes, consequences, and best practices. *International Migration*, 44(2), 182–203.

Schrecker, T. and Labonté, R. 2004. Taming the brain drain: A challenge for public health systems in Southern Africa. *International Journal of Occupational and Environmental Health*, 10, 409–15.

Skeldon, R. 2008. Of skilled migration, brain drains and policy responses. *International Migration*, 47(4), 3–29.

Staubhaar, T. and Vadean, F.P. 2005. International Migrant Remittances and their Role in Development, in *The Development Dimension: Migrant Remittances and Development*. Paris: OECD Publishing, 13–33.

Tanner, A. 2005. *Emigration, Brain Drain and Development: The Case of Sub-Saharan Africa*. Helsinki: Migration Policy Institute.

Teferra, D. 2005. Brain circulation: Unparalleled opportunities, underlying challenges, and outmoded presumptions. *Journal of Studies in International Education*, 9(3), 229–50.

The Herald. 2010. UZ faces critical staff shortage. *The Herald*, 16 February. [Online]. Available at: www.herald.co.zw.

United Nations. 2006. *International migration and development: Report of the Secretary-General*. Geneva: United Nations.

Williams, A.M. and Balaz, V. 2008. International return mobility, learning and knowledge transfer: a case of Slovak doctors. *Social Science and Medicine*, 67, 1924–33.

World Bank. 2011. *Migration and Remittances Factbook 2011*. Washington, DC: World Bank.

World Health Organisation. 2006. *Working Together for Health*. Geneva: World Health Organisation.

Yahirun, J.J. 2009. *Take Me 'Home': Determinants of Return Migration Among Germany's Elderly Immigrants*. California Center for Population Research Online Working Paper Series CCPR-2009-019. Los Angeles: University Of California.

Zinyama, L.M. 1990. International migrations to and from Zimbabwe and the influence if political changes on population movements, 1965–1987. *International Migration Review*, 24(4), 748–67.

# Chapter 18
# Conclusion:
# Healthy Development/Developing Health

Robin Kearns and Pat Neuwelt

As Phillips and Verhasselt (1994, 3) remarked in their edited collection, '... the health of populations and individuals is inextricably bound up with development'. The foregoing chapters have gone a considerable distance towards extending understanding of this assertion. As the majority of contributors are geographers, it is little surprise that scale has been an implicit theme: the personal and political have been shown to converge in the course of examining the health-development nexus at scales ranging from individuals and their behaviours to trans-national organisations and their policies. It is now quite literally a global world in terms of health and health care. Not only does the spectre of epidemics threaten global and personal biosecurity, but also the commercial decisions of pharmaceutical companies can influence the costs and availability of interventions to arrest the path of disease. New international trade agreements, as discussed by Lovell and Rosenberg in Chapter 15, threaten to take some nations into uncharted waters in terms of being beholden to decisions enacted far from their borders.

The complexity of influences on health outcomes reveals that both 'health' and 'development' can too easily be reduced to stereotypical understandings. They are, as Phillips and Verhasselt (1994, 3) noted 'beguilingly simple, defy(ing) concise and consistent definition'. We need to embrace this complexity for, as the World Health Organisation definition reminds us, health is more than absence of disease; rather it is a life-enhancing experience of multiple sets of wellbeing. Similarly, development must be understood as more than increased Gross National Product or the sum of activities and policies enacted by development organisations; rather it amounts to positive change in people's living environments.

While there are many examples of development initiatives positively contributing to wellbeing, we cannot presume that this link will always be evident. Indeed, few sights more deeply reflected the potential disconnection between development attempts and health outcomes than those that confronted us in 1987 when we visited Davis Inlet, on the Labrador coast in Canada. Here, previously nomadic Innu people had been urged to settle in a location where they could easily be reached by welfare services and encouraged to occupy western-style wooden dwellings. The 'backstory' was that their traditional hunting grounds were being overflown by NATO jets practicing low-level flying, scattering caribou herds and putting Innu people at risk (Wadden, 1991). At the time we visited this settlement, families were dismantling the houses and using building materials to support their traditional tents, erected nearby. Furniture was being burnt for firewood. As noted by Desai and Porter (2009), the complexities in attempting to intervene in favour of health and development are manifold. Tuberculosis, alcoholism and suicide were rife at Davis Inlet and, according to Scott and Conn (1987), these were not individualised health outcomes but rather should be seen as part of a wider 'socio-political morbidity' in which 'social, political, economic, and cultural alienation remain major causes of morbidity and mortality'.

A quarter-century later, Wilson, Rosenberg and Ning's (Chapter 5) survey of the health status of indigenous peoples in Canada reveals an example of the enduring disparities within ostensibly 'developed' nations. While the use of statistics is evocative, it is arguably time to strive for a strengths-based approach to health and development. This approach might start by profiling examples of community-based initiatives that have worked and that could be modelled by other communities. In the case of the Davis Inlet example, moving beyond a deficit model might involve asking how potentially different health and development outcomes might have been with sustained community engagement? Could a dialogue around housing and health and the meanings of their preferred nomadic lifestyle have led to small but significant steps to greater self-determination for the Innu? Paradoxically, perhaps, interventions led by the very communities that are marginalised have the best chances of success and can be, as hooks (1990, 342) has called them, 'sites of radical possibility'. As Margai and Minah signalled in Chapter 2, not only is disease (such as tuberculosis at Davis Inlet) deeply interconnected with the incidence of poverty, but so too community buy-in and engagement is connected with the likely success of health promotion and disease prevention. The co-promotion of economic and health-promoting policies thus constitutes a sensible, if challenging, way forward.

However, ways forward' are invariably challenging due to their complexity, a theme borne out in this volume. Oppong and Ebeniro (Chapter 3) contend that adverse events such as maternal death vary according to social and economic factors that prevail in the place of residence. Such places are commonly 'beyond the radar' of health and development agencies for practical as well as ethical reasons, or influenced by cultural beliefs that can – perhaps unintentionally — add to structural violence and the 'othering' of groups into marginalised status. As Hellen and Wadwa indicate in Chapter 4, there can be synergistically negative effects on health status wrought by social factors such as poverty and gender-based exploitation. These effects impact not only individuals, but also collectives such as families, communities and whole societies.

A particular paradox in considering complexity in the determinants of health is that the health system itself can create barriers to health care. As Dixon and Mkandawire point out in Chapter 6, the need for patients to make out-of-pocket payments for care can be a deterrent to health care utilisation, with a 'wait and see' attitude being a common response or, alternatively, an embracing of debt in order to access care. Too easily, accessibility can be thought of as involving only spatial barriers such as distance or transport limitations. In essence, paying for care individualises the transaction and moves health care further from the notion of health as intrinsic to the common good of the community, a view echoed by the WHO's Commission on the Social Determinants of Health (2008). The phenomenon of international medical migration, discussed with respect to Zimbabwe in Chapter 17, is another way in which the health system can be a barrier to health, with the movement of medical personnel potentially depleting expertise in the country of origin. When trained medical personnel leave their home countries they may be opting for enhanced personal and household development (e.g. better education for their children) but are depriving those who indirectly supported their education of the care they were trained to provide.

One theme introduced towards the end of the book is that the health and development connection is as relevant in the western world as elsewhere. This theme is a reminder that we who look out on countries afflicted by malaria, famine and poverty risk complacency in an era of such new and unprecedented challenges as climate change, the spectre of peak oil, and ecosystem degradation. Within crisis there can be opportunity, however. As Pennock, Poland and Hancock (Chapter 11) point out, the transitions needed towards lower-carbon communities and away from a century of cheap energy could in fact generate 'healthier, more vibrant and sustainable communities'. Too easily, narratives linking health and development such as the Millennium Development Goals get mired under the weight of unlikely change and impossible odds, yet this suggestion that peak oil may in fact lead to a world 'more consistent with public health's vision of healthier built environments' offers a welcome suggestion that geographies of hope may lurk within the spectre of crisis.

Arguably the emergence of such geographies of hope will be reliant on robust challenges to the conventional western scientific mind set which, despite manifold advances in technology and knowledge, has tended to isolate influences upon health and be too easily blind to connections that make sense but have yet to be statistically proven. Emergent ecological models of health suggest some sympathy with indigenous knowledges and see integration not separation in the determinants of health. By way of example, the 'hydrosocial system' discussed by Schuster-Wallace and colleagues (Chapter 12) signals the power of expansive thinking that can come with developing new vocabulary for the complexity and flows of influence that surround us. Too easily, perhaps, public health has embraced figures of speech but not looked far enough beyond the health system. The hydrological metaphor 'downstream effects', for instance, is commonly used but how often do health practitioners consider the importance of streams and waterways in potentially enhancing human wellbeing?

The figurative upstream determinants of wellbeing also matter. Chapter 12's authors point out that preventing disease in the community – that crucible of health development – can relieve the burden on clinics and hospitals. As Phillips and Verhasselt (1994, 9) advocate, there is a need to strive for 'sympathetic, effective health services'. But ultimately the 'elephant in the room' for exploring links between health and development is equity. In divided societies the line between the 'have and have nots' can determine life and death. For instance, as the authors of Chapter 14 indicate, tuberculosis had largely become the 'forgotten plague' 'because it had stopped bothering the wealthy'. This statement is as true in developing nations as developed ones. Research on transnationalism has identified that the resurgence of TB in urban New Zealand is primarily due to the embodiment of the negative impacts of migration on individuals and families. People migrate to developed nations in search of 'a better life' for themselves and their children. Yet, the impacts of resettlement from nations with a high incidence of TB, including the racism experienced in the new country can lead to the activation of TB disease (Littleton et al., 2008).

Many of the foregoing chapters have presented case studies of fairly grim health (and socioeconomic) realities in communities and nations, often far from the authors' current residential location. The gaze of the authors has been 'from a distance', and helpfully focuses on identifying needs and situations requiring attention, from a critical perspective. The danger of persisting with this perspective, however, is that it implicitly draws on a deficit analysis, reporting on trends over time that are, therefore, historical rather than future-focused. Populations inadvertently become framed as 'needy' unless balanced with a discussion of suitable interventions. Drawing on our positionality as transnational New Zealanders, we close this commentary with some reflections for a forward-looking gaze, which draws on a strengths-based analysis and incorporates a human rights perspective.

As highlighted in this book's case studies, colonisation is still a current reality globally. This is the case whether colonisation is defined in its traditional sense, or seen as the encroachment of neoliberal open-market ideologies on the economies of developing nations (e.g. through so-called 'global markets' trampling on local markets, thereby creating worsening inequities within poorer nations – see Chapter 15). Historically, under the guise of 'development', indigenous peoples across the globe were forced to assimilate with newer arrivals. Similar processes are recurring through contemporary international trade agreements. As highlighted in chapters 15 and 16, we are led to question the 'boundaries' of health and development in a global environment where trade and economic development trumps human development.

Looking to the future, we might consider the value of re-framing analyses of health and development in terms of human rights (e.g., indigenous rights, the right to health, the rights of the child). This move would identify strengths and opportunities for the future. For example, aboriginal peoples might be described in terms of their traditional knowledge (which has much to offer how we might adapt to the challenges of approaching peak oil – see Chapter 11), and their innovation in health service delivery in rural communities (which can speak to broader possibilities of 'people-centred approaches' – see Chapter 8). The next stage in scholarship is surely seeking out stories of meaningful local community and regional development that are comprehensive, people-centred, and equitable.

As contributors have emphatically shown, health and development are synergistically connected. The health status of a population in any place influences the economic and social development of the region; so, too, development initiatives can offer the economic traction needed to introduce health-enhancing interventions such as better sanitation or more widespread immunisation or health promotion. In reflecting on this book's themes, we are reminded of the enigmatic yet economical title of Gunnar Olsson's (1980) book: *Birds in Egg/Eggs in Bird*. What comes first: health or development? Perhaps it is neither. Maybe health and development are irrevocably implicated in each other; each cannot exist alone. This reality, explicit in the 1978 Alma-Ata Declaration on Primary Health Care (referred to in Chapter 12) remains true today. What, therefore, might be the implications if we are to consider health(y) development, or developing health, thus removing the conjunction 'and' that implies they are separate enterprises that need connecting? Such deliberation must wait until another collection of essays. For now this book has fostered further dialogue on development and health in a robust and wide-ranging way.

## References

Desai, V. and Potter, R.B. 2009. *Doing Development Research*. Thousand Oaks, CA: Sage Publications. .

hooks, b 1990. *Yearning: Race, Gender, and Cultural Politics*. Boston, MA: South End Press.

Littleton, J., Park., Thornley, C., Anderson, A. and Lawrence, J. 2008. Migrants and tuberculosis: Analysing epidemiological data with ethnography. *Australian and New Zealand Journal of Public Health*, 32, 142–9.

Olsson, G. 1980. *Birds in Egg/Eggs in Bird*. London: Pion.

Phillips, D.R and Verhasselt, Y. (eds) 1994. *Health and Development*. London: Routledge.

Scott, R.T. and Conn, S. 1987. The failure of scientific medicine: Davis Inlet as an example of sociopolitical morbidity. *Canadian Family Physician*, 33, 1649–53.

Wadden, M. 1991. *Nitassinan: The Innu Struggle to Claim Their Homeland.* Vancouver: Douglas & McIntyre.

World Health Organization. 2008. *Closing the Gap in a Generation: Health Equity through Action on the Social Determinants of Health.* Geneva: World Health Organization.

# Index